CHAPTER 1

HIGHWAY TO HUGENESS

started lifting when I was 14, and the results I'm after haven't really changed since then. I wanted bigger, stronger, better-looking muscles then, and that's what I want now. But I have changed my approach from time to time; I think every dedicated lifter does. In all, I've pursued six distinct belief systems about how to build muscle. Luckily for me, only one of them proved to be a dead end. The rest of the time I merged easily from one path to the next as I accumulated knowledge and experience.

Here's how you might experience the big six:

1. IF I FLEX THEM, THEY WILL GROW

When you squeeze a muscle, you feel it working. So it makes simple, perfect, and irrefutable sense to start out with the idea that you must work muscles to build muscles. For an absolute beginner, it's really all that matters. Lift the weight, lower the weight. It doesn't matter where you start, when you start, or what equipment you have. Your basic understanding of the process is as simple as a first-grade reader: "See Joe's muscles. See Joe flex his muscles. Flex, Joe, flex! Watch Joe's muscles get bigger. Grow, muscles, grow!"

That's exactly what happens when you stick with it for a few weeks.

Naturally, you assume that the mechanics of lifting matter more than anything. It's the most intuitive part of strength training. You look at the biggest guys in the gym or in your school's weight room. You observe what exercises they do, and you come away thinking that those exercises are all that stand between the body you have and the body you want. The idea gets reinforced every time you pick up a fitness magazine and see specific exercises recommended for specific benefits.

But, as with any self-taught skill, you quickly teach yourself into a corner. You gravitate toward exercises that offer the most squeezability, such as biceps curls and leg extensions. You avoid the ones that offer less immediate feedback, such as squats and other free-weight exercises that force you to coordinate the actions of several joints at once. Most of your time in the weight room gets allocated to exercises that allow you to watch your muscles being squeezed.

When you get home from a workout, you can't wait to strip off your shirt and flex in front of the bathroom mirror. You get so used to seeing your muscles one way—flexed and posed while pumped up from that day's workout—that you forget they don't look like that all the time, especially to other people. But you can't dodge reality for long. Maybe an old girlfriend who hasn't seen you for months fails to notice any difference. Or you bump into a co-worker at the gym where you've been a regular, and he asks if you're going to start a workout program.

It's a painful but important lesson, possibly the most important reality check you'll ever get: There's more to building muscle than flexing and unflexing. It's not just a mechanical process. The mechanics are crucial—make no

mistake about that. No matter how much you learn, you'll never get around the connection between muscle tension and muscle growth.

You will, however, begin to tell yourself that if some tension didn't do the trick . . .

2. MORE MUST BE BETTER

Since your progress stalled when you lifted two or three times a week, your natural instinct is to double down. You decide to train four times a week. Or five. Or six. Hell, you might begin to wonder why you need to take *any* days off. You learn more exercises, and you want to do them all—devoting entire workouts to your biceps and triceps, for example. If you walk into the gym with the goal of working your chest, you don't leave until you've hit it with barbells, dumbbells, machines, and cables. You do presses and flies and crossovers. You work with your torso upright, prone, inclined, and declined.

For a few weeks, or a few months, you feel like Superman, even if your perpetually stiff and slightly sore muscles make you move like the Tin Man. You love the feeling of working muscles from every angle, of pumping them until they're so fatigued and so engorged with blood that you can barely lift your arms or bend your knees.

Some bodybuilders train like this for years. But you aren't one of them. The breaking point is a little different for everyone. Maybe you first feel it in your elbows, which

Men'sHealth

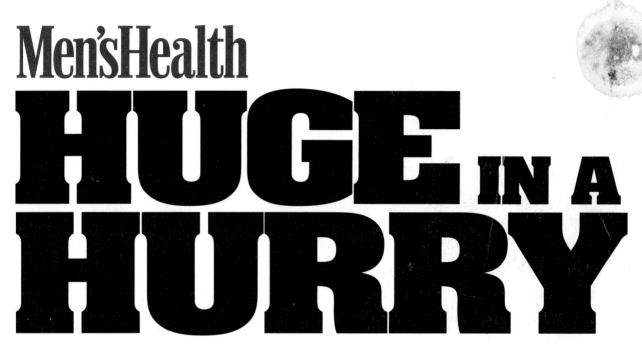

HUGE IN A HURRY

Get Bigger, Stronger, and Leaner in Record Time with the New Science of Strength Training

CHAD WATERBURY

RODALE®

NOTICE

The information in this book is meant to supplement, not replace, proper exercise training.
All forms of exercise pose some inherent risks. The editors and publisher advise readers to take full
responsibility for their safety and know their limits. Before practicing the exercises in this book, be sure that your
equipment is well maintained, and do not take risks beyond your level of experience, aptitude, training, and fitness.
The exercise and dietary programs in this book are not intended as a substitute for any exercise routine or dietary
regimen that may have been prescribed by your doctor. As with all exercise and
dietary programs, you should get your doctor's approval before beginning.

Mention of specific companies, organizations, or authorities in this book does not imply endorsement
by the author or publisher, nor does mention of specific companies, organizations, or authorities
imply that they endorse this book, its author, or the publisher.

Internet addresses and telephone numbers given in this book were accurate at the time it went to press.

Rodale books may be purchased for business or promotional use or for special sales.
For information, please write to:
Special Markets Department, Rodale Inc., 733 Third Avenue, New York, NY 10017

Men's Health is a registered trademark of Rodale Inc.

Printed in the United States of America
Rodale Inc. makes every effort to use acid-free ∞, recycled paper ♺.

INTERIOR PHOTOGRAPHS BY Mitch Mandel/Rodale Images and Brad Buckman (page viii only)
ILLUSTRATIONS BY Scott Halloday
BOOK DESIGN BY Susan Eugster

Library of Congress Cataloging-in-Publication Data

Waterbury, Chad.
    Men's health Huge in a hurry : get bigger, stronger, and leaner in record time
  with the new science of building muscle / by Chad Waterbury.
       p.   cm.
    Includes index.
    ISBN-13 978–1–59486–954–9 direct mail hardcover
    ISBN-10 1–59486–954–5 direct mail hardcover
    ISBN-13 978–1–60529–934–1 paperback
    ISBN-10 1–60529–934–0 paperback
    1. Bodybuilding.   2. Weight training.   I. Title.   II. Title: Huge in a hurry.
  GV546.5.W38 2008
  613.7'1—dc22   2008029457

Distributed to the trade by Macmillan

2 4 6 8 10 9 7 5 3 1 direct mail hardcover
2 4 6 8 10 9 7 5 3 1 paperback

LIVE YOUR WHOLE LIFE™

We inspire and enable people to improve their lives and the world around them
For more of our products visit **rodalestore.com** or call 800-848-4735

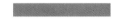

We all have someone in our lives who affects us immeasurably.

Maybe that person is a parent, teacher, or friend.

Maybe that person gave us just enough encouragement at a critical moment, even if at the time we didn't think it was enough.

Or maybe that person didn't always have our best interests in mind, but instead acted in ways that forced us to learn the rules of life.

Maybe what that person didn't give us made us who we are today.

This book is dedicated to my late father.

He's the reason I'm here.

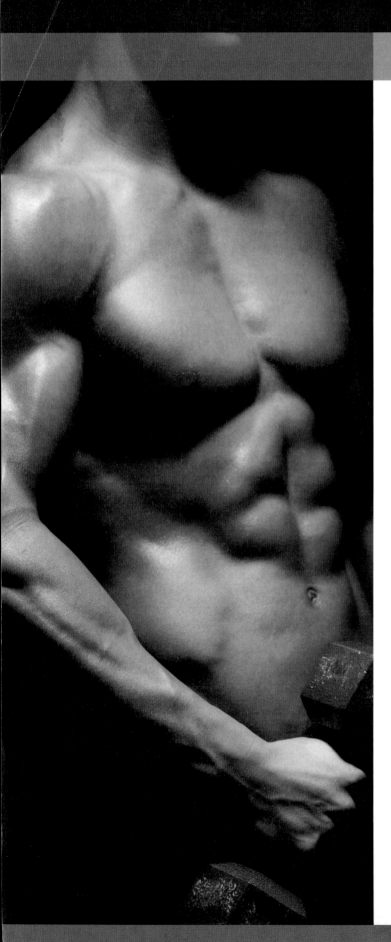

CONTENTS

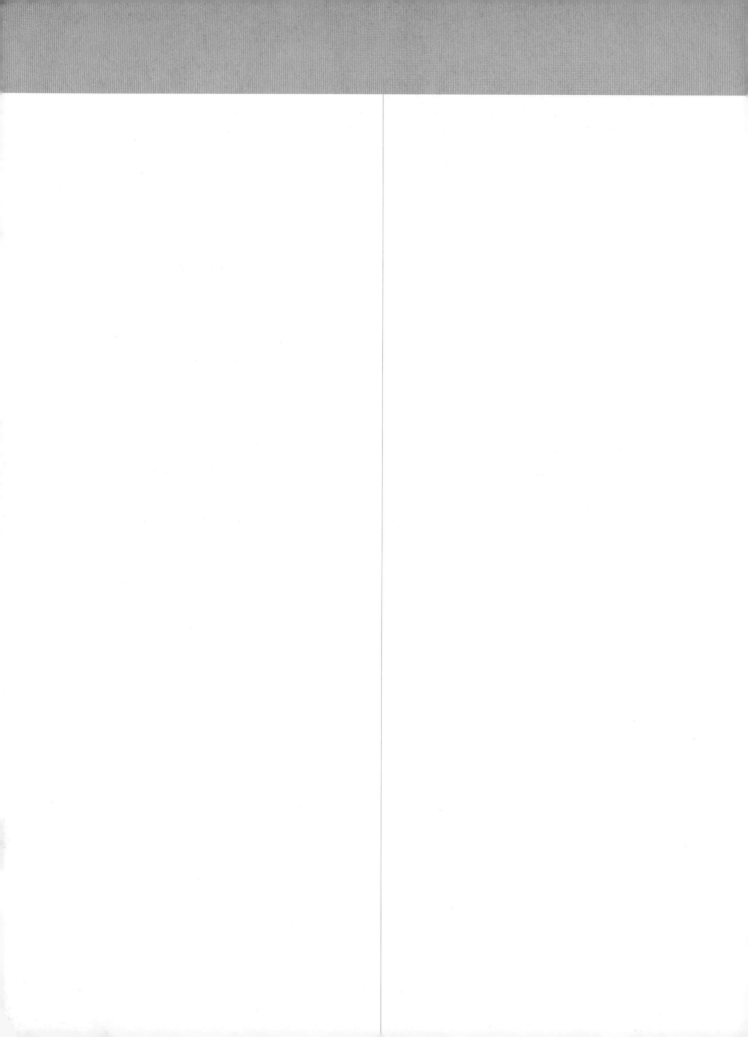

ACKNOWLEDGMENTS

First and foremost, I want to thank God for keeping me strong and healthy.

My mother is a close second. Thanks for your love.

Next up is the rest of my family: Lisa, for your abundance of joy, support, love, and even more support to top it off; Todd, for your wisdom and encouragement and for being unwavering in your honesty and integrity; Gary, for being as solid as a rock and for being such an incredible provider when I was a kid.

I want to thank my three best friends—Orbie, Stacey, and Telly—for the laughs and the beers. Thanks to TC, Tim, and Chris at T-Nation for your continued support; to Debbie for your encouragement; and to Bill Hartman for your help with the mobility and flexibility information. My sincere appreciation goes out to Rodale for the opportunity to write this book. I want to thank Lou Schuler, without whom this book would never have been possible. It was my honor and privilege to work with you. Last, I want to thank Leslie for your love and your incredible spirit.

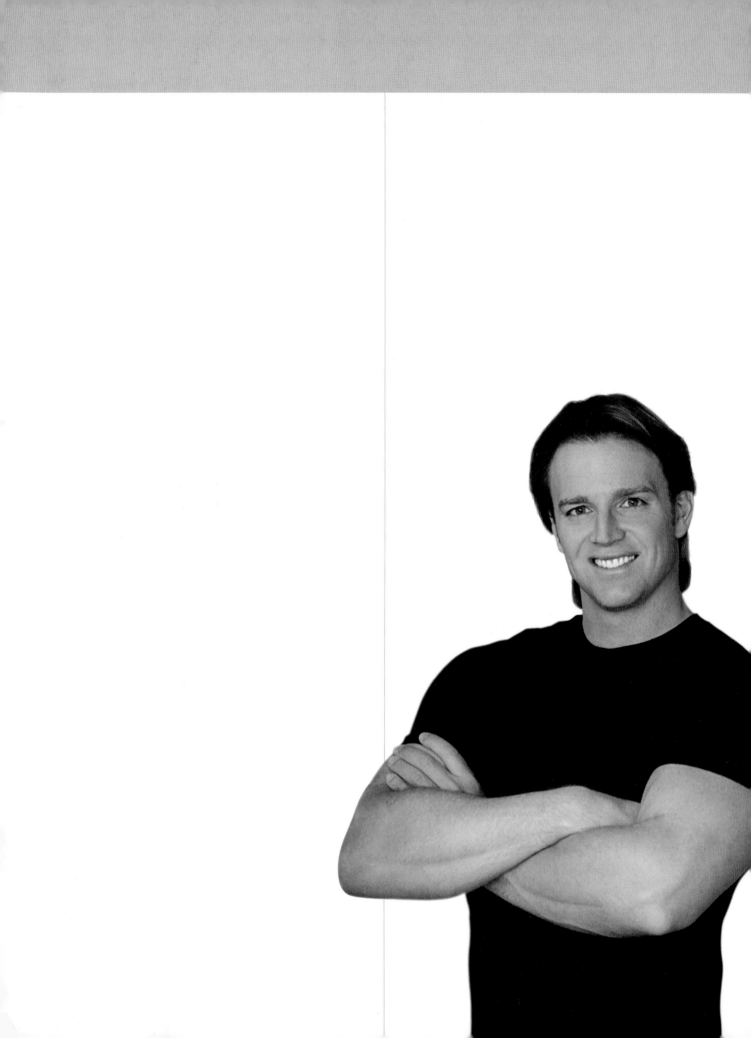

INTRODUCTION
THE NERVE OF THIS GUY!

I f you saw me walking down the street, your first thought wouldn't be, "Hey, that guy looks like a neurophysiologist." You'd probably guess that I'm a musclehead, which is fine. That's exactly what I am. And if you guessed that I make my living using my brawn as much as my brain, I'd still take it as a compliment. I used to work as a nightclub bouncer, asking belligerent drunks to leave the premises and not taking "no" for an answer. It's a tough job, and I feel fortunate to have gotten out with minimal scar tissue.

But I'm also a science geek who has a master's degree from the University of Arizona, with a focus on neurophysiology, the study of how the nervous system works in conjunction with the muscles to enable movement and improve human performance. My interest in the subject isn't remotely academic: I want to know everything I can about making the human body bigger, stronger, faster, and leaner. As soon as I think I've come across information that applies to those goals, I try it out in my own workouts. If it works for me, I try it with the clients and athletes I train for a living. And if it works for them, I write about it.

I've been writing for T-Nation, an online bodybuilding magazine, since 2000. If you had heard of me before you came across this book, that's probably why. Each article I write is typically seen by tens of thousands of readers, and some articles have generated hundreds of comments, as well as discussions that spill over to other sites that aren't affiliated with T-Nation. Those discussions can get heated, and some even turn vicious. But I've been around long enough to realize that heat and hate always accompany a genuine paradigm shift, even in something as apolitical as strength training.

When one of my articles gains traction, it's usually because I've challenged a long-practiced and long-accepted idea. A few years ago, for example, everyone agreed that the best way to build muscle mass was with sets of 8 to 12 repetitions of each exercise in your workout program. If you did fewer repetitions, you were building strength at the expense of muscle size. I flipped that around, showing readers that working with heavy weights and relatively low repetitions—3 to 5 per set—would build size and strength simultaneously. In fact, I argued, *heavy weights are the best tool for building muscle mass.*

That's not just my opinion; it's one of the most basic rules of exercise science. You can't pass a course in exercise physiology without knowing this rule. Yet, almost every trainer and strength coach ignores it as soon as he leaves the classroom.

It's called the *size principle,* which I explain in detail in Chapter 2. The executive summary is this: Muscle fibers come in different sizes and have different roles. But your body always uses them in the same order, with the smallest fibers going first and the biggest fibers only going into action when you absolutely need to generate all-out strength and power for a single, isolated action.

So I questioned the idea that the best way to build bigger muscles is with techniques that couldn't possibly employ all the fibers within those muscles.

Here's an analogy:

Imagine that you've bought a company, only to discover that a percentage of your employees sit around all day with nothing to do. And imagine that the previous owner of the company had done this deliberately, thinking it was a good idea to employ people who didn't have any actual work to perform. If you wanted to make that company succeed, the first thing you'd do is . . . well, to be realistic, most business owners would lay off all those workers. But you're smarter than most, and when you look at those workers, you realize they're incredibly skilled in one particular area

of your business, an area that the previous owner had neglected. When you give them work to do in that area, your business immediately generates more revenue, at the same cost. After all, you were paying the workers anyway. Now you're paying them *and* getting something in return.

The admonition to use heavy weights with low reps proved to be both popular and effective. For many lifters, the one thing they *hadn't* tried was working with heavier weights. I've heard this from more readers than I could ever count. They'd been told for decades that lifting near-maximum weights was both dangerous and ineffective for building muscle.

Why were they told that? The standard explanation—that heavy weights would make their muscles stronger but not bigger—is a truly breathtaking misunderstanding of basic exercise science. Why wouldn't stronger muscles also be bigger, all else being equal? Or, put another way, why would muscles get bigger unless they needed to get stronger? Why would your body add muscle tissue unless there's a functional reason for it to be there?

I wasn't the first lifter to see the light, of course. Not even close. Coaches and trainers and athletes have observed throughout history that lifting heavy things makes humans bigger and stronger. If the Neanderthals had invented gyms before they went extinct, they might very well have figured it out before humans did.

That said, the pursuit of muscle size has always been the bastard stepchild of exercise science theory and practical application. There's a reason why thousands of scientists today work to expand our knowledge of *strength* training, while there's no recognized discipline called *size* training. In the lab, an increase in muscle size is regarded as the by-product of an increase in strength. In the gym, an increase in strength is seen as the by-product of an increase in size. And in the places where the best strength coaches work with the best athletes, size and strength are both by-products of improved performance. If the process of making a sprinter faster also makes his muscles bigger and stronger, that's fine—as long as the athlete keeps getting faster.

The three groups I've just described—lab rats, gym rats, and performance rats—don't talk to each other. Or maybe I should say they tend to talk past each other. They're all concerned with the same things. They just talk about them in different ways.

Which brings me back to my breakthrough as a popular giver of advice. I told readers to do something that many, many people before me had figured out. It wouldn't be basic science if everyone who studied science weren't aware of it. But nobody was telling the gym rats what everyone in the labs and high-performance training centers knew, understood, and sometimes even implemented. In fact, for the past 4 decades, if not longer, aspiring bodybuilders and muscleheads have been told to do the opposite.

That's why most of the lifters you see in gyms, and a lot of the people reading this book, believe that the best way to build muscle is with moderate weights used in high-volume workouts involving lots of sets and reps of lots of different exercises. (Chapter 3 gives the full story of why so many people are so confused about the best way to build muscle.)

On one level, what I'd told readers was ridiculously simple, and I could have retired right then, knowing I'd left my fellow muscleheads with enough information to make real improvements.

But on another level, I knew there was more for me to learn, and more to share. That's where the neurophysiology comes in. The more I learned about the way the nervous system works, and how it recovers from the work it does, the more I realized that this was some of the most important information a musclehead should have.

Specifically, I started thinking beyond the relationship between the amount of weight you lift and the size of the muscles you build. I focused on the speed at which you lift, and how it affects the parts of the nervous system that control your favorite muscles. The more I looked into it, the more I began to suspect that maybe we had this whole thing backward: Instead of thinking mainly in terms of the weight on the bar, maybe we should redirect our attention to how fast we can move it. After all, the weights are tools for building muscle, no more, no less. It's how we use the tools that determines the results we get from our workouts. And the basic science seemed pretty clear that the best way to use the tools was at the fastest speed possible.

I talked to others in my field—people who, like me, were muscleheads first but lived double lives as scientists or performance specialists. They agreed that the idea made sense. So I wrote an article for T-Nation called "Everything Is About to Change."

In retrospect, the title was a bit overenthusiastic. As many helpful Internet experts pointed out, my argument about the importance of lifting speed is not new to power athletes. Weightlifters, discus throwers, sprinters, and many others whose performance depends on a high-speed application of strength have known for decades that they have to train fast to get fast. A guy who aspires to Olympic gold in the shot put would never waste his time lifting weights at slow speeds, just as an elite sprinter wouldn't be caught dead jogging. To get fast you have to train fast. You also have to avoid training slow. These guys have magnificent physiques—hell, the women in those pursuits are more muscular than most guys you see in gyms—so, clearly, they were way ahead of me on this one.

The problem, as I explained earlier, is that the coaches and athletes who understand the muscle-building benefits of fast lifts don't talk shop with bodybuilders. They don't hang out in Gold's Gym offering free advice. And frankly, it's hard to imagine the average musclehead taking them seriously if they did.

So a better title for that article might have been "Your Concept of the Ideal Lifting Speed as It Applies to the Size of Your Muscles Is About to Change." It wouldn't have been catchy, but I'd have gotten more points for accuracy.

HOW TO USE THIS BOOK

I could sum up the training programs in *Huge in a Hurry* in just four words: "Lift heavy stuff fast." And, to tell you the truth, I kind of like the idea of writing the world's shortest book. But I wouldn't be doing you any favors. For starters, my workouts require you to do two things that are very much outside the norm in a typical commercial gym:

1. Lift heavy stuff.

2. Lift fast.

When your gym's employees are encouraging their customers to lift light weights slowly, and to use machines instead of free weights in the process, I think you need more than four words before you turn your workouts upside down. So I've provided the theory as well as explicit instructions on how to put it into practice to build the biggest, strongest, leanest body possible.

The book, as you'll see, is divided into five parts.

Part 1 gives you the science behind my ideas. The first two chapters show you why I advocate lifting heavy things fast, and they're followed by a chapter that explains why I reject other popular systems for building muscle.

Part 2 introduces the application of the science. One big difference between my workouts and most of those you see in other books and magazines is that I advocate total-body training. That is, I think you should train all your major muscles three times a week. And if you want to get really big and are willing to devote some serious time and energy to the task, I explain in Chapter 5 why high-frequency training—working selected muscles up to seven times a week—might work for you.

Part 3 is the meat of the book. It's built around three 16-week programs. The first focuses on size, the second on strength, and the third on fat loss. But those are by no means the exclusive benefits of those programs. You'll get much stronger on the size program,

you'll build size on the strength program, and you'll probably increase muscle size while preserving your strength on the fat-loss program. (Your actual gains or losses depend on your diet, although I'm getting way ahead of myself if I get into all that here.) I've also created an advanced 16-week program for strength—which, of course, will also lead to gains in muscle mass for just about anyone who does it—along with two sample high-frequency programs for the most serious muscleheads.

The exercise photos and instructions appear in Part 4. The nutrition program follows in Part 5, showing you how to eat, as well as how much to eat, to reach your goal of building a bigger, stronger, leaner body. That section concludes with my tips on how to get into peak condition for a special occasion. It'll come in handy whenever you need to look your best, whether it's something as important as a bodybuilding contest or a mixed-martial-arts fight, or just some silly thing like your wedding day.

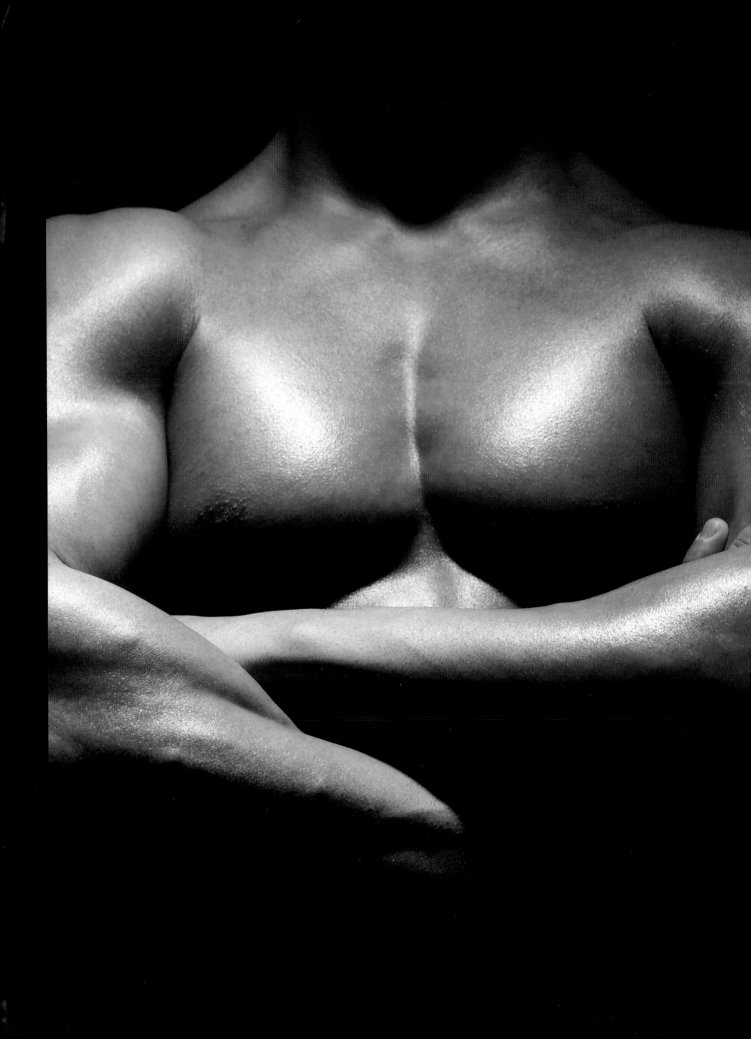

PART 1: THE BRAINS

start to ache one day and don't stop. Or maybe, with no warning, you feel sharp pain in one shoulder when you do an exercise that never hurt before. Or it could hit you in your knees or back. Whatever it is, your first instinct is to soldier through the pain, to "work around" the injury. You strap your belt on tighter, use wrist straps to help you grip the weights, and buy neoprene compression sleeves for your elbows and braces for your knees. When the mechanical props don't stop the pain, you turn to ibuprofen. Soon you're popping a handful after every workout, and sometimes a few more at night to help you fall asleep.

Then again, it might not be an injury that gets you. It could be a job change that makes it impossible to work out almost every day. What's the point of doing every chest exercise in the book in today's workout when you don't know when you'll be able to hit all the other body parts?

Some guys just quit lifting at this point. They get too frustrated by their injuries, or schedule conflicts, or whatever else forces them to work out less often than they'd like. You consider that option. But then you bump into a guy who has a completely different training philosophy, one that's based on the most counterintuitive idea you've ever come across. Any other time, you wouldn't have given his idea a second thought. Right now, however, you're willing to consider just about anything that allows you to keep lifting. Even something as crazy as this.

3. LESS IS MORE

Usually, the guy is a trainer, someone who has a good physique and comes off as smart and sincere. Or he could be a gym rat like you, probably older and presumably wiser. The pitch is the same either way: "I used to be like you. I did all kinds of crazy stuff to build as much mass as I could, as fast as I could build it. And it worked for a while—I even won the Southeastern New Jersey Junior Bodybuilding Championship, light middleweight division. But that's before I figured out the *real* way to train."

It's called "high-intensity training," or HIT. He warns you that it's simple, but not easy. It involves doing a single set of 8 to 12 exercises per workout. The simple part is that the workouts are short, straightforward, and infrequent—twice a week to start, going down to once a week if necessary. The not-easy part is that it only works if you do each set until your muscles "fail." That is, they're so completely fatigued that you can't do another repetition. There's even an advanced version in which you go beyond failure, with the trainer or a lifting partner helping you complete repetitions after your muscles have given up.

The first workout is amazing. You thought you knew what it meant to work hard, but this was double the effort of your past workouts, in half the time.

Two days later, you realize why you can't do this type of training more than twice a week. You aren't just sore in the typical places—your biceps, pectorals, quadriceps. Your glutes are sore. Your traps are sore. Those fingerlike muscles on the sides of your rib cage are sore. You're sore in muscles that, before now, you didn't even know you had.

The crazy thing is, it works. After the first month, you're bigger and leaner than ever. Your trainer says this is proof that you were "overtrained" before, and that this is the only way anybody should work out. The extreme soreness is still annoying, and those nagging injuries that drove you away from your last workout system aren't really gone, even though you only have to worry about them twice a week. But, all in all, the rewards make it seem like a reasonable trade-off.

Four weeks later, though, you aren't so sure. Your muscles aren't as big or full as they were, and you notice a layer of fat on your stomach that wasn't there before. When you tell your trainer, he says that it sounds like overtraining to him, and he suggests working out once a week, instead of twice.

You still trust him, so you try it for a few weeks. Your injuries become less of an issue— he was right about that—but your muscles are still shrinking while your waistline, if anything, looks bigger.

When you try to tell him you think you aren't working out often enough, he snaps at you. The problem isn't the system, he says. It's you. You aren't working out hard enough, and as a result you're losing sight of the true path. You're listening to people who aren't smart

enough to know how great high-intensity training really is.

You wonder what brought that on. Whatever it was, you realize your trainer, sincere as he is, isn't particularly objective about strength training. So you talk to another trainer. At first you feel like you're cheating on your HIT trainer, but soon enough you're glad you did. The new trainer listens carefully to your story, and then asks a question: "This trainer, is he in really good shape?" You nod. "Was he in better shape before he started doing HIT?" Well, yeah, he was a bodybuilding champion. "But he told you his new system was better, even though he didn't use it to build his own body?"

That's when you realize you've hit a dead end with HIT, and it's now time to make a U-turn and get back on the road to bigger, stronger muscles.

4. THE BEAUTY OF BALANCE

The new trainer gives you a no-frills program you can do two or three times a week. At first it looks too easy to work. Instead of five chest exercises, you do one. And instead of working the muscles you can see in the mirror more than the ones you can't, you spread the work around—front to back, pushing and pulling, upper body and lower body. Nothing is overtrained or undertrained.

You tell yourself you've gone back to basics, but in truth this is the first time you've actually done the basics. Your muscles start to grow again, you lose the extra flesh around your middle, and joint pain is an increasingly distant memory. Now you sense that you're ready for something new, something more aggressive. For the first time, the change isn't motivated by lack of results, boredom, or pain. You're ready to move on because you feel good, and you feel like it's time to challenge yourself.

As luck would have it, one of your co-workers is a pretty big guy, and a serious lifter. You ask him about his workout, and he invites you to join him after work one day. That's when you discover there's a whole new way to build muscle that you'd never considered.

5. LIFT BIG TO GET BIG

When did it happen? When did the phrase "three sets of 10" get implanted into the part of your brain that stores weight-lifting advice? And why didn't you notice it before? Because everyone around you was doing 10 reps, give or take a couple, on every set of every exercise? Now you see your co-worker and his lifting buddies doing the opposite—10 sets of three reps on the main exercises—and you wonder why no one ever suggested this to you before.

Another difference: They spend most of their time on basic exercises—bench press, squat, deadlift, row. Other than an occasional exercise using the cable stations, it's all free weights, all the time. They don't use belts or

wrist straps, and they laugh the first time they see you wearing workout gloves. "Time to build some calluses," your co-worker says.

But by far the biggest change is the amount of weight on the bar. You've been lifting for 3 years so far, and you've seen your body change. Your arms and legs are thicker, your shoulders are wider, you weigh more, and you've outgrown some of your favorite shirts. You've gotten stronger, too, compared with those first few months in the gym, but you've never really given much thought to the pursuit of strength.

Until now.

At first, you're embarrassed. The other guys do their warmup sets with more weight than you can lift for a single rep on your best day. When it's your turn on the bench, the spotters pull more than 100 pounds off the bar. You do your set, and then they put the weight back on for the next guy. It's even worse in the squat rack. You've never done a real squat before, with the tops of your thighs parallel to the floor, and the most you can use with decent form is a pathetic 95 pounds. Nobody else in the group trains with less than 225.

Then you stop being embarrassed, because it doesn't bother your new lifting buddies, who never expected you to be able to lift as much as them. In fact, they seem to enjoy having a new guy in the club. They work with you on your form and encourage you on every rep. Helping you get "stronger" isn't important to them; they want you to be *strong*.

Week after week, month after month, you indeed get stronger. You're also getting bigger. For the first time in your life, you don't have to flex your muscles in the mirror to make yourself look like a lifter. You look that way before you flex. Sometimes you see your reflection and, for a split second, don't even realize the guy with the muscles is you. People who haven't seen you since you started lifting big iron invariably mention this transformation.

Curiously, though, the muscle sometimes seems like an afterthought. The pursuit of strength is the most interesting athletic challenge you've ever attempted. It's so absorbing, in fact, that it has become an intellectual challenge as well as a physical pursuit. You read more about training, gaining a working knowledge of anatomy, physiology, and biomechanics. "Endocrinology" was never in your vocabulary, but now you're starting to understand how hormones like testosterone and insulin affect your training and recovery. You marvel at how much there is to learn and you laugh at some of the crazy notions about building muscle that used to make perfect sense to you.

In fact, you're becoming so knowledgeable that your lifting buddies sometimes ask you for advice. They still lift more than you, but you're getting closer all the time.

Injuries are minor and rare, thanks to your growing awareness of how hard you can push yourself and when it's best to take it down a notch to let a tweaked muscle recover.

The changes go beyond the gym. For the first time in your life, you understand how your diet affects your results, and you want to kick yourself for not taking nutrition seriously before now. You eat more protein and fewer carbs, invest in some high-quality supplements, time your meals around your workouts, and indulge in fast food so rarely that you can't even remember which chain has the best drive-thru.

It's all coming together for you: You take yourself seriously as a lifter, and people you meet can tell that's what you are without asking. You'd appreciate it if strangers wouldn't ask how much you can bench, but that's only because you're strongest in the deadlift, and nobody ever asks you about *that*.

Then one day, without meaning to, you come across the information that completes your evolution as a lifter.

6. IT TAKES A LOT OF NERVE

Scientists who study the brain know it. The top strength coaches in the world know it. And those who want to get bigger, stronger, faster, and leaner will eventually realize this basic fact of human physiology: Your nervous system is the key to reaching your ultimate potential.

Everything you do starts in your brain. This doesn't come as a shock, but you begin to see that it's the most often overlooked component of the muscle-building process.

Think of a simple dumbbell curl: Three key parts of your brain—your cerebellum, association cortex, and basal ganglia—meet to decide how many muscle fibers you're going to need to lift the load. Once this brain trust has made its final decision, it sends an electrical signal down your spinal cord to a specific set of neurons. Those neurons then tell your biceps what it needs to do.

If the brain gets it right, you lift the weight without giving the neural process any special thought. But your brain sometimes gets it wrong. If the weight is heavier than you thought it was going to be, you can't lift it with your normal form, the smooth athletic grace that comes with repeating such simple lifts thousands of times over the years. (Or over the weeks, if you're doing the latest biceps-blasting workout you found in a bodybuilding magazine.) Conversely, if the weight turns out to be much lighter than you expected, you could pull so hard you throw yourself off-balance.

Nobody thinks about their brain, spinal cord, and nerve fibers while they're lifting. Even though you are lifting heavier weights than ever before and have far more knowledge and insight into the way your body works, you still focus on what you can feel and see.

Still: If your nervous system controls and regulates muscle contractions, it must have some control over your ability to build bigger, stronger muscles, right?

FROM BRAIN TO BICEPS

You probably know that muscle fibers come in different sizes. For simplicity, let's call them small, medium, and large. Even if you didn't know anything else about exercise physiology, you could probably guess, going on nothing more than intuition, that small muscle fibers are used for small tasks involving fine motor activities—blinking your eyes, working your fingers, turning that frown upside down. And the big muscle fibers? Of course they're in charge of doing big things, like lifting heavy weights. You might not know that each muscle group includes a mix of fibers of all sizes, but it makes sense that they do; after all, you don't have any parts of your body that do only big or small tasks. Your fingers, for example, would be pretty useless if they couldn't grip a barbell as easily as they can hold a paintbrush.

If I told you that the nerves controlling muscle fibers—the motor neurons—also come in different sizes, you could also guess that small neurons control small muscle fibers, with the big ones working the big fibers.

And it wouldn't be a bad guess. You'd be partially right, especially about the way nerves and muscle fibers match up according to their relative size. That's important to keep in mind: Big muscle fibers are controlled by big nerve cells; they combine to allow you to lift big weights, and that's how you end up with big muscles.

But it's not *entirely* right, and the part you'd never guess holds the key to building the best physique possible.

If you were going strictly on intuition, you'd expect the small muscle fibers to contract fast, while the biggest ones contract slowly. But the opposite occurs. The small fibers are designated as "slow," and the big ones are "fast." The benefit of a slow contraction speed is that those fibers can keep working for a long time. That's why you depend on your small muscle fibers and nerves during endurance exercise, even though you're using your body's biggest muscle groups when you run a marathon.

What you gain in endurance you lose in power. Slow fibers can take you from zero to 30, but when you want to get up to top speed, you need those big fibers. Problem is, those big fibers aren't good at endurance. The biggest ones poop out in 15 seconds or less. That's the difference between sprinting and jogging.

Now you see the limits of intuition when it comes to building your body. If you just looked at muscles from the outside, you'd think that running is running, and suppose that because the same parts of your body are moving, the same muscles must be involved. So the difference between sprinting and jogging must involve something beyond the muscles—the heart and lungs, probably. You can't sprint longer than 15 seconds because you run out of wind.

You'd be partly right, but once again the part you wouldn't guess is the most interesting. The science tells us that within your muscles you have all types of fiber, from small to large, and those fibers go into action when your brain tells them to. Furthermore, they go into action in a fixed, orderly system, from smallest to largest. This is called the *size principle*, and it's the key to everything you do to build your body.

CHAPTER 2

THE SIZE PRINCIPLES

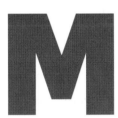uscle fibers are arranged in bundles that can consist of several fibers, several thousand, or anything in between. The smallest fibers end up in bundles with the fewest total fibers, which makes all this easy to remember: small fibers, small bundles. These are the fibers that get called into action to perform the tasks that require the least amount of strength and power. So when small bundles of small fibers are activated, there's a relatively modest change in muscle tension. But, as I explained in Chapter 1, those small fibers can maintain that modest increase in tension for a long time.

That comes in handy when we're talking about hands. The bundles of fibers in your hands, as you could probably guess, are generally small, allowing your fingers to perform fairly intricate tasks, like typing or drawing, and to go much of the day without getting exhausted.

Conversely, the largest muscle fibers end up in the largest bundles—that is, the bundles with the most fibers. Your hamstrings are a good example: big fibers, big bundles. They can perform tasks requiring all-out strength and power. The only drawback, as I noted in the first chapter, is that the biggest fibers can only generate this extreme muscle tension for 15 seconds, tops.

Each bundle, no matter how big it is, is triggered by a single nerve cell, or motor neuron. Once again, size is relevant. A small bundle has a small motor neuron calling the shots, while a big bundle has a big neuron.

The combination of one motor neuron and the bundle of fibers it controls is called a motor unit. I don't mean to bog you down with a lot of terminology, or lose you in the tall weeds of science. My goal is for you to understand what I mean when I talk about size. Small fibers end up in small bundles controlled by a small neuron. The combination is a small motor unit. Large fibers end up in large bundles controlled by large neurons. Those are the big motor units. The biggest of the big motor units are the ones that generate maximum strength and power, but with minimum endurance. The smallest motor units generate the least amount of muscle tension, but continue to provide it for the longest possible time.

So that's what I mean by "size." Now let's move on to principles.

STARTING SMALL

When muscles contract, the small motor units fire first, producing tension that increases in small increments. As more force is needed, larger motor units are recruited, each contributing progressively more tension, with that tension increasing in progressively larger increments.

That's what we call the size principle.

I want to emphasize that this is an orderly, efficient process. Most of the time, there's no need to think about it. Your body knows it's supposed to use small motor units for easy tasks that don't require much muscular tension. Typing, for example, requires small amounts of tension in your hands, so your body delegates small motor units to handle the job. If you're in the gym doing squats with a near-maximum weight, your body needs extreme muscle tension, and it needs that tension in its biggest muscles. So your brain sends almost everything it has into the fray, from the smallest motor units to the largest.

In both cases, though, *the smallest motor units go into action first.* The biggest motor units go in last, if they're needed at all. If your body recruited the big motor units first and the small ones last, you'd have no coordination, since you'd produce power first and fine movement control last. This is why you type with your fingertips instead of your knees, and why maximum efforts always start with your fingers and toes.

Here's a fun fact to remember: When you walk or run, the first muscles to go into action are in your big toe. When you lift, the first muscles to contract are usually those in your fingers. So, while the size principle, as a scientific concept, tell us that small motor units precede larger motor units in any action performed by your muscles, you can expand the idea into what I call "size principles": Small parts of your body, like fingers and toes, start the action that you think of as being performed by big parts of your body.

But even that fact is deceptive, since all muscle contractions start in your brain. Once you decide to perform a movement, your brain sends an electrical signal down your spinal cord and out to your muscles. How many motor units are recruited depends on how strong the signal is.

Once again, it's helpful to think of multiple size principles. Small motor neurons respond to small signals, whereas large motor neurons won't go into action unless the brain sends a signal that's proportionally large. Sending a small signal, thus activating small motor units, is easy for your body to do, and comes with little risk. Your body won't expend a lot of energy, and it will quickly recover from whatever exertion was involved.

On the other hand, it's risky and metabolically expensive to use the biggest motor units. It takes a lot more effort, and a lot more recovery after the effort. That's why your body waits as long as possible before using its biggest, most powerful tools.

MAKE THE FORCE BE WITH YOU

Here's something that all lifters can relate to: You're doing seated rows at a cable station in your gym. After finishing a set with 60 pounds, you get up to get a drink at the water fountain. When you return to the cable station, you sit back down, grab the bar, pull . . . and it barely moves. Someone has changed the weight to 90. Your brain knew how much power your body needed to do a repetition with 60 pounds, but it wasn't prepared to pull 90.

Now imagine a slight variation on this example: Let's suppose that you were merely warming up with 60 and deliberately changed the weight to 90 for your next set. Your body

would know what to expect, and chances are you'd move the heavier weight smoothly. Someone watching you might not know you were using a heavier weight in the second set. Your form and repetition speed would be about the same as with the lighter weight, even if you were working a lot harder.

A logical question: In the first example, why didn't your body simply adjust to the heavier weight by recruiting bigger motor units?

To answer, let's look at an equation you might remember if you've ever taken a physics class:

$$\text{Force} = \text{mass} \times \text{acceleration}$$

To produce more force, you must increase either mass or acceleration.

In the first example, mass has been increased without your knowledge. *Mass,* I should note, isn't synonymous with *weight* in physics. The mass of a balloon filled with water could be the same as a balloon filled with air, but the first one would weigh more. And the weight of either object could change if there were an increase or decrease in gravity, even though the mass would remain the same. For lifters, though, the two terms are functionally synonymous: A bigger weight has more mass. Since gravity doesn't change (unless your gym is a lot more interesting than mine), the weight with more mass is heavier.

You sat down planning to apply enough acceleration to move 60 pounds, which turned out to be less than you needed to move 90 pounds. If you'd intended to move 90 pounds, as you did in the second example, then you would've applied more acceleration. When I say "acceleration," I don't mean the actual speed the weight moves, since the heavier weight will probably move at the same speed, if not a bit slower. I mean the strength and power you apply as you move the weight. The result is the same: A heavier weight moved at the same speed means you're producing greater force.

Force and muscle fiber recruitment go hand in hand. (They're "positively correlated," a scientist would say.) As one goes up, so does the other. When all else is equal, you'll recruit more muscle fibers when lifting a heavier weight because you're generating more force.

Which, of course, is stupendously obvious to a lot of you reading this.

HOW YOUR MUSCLES FATIGUE

In Chapter 1, I suggested we keep things simple by classifying muscle fibers, and by extension motor units, as small, medium, and large. I noted that the biggest ones fatigue the fastest, but I didn't explain why.

The key is the energy supply. The biggest fibers use a relatively small energy pool called the *creatine phosphate system.* It runs out fast, and it takes much longer for your body to replenish it than to use it up. Your smallest fibers, on the other hand, can use virtually all the energy supplies your body has to offer, from the glycogen in your blood, liver, and muscle cells to the fat that's stored just about everywhere. Altogether, you have pounds of available energy, and your small fibers can dip into it.

Your medium-sized muscle fibers combine characteristics of big and small. They can't tap into all those juicy pounds of fat, but they can use glycogen efficiently enough to keep your body moving for a few minutes.

The most efficient way to convert stored energy into fuel for physical action is with oxygen, which your smallest muscle fibers can use throughout the day to burn a combination of fat and glycogen. The less effort an activity takes, the easier it is for your body to tap into your fuel supplies to keep you going. The more effort you have to put out, the harder it is for your body to provide the fuel you need.

That's why you can lie around and watch TV all day, you can walk for hours, you can jog for less than an hour, you can run fast for less than 2 minutes, and you can only sprint for 10 to 15 seconds. The fuel is there to go longer; you just can't tap into it on the fly.

But acknowledging this basic fact of exercise physiology and applying it are two very different things.

Imagine you're in the gym, and you're watching someone lifting a really heavy weight for two or three fast, full-effort repetitions. Then you watch another guy lift a medium-sized weight for 10 or 12 slow, grinding reps. Which guy appears to be working harder? The first one, who strains and grunts but finishes his entire set in 10 seconds? Or the second, whose face is contorted and whose muscles are shaking uncontrollably by the end of his 45-second set?

I'll concede that the second guy has certainly worked his muscles to exhaustion. But which lifter has used more muscle fibers, assuming both are doing the same exercise?

The size principle tells us that the first lifter, working with near-maximum weights, has used more muscle fibers, which is to say he's employed more motor units.

But if the second guy used fewer motor units, why does he look so much more fatigued after his higher-rep set? Because he *is* more fatigued. Using a lighter weight means you're using fewer motor units to begin with. Then, as those motor units get exhausted, some of them drop out of the action. That leaves you with an even smaller number of motor units doing all the work by the time you get to your final repetitions. So of course the lifter's muscles are shaking by the end of the set. He's burned out a lot of motor units, and some of the neurons are misfiring as a result.

A lot of trainers and gym rats would tell you that the second guy, the one with the shaking muscles, is the one who's getting the better workout. The size principle, though, tells us the first guy has the right idea. He's used more motor units and generated more force.

There is, however, a catch: No one can lift superheavy weights in every workout. The risk of injury would be too great, and burnout would be practically guaranteed. Fortunately, the combination of the size principle with basic physics gives us a way to increase the number of motor units we use with lighter weights.

Remember the equation: *force = mass x acceleration*. It tells us that we can generate more force by lifting a lighter weight faster. We're still generating more force, which means we're recruiting more motor units.

Now we have two ways to use more motor units with the goal of building bigger muscles:

1. Lift heavier weights

2. Lift lighter weights faster

You wouldn't be able to build an effective, sustainable muscle-building system out of one or the other. But combining the two techniques in alternating workouts gives you just about everything you need to build the body you want.

THE NEED FOR SPEED

No matter how heavy or light the weight, I want you to lift it as fast as possible when you do the *Huge in a Hurry* workouts. Well, let me modify that a bit: I want you to lift at the fastest speed at which you can still control the weight. The actual speed the weight moves doesn't matter as much as your *attempt* to move it as fast as possible. Your goal is to send the strongest possible signal from your brain to your muscles, activating the biggest motor units. Effort is everything.

Here's what I mean: Let's say you've just read the latest "get huge" article in a body-building magazine, and you can't wait to get to the gym to take the advice in the article for a test drive. It tells you to do three sets of 12 reps, using a slow, controlled tempo. Certainly, it *feels* harder to lift this way. By the end of each set, your arms shake on the outside and burn on the inside. You have an incredible pump, having forced so much blood into the muscle bellies.

You can see why so many trainers and recreational bodybuilders think this is the best way to build muscle.

Now let's imagine a different scenario. You're going to do the same exercise with the same weights, for the same number of total repetitions. But instead of lifting the weights slowly, you're lifting them as fast as possible, stopping each set (as I'll explain later in this book) when your form changes or when your rep speed slows. Instead of doing three sets of 12 reps, you end up doing six sets, averaging 6 reps per set.

Which workout is better for your goal of building bigger muscles? The size principles tell us that it's better to recruit more muscle fibers, all else being equal. And basic physics tells us that in the second example you did, indeed, recruit more muscle fibers. You applied more acceleration to the same mass, so you employed more motor units per repetition.

I'll grant that the muscle magazine workout looks harder and feels harder. Two days later, your muscles would feel stiff and sore, which most of us are conditioned to equate with an effective workout. My version, though far from easy, won't feel as exhausting at the time you're doing it, and it won't make your muscles feel as sore a day or two later.

Take a look at the graph on the opposite page. On the horizontal axis, you can see that your brain recruits more muscle fibers as the difficulty of the action increases—you need just a quarter of your motor units when you're standing, half of them when you walk, and almost all of them when you jump. The biggest motor units don't get involved until you need them for running and jumping. But the smallest motor units are involved in every action—once they're recruited, they can't be unrecruited. They work to help you stand, walk, run, and jump.

Now look at the vertical axis. That shows

THE RELATIONSHIP BETWEEN FORCE, MOTOR UNIT RECRUITMENT, AND SPEED OF MOVEMENT

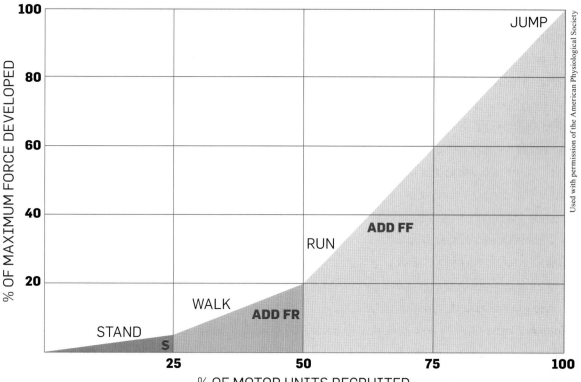

you how much of your maximum force goes into each action. You'll notice that the percentages aren't the same. You might use 50 percent of the motor units in your working muscles when you walk, but barely 20 percent of the force those muscles are capable of generating. To make the percentages equivalent, as they are in the upper-right-hand corner of the chart, you have to employ almost all your motor units, to produce almost all the force possible.

There's one more important lesson found in this chart: *You can't selectively recruit your largest muscle fibers.*

This is actually one of the most beautiful aspects of the size principle: When you recruit the largest muscle fibers you're also recruiting *all of the other muscle fibers.*

Your goal on almost every repetition is to get up toward the upper-right-hand corner of the graph. That's the point at which you're using the most muscle fibers to generate the most force.

You could start doing this today, without reading any farther in this book, simply by going into the gym and lifting as fast as possible. You'll recruit more muscle fibers because you'll be generating more force.

However, it's not quite as simple as that. The size of the weight does matter. If it didn't, baseball pitchers would look like powerlifters (on one side, anyway). And powerlifters, by extension, would be able to throw harder than the relatively lanky pitchers who actually generate the highest velocity.

Your brain senses the weight of the object you're holding, and prepares itself to recruit a commensurate number of muscle fibers.

Picture yourself in the gym holding a 5-pound dumbbell. No matter how fast you curl that dumbbell, your brain can only recruit a limited percentage of motor units. Sure, it'll dispatch more muscle fibers for a faster lift, but not enough to make any kind of difference to your physique. You'll finish the repetition before your brain senses the need to send in the biggest motor units. The smaller motor units are enough to move the weight as fast as it can be moved within the limited range of motion required by the exercise.

Now imagine yourself holding a 50-pound dumbbell. Before you even start the movement, your brain has already decided it's going to need a higher percentage of your motor units. Moving the weight as fast as possible will bring almost every available motor unit into the action. And, because you can't move the 50-pound dumbbell as fast as you moved the 5-pounder, there's more time available for this to happen.

SPEED, RANGE OF MOTION, AND TECHNIQUE

If you're going to lift with the goal of using as many muscle fibers as possible with each repetition, you want to stop the set when:

1. Your speed slows down.

2. Your form changes.

3. Your range of motion shortens.

Speed is easy enough to judge, most of the time. If you think your reps are slowing down, they probably are. But it's also possible to lift at the same speed with fewer motor units. That's why it's important to pay attention to your technique and range of motion.

Picture this: You're watching a Strongman competition on ESPN. A massive guy named Magnus steps up to deadlift the back end of a wagon that's filled with iron, with the goal of completing as many reps as possible.

The first lift goes up easily. He pulls hard with his hamstrings, lower back, and gluteals, and locks out the repetition. You'd consider it textbook form, if there were actually a textbook describing how to deadlift one end of a wagon filled with iron. The second rep looks like the first. The third looks similar, but you notice Magnus takes longer than before to lock it out. By the fourth rep, his form has changed. His hamstrings are fried, and he's relying more on his back. But he still completes the lift. The fifth rep is worst of all. It's slower than the others, his form is even worse than it was on his fourth rep, and after all that he fails to lock it out at the end.

You can't know this for sure, but you can guess that after the second rep his biggest motor units got fatigued and began to drop out of the action. The first sign was the slower rep speed. Then he changed his form to compensate, which brought in some other muscles that he hadn't used before. Finally, his range of motion shortened—without his biggest and strongest motor units, he couldn't produce enough force to finish the repetition.

None of this is a secret to Magnus. He could tell his muscles were hemorrhaging motor units by the third repetition, but because he was in the middle of a contest, he had to keep going anyway. If he'd been doing the *Huge in a Hurry* workouts, he would've stopped after completing a rep that was noticeably slower than the one that preceded it. He wouldn't have needed to wait for his form to change or for his range of motion to shorten.

Most of the time, then, speed is the key—but not always. Let's go back to the example of the cable row I used earlier in this chapter. Cable machines just aren't designed for fast lifting. You can still lift faster than most others, but if you pull as hard as you can, you might break the machine, or at least knock something off track. Even if you don't break it, you'll annoy the hell out of everyone when the weight plates slam up against the top of the machine.

So instead of using rep speed as your only

criterion, you also should watch out for subtle changes in your form—for example, instead of staying upright throughout the repetition, you find yourself bending forward to start the rep, and then leaning back to finish it. Your rep speed might be about the same, but now your form is different.

Even that cue might not be enough, especially on a more complex lift such as a barbell squat. With all those moving parts, and all the effort and concentration it takes to maintain your balance, you might not notice a change in rep speed or a minor shift in your form.

But you should be able to tell when your range of motion shortens. In the squat, the change will come on the descent; you won't go down as far before you reverse direction. That's your body's way of telling you it's fatigued and can't do this rep the same way it did the others—not with any hope of returning to the starting position.

Range of motion is also a useful gauge of motor unit recruitment on exercises in which the form is deceptively simple. Take chinups, for example. You might not notice changes in speed or form, but when your chin no longer goes over the bar, there's no better sign that your top motor units are cooked and it's time to end the set.

Now, having staked this position, I'll concede that a lot of experts would tell you to keep going even with slower reps, altered form, and a shorter range of motion. Even if they concede that you're no longer working all your motor units, they'll argue that you're still using enough of them to make those reps worth the effort. After all, all your fibers have growth potential.

I agree that you can still build good muscle with bad reps. I just don't think it's worth the effort. On some lifts, I'll argue that it's dangerous to keep going. See, the high-threshold motor units that are dropping out aren't just in your primary muscles, the big ones that you're targeting with the lift. The ones in your smaller muscles are getting fatigued as well.

Consider the four muscles in your rotator cuff. They help stabilize your shoulders during pressing exercises. When they fatigue, your shoulders lose some of their protection against injury.

Or consider the reverse: Suppose the high-threshold units in your big muscles fatigue first. Your smaller muscles start acting as prime movers, which diminishes their ability to stabilize.

Maybe all of this could be summed up in five simple words: Never choose quantity over quality. Conveniently enough, that's the major theme of Chapter 3.

KNOWLEDGE IS POWER…
AS LONG AS IT'S ACCURATE

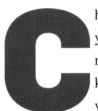hapters 1 and 2 focused on what you don't know—particularly the ways in which your nervous system controls the muscle-building machinery and how to use it to make bigger, faster gains. This chapter is the opposite; it's about what you *do* know—knowledge that just happens to be inaccurate and that might be holding you back.

MYTH #1: NO PAIN, NO GAIN

As a fitness professional, I've heard this one a lot. The problem with this myth is that it *seems* true. All of us, no matter how much education and experience we possess, use postexercise soreness as a sign of a successful workout. It means we did something that was different from what we'd been doing before. It means we worked out harder or longer, or we hit some of our muscles in a new way.

But even though all that is true, as far as it goes, it doesn't mean that there's any actual connection between the degree of pain you endure and the amount of muscle you build. It's entirely possible to make the same gains, or even bigger gains, with minimal postworkout suffering.

You can't avoid soreness entirely if you're doing an effective program. A good workout breaks down muscle tissue, which is the cue for your muscles to add new protein to those areas, resulting in a net gain in muscle size. But more damage—and the excess pain that comes with it—does not lead to more growth. If that were the case, you could add an inch to your upper arms in one day by doing 100 sets of biceps curls and triceps extensions. Your goal is to *minimize* this kind of damage, not seek it out. The more damage you do to your muscles, the longer it takes for them to recover fully. That's why excessive muscle breakdown is detrimental to your success.

Our trust in postworkout soreness feeds into another belief: Extreme results require extreme workouts.

This idea is reinforced everywhere you look. Take muscle magazines, for example. A typical workout feature might include a picture of a gargantuan bodybuilder, with legs as thick as mature sequoias, doing a leg press on a machine loaded with ten 45-pound plates on each side. You do the math and see he's lifting 900 pounds. If you only saw his contorted face, with pain etched into every square centimeter, you'd swear he was giving birth to 900 pounds of iron rather than lifting it.

The connection between big pain and big muscles seems obvious and inarguable, and the articles that accompany the photos reinforce the point. They tell you that every set of every exercise has to be taken to "failure"—the point at which you can't move the weight another inch. If you don't pulverize your muscles, you can't expect them to grow to the size of a bodybuilder's.

So you pulverize them and find that you're rewarded with pain three times over: The workout itself is an exercise in physio-masochism. You feel drained for the rest of the day, which further reinforces the idea that you didn't hold anything back—you left it all in the weight room. Then the postworkout soreness that kicks in the next day, and might last the better part of a week, seals it for you. You suffered for your muscles, and now you can't wait to see the rewards.

Before I get to that part, let me clear up a few things that I skipped over earlier. You know that picture of the bodybuilder straining to leg-press 900 pounds? Chances are, that's a lot more weight than the guy could actually lift. And even if he really is that strong under normal circumstances, a photo shoot isn't a normal circumstance. The bodybuilder is in "contest condition," meaning he's at the end of a crash diet that allowed him to reduce his body-fat percentage to the low single digits. He might be weaker than his little sister at the time of the shoot, despite his cartoon-superhero appearance.

What he's really doing, in all likelihood, is *lowering* 900 pounds, not lifting it. The foot platform on a leg-press machine starts in the "up" position. So if the photo crew loads up the machine with 20 plates, all the bodybuilder has to do is release the supports and lower the weight. In a photo, it all looks the same, and readers never see how many people it takes to lift the weight back up to the starting position.

And that assumes the plates themselves are real. They might be hollow aluminum shells painted to look like the real thing. A friend who used to work for a bodybuilding magazine told me that the skinniest editor or photographer could easily lift the 100-pound dumbbells shown in muscle-mag photos. In fact, one of their favorite jokes was to use the fake weights to initiate each new member of the photo crew. Someone would pretend to grunt and strain while lifting a massive dumbbell, then without warning hand it off to the newbie, who had no idea it didn't really weigh 100 pounds. My friend said it was harmless fun, and no underwear was actually ruined in the initiate's moment of sheer terror.

But the artifice doesn't end there. The article itself, with its exhortations to take each set to the limit and revel in the pain it causes, probably wasn't actually written by the bodybuilder. The bodybuilder might not even speak the same language as the editor writing the story under his name.

Competitive bodybuilders, in my experience, rarely do the things you see in magazines. When I see them at Gold's Gym in Venice, California, where I work out, they're doing ordinary routines with ordinary weights. But the magazines don't want you to see that. The top bodybuilders are under contract to the magazines that feature them, and the publishers of those magazines know that readers don't want to see their heroes doing curls with 30-pound dumbbells.

If you want to see guys lifting huge weights for real, check out a powerlifting contest. Take note of the enormous belts the powerlifters wear, the special shirts they use for bench presses, and the suits and knee wraps they use for squatting. Finally, take note of the physical proportions that allow for superheavy lifts. You'll see barrel chests instead of six-pack abs.

You'll also see quite a bit of pain on the lifters' faces. Take my word on this: The pain is real. If you want to compete at this level, pain is necessary. But in the pursuit of bigger muscles, it's highly overrated.

MYTH #2: SLOW LIFTS ARE SAFER AND MORE EFFECTIVE THAN FAST REPETITIONS

For most of the history of strength training, it was just accepted that weights had to be lifted quickly. That's because the focus was on strength and power, and you can't develop those qualities by lifting things slowly.

But starting in the early 1970s, a strength-training guru named Arthur Jones came up with an entirely new way to train. Jones was a bodybuilding enthusiast and inventor who'd developed a line of exercise machines to accommodate his new training philosophy. The name of the company he founded, Nautilus, eventually became synonymous with his system: Each exercise was performed for just one set of about eight repetitions, and each of those repetitions was supposed to last about 8 seconds. The set didn't end until "failure," the point at which your muscles were completely exhausted. Entire workouts might last just 20 to 30 minutes, and the resulting muscle damage was so severe that you couldn't work those muscles again for another week. Jones started off advocating three workouts a week, but his disciples often recommended just two or even one workout a week. That's not "one workout per muscle group per week," a protocol many bodybuilders use. It's one or two *workouts* per week, total.

This was revolutionary, since it came in the golden age of bodybuilding, when increasingly popular musclemen like Arnold Schwarzenegger were telling their fans to work out for hours a day, 6 or 7 days a week.

Some of Jones's ideas made sense. Mainstream fitness experts soon figured out that less training could yield better results for most exercisers. Elite strength coaches realized that pushing their athletes to work harder instead of longer was a better use of everyone's time and energy.

That's where we are today—most fitness advice suggests 3 or 4 hours a week of strength training as the upper limit for even the most dedicated gym rats. Those who feel that's not enough are typically advised to work harder in those 3 or 4 hours, rather than adding more time in the gym.

However, one of Jones's worst ideas also made it into the mainstream, and it has become so entrenched in so many circles that it's impervious to actual science. I'm talking about the value of slow repetitions. Bodybuilders like them because they want to "feel" the muscle working, to make a "mind-muscle connection." (Actually, though, bodybuilders would create a better connection if they improved the neural drive to their muscles. And a great way to do that—surprise!—is by lifting fast.) At the opposite end of the iron hierarchy, trainers who work with beginners and other nonathletic clients are convinced that fast lifts are dangerous, and believe slow reps are safer.

I disagree with them about the safety issue; if your body is perfectly capable of running, jumping, and throwing, all of which involve accelerating as fast as possible, why is it dangerous to lift fast? But let's look at it from the musclehead's point of view:

When you lift a weight slowly—really, at any speed less than the fastest possible—you're limiting the number of muscle fibers you can recruit. Typical advice these days is to take 6 seconds for each repetition, and to do a relatively high number of repetitions per set, usually 10 to 12.

Let's attach some numbers to a typical workout recommendation. Say your routine calls for three sets of 12 reps of biceps curls. You load the barbell with a weight you're pretty sure you could lift that many times at a deliberate speed—2 seconds to raise it, 4 seconds to lower it. That weight is probably in the neighborhood of 60 percent of the amount you could curl for a single repetition.

Just for the sake of this example, let's say that these numbers equate to percentages of muscle fibers used during the set: 100 percent of your one-rep max uses 100 percent of your fibers, and 60 percent of your max recruits 60 percent of your fibers. Of course, you could use a higher percentage of fibers if you lifted this weight as fast as you could. But once you

FAILING UPWARD

True confession: I sometimes oversimplify my own ideas. (Some would say I often do, especially in my online articles.) I've already done it twice in this chapter, first when I suggested that training to "failure" is overrated, then when I said that you should stop your sets when your reps slow down, an indication that your biggest muscle fibers are fatigued. Neither "failure" nor "fatigue" is as simple or predictable as I sometimes make them sound.

Let's say you're doing sets of three repetitions with a weight that's close to the most you could lift for a single rep. Chances are, your second rep would be faster than the first rep, due to some momentum coming into play. But your third rep could be much slower than your first or second. That doesn't mean you shouldn't do that third rep, or that you should stop in the middle of the rep when you feel the bar slowing down. Completing that third rep, at any speed, is important. Fatigue is an important stimulus for muscle growth, so you can't stop the set until you've seen clear evidence that you've fatigued the muscle fibers you're targeting.

Now let's look at failure.

You might reach the point of failure on a low-rep set. That is, you might start your third or fourth rep thinking you can complete it, but your muscles have other ideas, and the bar stops well short. You've just trained to failure, and that's fine. You have to push toward your limits to get the results you want, and in this case you've reached a limit without intending to. Now you'll have the pleasure of blasting past that limit in future workouts. I don't have to tell you how gratifying that is; for muscleheads like us, knowing we're stronger today than we were last week is proof that the world is working the way it should.

If you're looking for a guideline to follow, just remember that your biggest muscle fibers fatigue in about 15 seconds. A low-rep set won't go beyond 15 seconds whether you hit failure or not. But if you're doing more reps with a lighter weight and going beyond 15 seconds, pay close attention to the speed of your reps, and stop after you finish a repetition that was clearly slower than its predecessor.

made the choice to do all your reps *at a deliberate pace*, you restricted yourself to this otherwise unchallenging weight, and left your biggest, strongest muscle fibers out of the action.

I've heard advocates of slow lifting say that bigger muscle fibers do indeed come into play as the smaller ones get tired. It kind of sounds like the size principle, in that bigger fibers are activated when your brain realizes the smaller ones can't complete the task. But it's not at all the way the size principle actually works.

What really happens is that your smaller fibers get recruited and stay recruited. Your bigger fibers start on the sidelines and stay there. If bigger fibers actually came to the rescue in the middle of a set, you'd get stronger, and be able to move the weight faster. Instead, the opposite happens: Some of the fibers get exhausted and shut down, and you become weaker toward the end of the set. You start out lifting the weight slowly and deliberately out of choice. You end up lifting the weight slowly because you couldn't move it faster even if you wanted to.

But it's even worse than that: Bigger fibers get exhausted before smaller fibers. So when you start to slow down and struggle on the eighth or ninth rep, the bigger fibers are dropping out, leaving the smaller ones to keep going. You already know that you haven't recruited the biggest fibers, so the ones dropping out are only "bigger" when compared to the ones that are left to do the rest of the work. And those are the smallest ones you have.

Think of it like a football game: You benched your first string before you even started the set. And now, as you struggle through your final reps, you've lost your second string as well. You're trying to win the game—to build the best possible physique—with your best players on the bench and your scrubs on the field. It's better than sending in the marching band, but not by a lot.

Really, the argument against slow lifting teaches us two important lessons:

»Starting a set without recruiting the maximum number of muscle fibers is a poor use of your time and energy. For the same effort, you could use more muscle, and thus build more muscle.

»Continuing a set after your muscles are exhausted means you're working with even fewer motor units than you had at the start of the set. That's why I want you to stop each set in the *Huge in a Hurry* workouts when your reps start to slow down. Your goal is to work with as many motor units as possible as often as possible.

MYTH #3: SPECIFIC EXERCISES CAN CHANGE THE SHAPE OF THE MUSCLES THEY TARGET

I'm going to pick on bodybuilding magazines again, because that's where I first got the idea that certain variations on the biceps curl could give my biceps a better "peak." I think I was 15 at the time, and like every 15-year-old (not to mention every 25-, 35-, 45-, and 55-year-old), I wanted that very thing.

So I followed the advice as written. I'd use three or four different types of curls, each from a different angle, to make the middle part of my flexed biceps look more like mountains and less like Indian burial mounds.

The idea made some sense to my teenage mind. The biceps, after all, has two parts, or heads. They start at the same tendon just above the elbow joint. But the two parts attach to your shoulders in different spots. The "short head," the inner half of the muscle, has a tendon that attaches to the inside part of your shoulder blade. The "long head," the outer half, has a tendon that crosses the ball and socket of your shoulder joint. To look at them in an anatomy textbook, you would assume that they must serve separate functions. Otherwise, why would they split off from each other? If they did different things, then it must be possible to work one side or the other preferentially. And if I could make one side—the long head—grow more than the other, I'd have a better "peak."

At least, that's what the bodybuilding magazines said would happen.

Did it work that way? Nope.

I gave up on curls altogether after a few months, and focused instead on pullups. I figured if I had a bigger upper back, it would make up for having unimpressive upper arms.

But then a funny thing happened: My biceps got bigger along with my upper-back muscles. The shape never changed, but I discovered they looked just fine in their new, larger size.

I didn't give it much more thought until I got into college and studied biology and exercise science. That's when I learned that you can't activate the fibers on one side of the biceps without activating the fibers on the other side. (Okay, technically, you can fire up whichever side you want with electrical stimulation. You just can't do it with barbells and dumbbells.) The two heads are designed to work together, which means they grow together.

This basic fact of physiology hasn't stopped bodybuilding gurus from inventing exercises to emphasize one side or the other. The classics:

>> *Elbows in, hands out.* By curling with your elbows against your sides and your hands beyond shoulder-width apart, you'll allegedly work the short head more than the long head.

>> *Elbows out, hands in.* Curl with a more narrow grip and elbows flared out and, according to legend, you'll hit the long head more.

The truth is, no matter where your elbows and hands are positioned, both heads of your biceps will fire to curl the load. Even if one fires more than the other, the results wouldn't be visible from the outside, which is all that matters in the sport of bodybuilding. I've been intensely interested in muscles since my early teens, and in all my years of practice and observation, I've never seen a single example of someone's muscles changing shape. *Bodies* change shape over time, getting bigger and/or leaner. But, as I said, I don't know of any lifter who has changed the shape of a specific muscle by doing specific exercises.

Even if that were possible, the biceps would be the least likely candidate, due to their relatively small size and limited functions.

That said, a really dedicated bodybuilder can change the size of certain muscles in proportion to others, giving the illusion of an altered shape. For example, there's a thick, flat muscle beneath the biceps called the brachialis. It generally works along with the biceps on elbow-flexing exercises, but you can make it work proportionally harder by changing your grip. You've probably heard of hammer curls, in which your palms are turned toward each other. That puts your upper arms in their strongest position, since your brachialis and biceps are engaged together. If you use a palms-down (pronated) grip, as you would on pull-ups, you engage your brachialis at the expense of your biceps. The effect of that, over time, would be a thicker brachialis. That pushes your biceps up higher when you flex your arms, and could create the illusion of a better peak.

The quadriceps is the best example of a group of muscles in which you can selectively emphasize one part over others. The four-muscle group has one main function—straightening your knee joint—with lots of fine print. If you look at speed skaters, cyclists, and downhill skiers, you can see the difference with untrained eyes. They all have distinctive development of the vastus lateralis, the part of the quadriceps on the outside of the

thigh. That's because their sports require their knees to bend and straighten through a relatively short range of motion, which gives the vastus lateralis more work in relation to other parts of the quadriceps.

Conversely, athletes who have to use deep knee bends—think of Olympic weightlifters, who squat ass-to-calves in the bottom positions of cleans and snatches—will have pronounced development of their vastus medialis, the teardrop-shaped muscle on the inside of the thigh, just above the knee. That part of the quadriceps has more of a role in stabilizing the knee joint, and it works hardest when the knee is in its most vulnerable position.

So you can change the overall shape of the quadriceps group by doing exercises that selectively target a function of one part of the group. You can also selectively avoid development of a part. This is important for athletes, who might hinder their performance if the wrong part of the muscle group becomes too strong and throws off the firing pattern of the motor units that are most crucial to success in their sport. But it also matters when the goal is purely aesthetic. I've trained several figure competitors in recent years and found that subtle changes in the quadriceps—emphasizing the outer part especially—can make a big difference in how my clients look onstage.

In any case, the shape of the muscle isn't changing. What's changing is that one part of a collection of muscles has grown due to the specific demands imposed upon it.

MYTH #4: YOU CAN'T BUILD A GREAT PHYSIQUE WITHOUT MUSCLE-ISOLATING EXERCISES

Most exercises we do in the weight room fall into one of two broad classifications:

>> "Isolation" movements, such as biceps curls and knee extensions, are designed to work a single muscle or group of muscles by restricting movement to a single joint.

>> "Compound" movements, such as bench presses and squats, work more than one joint and thus more than one muscle or muscle group.

In the real world, there's almost no such thing as an "isolation" movement. The human body is a system of integrated parts. Simply reaching for your coffee cup involves movement at the shoulder, elbow, and wrist joints. Any bending, twisting, or leaning you have to do will engage the joints of your spine, and possibly your hips as well.

Bodybuilders and equipment designers try to get around this basic human tendency to move in a coordinated fashion, and in one sense they probably do succeed. They can certainly alter a person's natural coordination by forcing muscles to work in ways that depart from the muscles' functional purpose.

That, of course, is one of the problems I have with isolation exercises. But it's not the biggest problem.

My main argument against more than occasional use of isolation exercises is that the practice is based on misunderstood science and false premises.

I've already discussed two examples of bad science. First, muscles can't be "shaped" with specific movements. They can be made bigger or allowed to get smaller. That's it. Second, specific sections of muscles can rarely be isolated in any meaningful way.

The false premise is that muscles *need* to be isolated. A typical argument I've heard goes something like this: Compound exercises emphasize your strong points and minimize your weak points. If you're doing chinups and your back is strong relative to your biceps, your back will do more work than it ordinarily would and your biceps will do less than they need. So, if your biceps are already small and weak relative to your upper-back and shoulder muscles, the imbalance will only get worse unless you do exercises designed to make your biceps bigger and stronger.

I've heard similar arguments about the bench press, which mainly involves the chest, shoulder, and triceps muscles. Most guys are going to be stronger in one or two areas and proportionally weaker in the others. If your triceps are too strong, they'll do too much of the work, and your pectorals won't grow as much as they should. And if your triceps are too weak, they'll prevent you from working with weights heavy enough to give your pecs the kind of workout they need.

The answer to this dilemma is simple: Change your angle and grip to emphasize the muscles you're trying to build. A wider grip shortens the range of motion and reduces the amount of work your arm muscles have to do. If you're doing a bench press with a wide grip, you emphasize your chest and shoulders. If it's a row or chinup, you create more work for your lats and the other muscles acting on your shoulder joints, and less for your arm muscles. Move your hands closer together, and the range of motion lengthens. That gives your arm muscles—the ones that bend and straighten your elbows—more to do.

That answer, though, raises a follow-up question: Why not just do a combination of compound and isolation exercises, with the compound exercises focusing on the biggest muscles and the isolation exercises targeting the smaller ones?

My response: Because you can give smaller muscles a better growth stimulus with compound exercises.

Think of the biceps exercise that allows you to use the heaviest possible load. It's a standing barbell curl, right? Let's say you weigh 180 pounds and you can do sets of curls with 90. But if you do close-grip chinups instead, you're working with your entire body weight, which is double what you could use for an isolation exercise. Who could argue that working with 90 pounds would yield better results than working with 180? It doesn't matter that your back muscles are also involved in the movement. They can't pull your chin over the bar by themselves. Your biceps have to carry a lot of the load.

Same thing with triceps. They'll get a lot

more work helping your chest and shoulders lock out 200 pounds on a bench press with a narrow hand position than they would doing extensions with less than half that much weight.

Finally, there's the original point I made in this section: If you have a choice between a great-looking body that's functional and well coordinated and a great-looking body that's not as strong or graceful as it looks, why would you choose the latter? Who wants to be weaker and clumsier?

MYTH #5: THERE'S AN INVERSE RELATIONSHIP BETWEEN REPS AND REST PERIODS

Sometimes, knowing a little about how the nervous system affects exercise performance can be worse than knowing nothing.

Like everyone else, I assumed that low-rep, heavy-load sets required long rest periods to allow your nervous system to recover. So, if you were doing 10 sets of three reps, you'd need to rest 3 to 5 minutes between sets. Old-school powerlifters used to take even longer than that; one *really* old-school lifter said he used to sit down on a bench and read the newspaper in between sets. The longer they rested, the more time their nervous systems had to recover, and the more they could lift in their next set.

The flip side is that if you're working with relatively light weights and doing relatively high reps—12 to 15, say—you can get away with just a minute in between sets, since they're not as taxing to the nervous system.

It's easy to figure out the problem with this formula. Next time you're in the gym, do a set of 20 squats. Then try to do another set of 20 a minute later. If you aren't still hugging the floor 60 seconds after finishing that first set, with your heart beating so hard it's setting off seismometers a mile away, you're a better man than most.

Conversely, if you've ever done a heavy-weight, low-rep workout, you probably found that you were ready for your next set within 2 minutes. Holding off for 3 to 5 minutes, as many programs recommend, turns the weight room into the wait room. It's as much fun as a day at the DMV. But it's also unnecessary. Even with a really heavy set of two or three reps, the heart-pounding fatigue lasts only a minute or so. After 2 minutes, your heart has slowed down and your muscles and nerves are ready for the next set.

As for the notion that your nervous system requires a longer recovery, that's only true if we're talking about an attempt at a personal-record lift, or some type of competition that involves a surge of adrenaline. The nervous system, as we currently understand it, doesn't take very long to recover from a less exciting short-duration challenge, such as a set of two or three reps in a normal workout. The processes take less than a minute, and then you're good to go.

A high-rep set of compound movements such as squats or deadlifts will crank your heart rate up so high that it takes several minutes for it to come back down. Your only choice is to wait it out. That's why I put less emphasis on the nervous system as it relates to this particular aspect of training and more on cardiovascular recovery.

And yet, if you look at just about any workout program in a book or magazine, you'll see long rest periods following low reps and short ones for high-rep sets.

How did we get this backward? It's hard to say for sure, but I'll take a stab at it.

Back in the 1980s, when most of our popular ideas about training were migrating from the bodybuilding culture to mainstream health clubs, typical workouts included both compound and isolation movements. Compound movements were for building mass; isolation movements were for shaping muscles. Remember what I said earlier about the "mind-muscle connection"? The idea was that you made that connection with higher-rep ranges, literally squeezing your muscles into the shapes you wanted them to attain. A set of 12 biceps curls is certainly taxing for your upper arms, but it's not a major challenge to your cardiovascular system. So you wouldn't need much recovery.

When bodybuilders did lower-rep sets, they tended to use compound exercises, and of course they realized that they needed more recovery from squats than they did from biceps curls.

Somehow that formula came to be codified into "longer recovery for low-rep sets, shorter recovery for higher reps." But, really, it only works that way with specific exercises. Low-rep sets of biceps curls require less recovery time than high-rep sets of squats or lunges. Even if you didn't see it in writing, you'd figure it out pretty quickly in the gym.

MYTH #6: ECCENTRIC-FOCUSED TRAINING IS NECESSARY TO BUILD BIGGER, STRONGER MUSCLES

This myth, like #5, may be a bit esoteric for some of you. If you've only been lifting for a year or two, or if you've never spent any quality time reading books and magazines about our favorite pursuit, you probably wonder why this myth you've never heard of is important enough to debunk.

But even if the phrase "eccentric-focused training" is new to you, I'll bet you've been exposed to the idea it represents. Before I get to that, let me explain the words themselves.

Your muscles have three types of actions. Most of us think of our lifts in terms of the primary action, which shortens the muscle. On a curl, for example, the biceps muscle bulges because it's shortening. This is called a *concentric* muscle contraction. When you lower the weight, you're lengthening the muscle; that's called an *eccentric* contraction. (Never mind that the word "contraction" doesn't really fit when we're talking about

your muscles doing the opposite.) If you simply hold something in an unchanging position, that's called an *isometric* contraction.

Every lift has concentric and eccentric phases, in which you shorten muscles and then allow them to lengthen. (Some training systems also include isometric holds.) You work against gravity when your muscles are shortening, and you're assisted by gravity when they're lengthening. You can't, however, let gravity take total control during the lengthening phase. That would involve simply dropping the weight from the top position. If it's a deadlift in a crowded gym, the racket will make you exceedingly unpopular. If it's a bench press . . . well, let's just say it's never a good idea to let a loaded barbell fall onto your chest.

Lowering a weight under control, on the other hand, forces you to resist gravity. That means you're making your muscles work during the lengthening phase as well as the shortening phase.

Of course, there's no comparison of the effort involved in these two phases. It's much harder to lift a weight against the force of gravity than it is to control its descent. That's why you can lower weights that are much heavier that any you could lift (see my leg press example on page 22, under Myth #1).

But exercise scientists figured out something kind of interesting: In experiments, they sometimes demonstrated that people who did nothing but eccentric contractions gained more muscle than people who did concentric-only versions of the same exercises.

The impracticality of this information is self-evident: Nobody can just walk into a gym and do eccentric-only contractions. Once you lower a bar loaded with more weight than you could lift, how do you do the next repetition? And how do you do an eccentric-only bench press without trapping yourself beneath a loaded barbell?

Strength coaches were intrigued enough by the performance-enhancing possibilities of eccentrics that they came up with two basic techniques:

➤➤ *Eccentric-only contractions*. On a bench press, two spotters would help you get the bar off the supports. You'd lower it to your chest, and then the spotters would lift it back to the starting position. If the lifter didn't help the spotters push the weight back up, the concentric phase could be eliminated entirely.

➤➤ *Eccentric-overload training*. Your spotters put extra plates on the bar for you to lower, then take those plates off so you can lift it under your own power.

I'll talk about the real-world results of these techniques in a moment. First, though, I want to hit on something that's universally agreed upon: Eccentric training causes more muscle damage than traditional lifting. A *lot* more. You might be able to guess the reason by now.

Earlier in this chapter, I noted that doing long sets of slow reps is popular in some circles because of the soreness it induces, since many believe that excess pain will produce oversized gains. (It won't, but as I said, it's difficult for any lifter to shake off the idea.) The pain comes from taking relatively small muscle fibers beyond their limits—in effect, punishing them for the fact they're capable of more endurance than your biggest fibers.

Eccentric training produces deep soreness for the same reason: Your brain recruits smaller motor units to handle bigger weights when your muscles are lengthening. That means it also recruits *fewer* motor units for eccentrics, since it always recruits them in order, from smallest to biggest.

This may seem like a contradiction, since the whole point of eccentric reps is to work with heavier weights. Why would your body use fewer motor units when the weight is heavier? You can probably guess the answer to this one as well as the question about soreness: When you do eccentrics, the goal is to lower the weight slowly, to extend the muscle action. Deliberately slow movements always involve smaller motor units. Thus, you induce lots of trauma in smaller fibers when you do eccentrics, producing profound muscle soreness for up to a week afterward.

Unfortunately, after the pain has subsided, you discover you haven't really done anything to make yourself bigger and stronger. I mean, I could beat on your hamstrings with a baseball bat and make them sore as hell, but it wouldn't do anything to improve your vertical jump or the amount of weight you can pull on a deadlift. The swelling might make them bigger, but once it goes down, you're left with muscles that are now undertrained because you had to take so much time off to recover from the soreness.

All that said, I admit that there's some logic involved in eccentric-focused training. A good strength coach can use the technique selectively, neither seeking out nor inducing massive soreness. His goal would be to train his athletes to work with heavier weights, with the hope that an increase in strength in the lengthening phase will transfer to strength in the shortening phase.

It's not a bad idea, and it's backed up by some research, with studies using subjects ranging from novices to elite Olympic weight-lifters. That's why I experimented with eccentric-focused training for more than a decade, in my own workouts and those of the athletes and clients I trained. But I just couldn't make it work. In my experience, there's minimal carryover from strength you build in the eccentric phase to performance in the concentric phase. What looked good on paper didn't pan out in the gym.

I think it fails to translate because it violates a well-known scientific principle: *Specific Adaptations to Imposed Demand*, or *SAID*. SAID tells us that you won't improve your squat by jogging. And, in this case, you won't increase your ability to lift a weight by teaching your body to lower it. The only way eccentric-focused training will give you an edge is if you plan to compete in a weight-

lowering contest. In that case, eccentrics are your ticket to the winner's circle.

Before I wrap up this topic, I want to emphasize that the eccentric phase of a repetition isn't useless. Your body needs to be able to lower anything it can lift. If your neighbor asked you to help him move his couch, you wouldn't just lift and carry it to the designated spot, and then drop it on his hardwood floor. (If you would, it's only polite to let him know that in advance.)

In the gym, your muscles do get some work on the eccentric phase of each repetition, since they remain under tension. It's not anything you need to focus on, but it's not something you'd want to eliminate, either. Lowering a weight under control helps teach your muscles to protect your joints when they're the most vulnerable. "Under control" doesn't have to mean "slow." It just means that, after lifting the weight as fast as possible, you control its descent, protecting your joints and getting your body into position for the next rep.

Each lifter will have a slightly different way of controlling the weight. Less experienced lifters will go more slowly on both phases of the repetition. Older lifters will probably be more cautious on the eccentric phase. But younger lifters with experience can lower the weight at any speed they can control. In fact, some recent research—including an often-cited University of Saskatchewan study published in 2003 in the *European Journal of Applied Physiology*—has shown that faster eccentric contractions result in more strength and muscle growth than slower ones. Why? Another study, published in 2005 in the *Journal of Applied Physiology*, suggested that the faster eccentric reps caused more muscle damage, resulting in more protein being added to compensate.

MYTH #7: YOUR MUSCLES NEED AT LEAST 48 HOURS TO RECOVER BETWEEN WORKOUTS

I'm not minimizing the importance of recovery. You need to treat your muscles well if you want them to grow, and making sure they get enough time to recuperate between workouts is mandatory. But I am questioning the cookie-cutter approach to recovery. The standard advice these days is that you should give yourself at least 48 hours in between full-body workouts, and 72 hours in between workouts that focus on specific muscle groups. So if you do an upper-body workout on Monday, you shouldn't do another upper-body workout until Thursday at the earliest.

I say this knowing full well that the standard formula might work perfectly for you. But it might just as easily give you more recovery than you need, or less. It all depends on the way you train and how often you want to train.

If you're a busy guy with a family, a full-time job, and a secret life fighting crime, you probably don't want to work out more than three times a week. So if I tell you to do three total-body workouts every 7 days, you're not even tempted to ask whether it's okay to train more often.

But let's say you are 25, work an entry-level job with minimal stress, and are highly motivated to build the best physique you can while you have the time and energy. Do the 48- and 72-hour rules apply to you as well? Will you sabotage your results if you don't let your muscles rest for multiple days between workouts?

The SAID principle tells us that a body will adapt to the demand that's placed on it. If your muscles always have at least 72 hours to recover between workouts, that's how long the process will take. Why? Because you haven't given your body any reason to make those muscles recover faster. You don't know if they could recover in less time because you haven't tried imposing that particular demand on them.

Consider athletes who work the same muscles every day, or multiple times each day. Do gymnasts have puny shoulders and upper arms because they don't give those muscles 72 hours to recover after using them on the rings or parallel bars? Do speed skaters or downhill skiers have skinny thighs from daily sprints and training runs?

I think this subject is so important that I use all of Chapter 5 to explain how you can benefit from working out more frequently, if you have the time and desire to do so. For now, I'll just leave you with this: There's no single recovery protocol that applies to every lifter and every type of training.

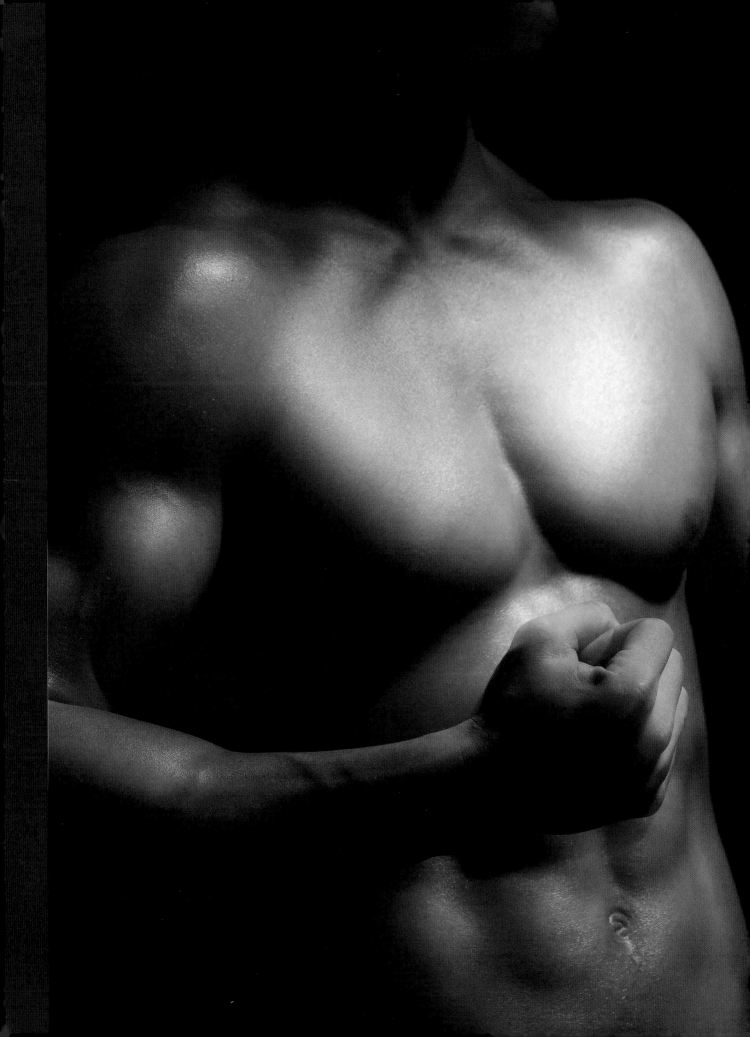

PART 2: THE BRAWN

CHAPTER 4

TOTAL-BODY TRAINING

n the Introduction, I noted that I first got attention on the Internet for recommending heavy weights and low reps for bodybuilders. It was hardly a revolutionary idea, as I said; it just happened to be the opposite of what fitness magazines and bodybuilding experts were telling gym rats to do back then. The whole point of T-Nation is to share information that lifters aren't getting from the mainstream, and that particular advice was a hit with readers.

My next attempt to change the bodybuilding paradigm came when I recommended total-body workouts instead of body-part splits. That was a much harder sell, even though it has a long and respectable history in muscle lore.

Pre-1960s bodybuilders did total-body workouts for a variety of reasons. If you go back far enough, way before the invention of the Universal machine and all the industrial horrors that followed (I'll explain why I'm so down on machines later in this chapter), lifters didn't have benches or squat racks. Almost everything they lifted started on the floor. Total-body workouts were a necessity in the first half of the 20th century.

If you wanted to do squats, for example, you first had to lift the bar off the floor, over your head, and onto your shoulders. And then you had to lift it back over your head before you could lower it to the floor when you were finished with your set. You couldn't work lower-body muscles without also activating all the mid- and upper-body muscles needed to get the bar into position.

The same problem applied to upper-body exercises. For shoulder presses, you had to get the bar to your shoulders before you could press it overhead. Bench presses didn't exist, since there weren't any benches. A lifter who wanted to work his pectoral muscles would lie on his back on the floor with the barbell behind his head. From there, he'd pull it up over his chest. One version of the exercise involved a severe back arch, which brought his thighs and gluteals into the action.

That's why lifters, by default, worked most of their major muscles every time they hit the gym. And it's why, for most of the history of strength training, there was no such thing as "leg day" or "arm day." If a lifter had walked into a gym in the 1930s or '40s and told his buddies, "I'm working chest and tri's today," nobody would have understood what he was talking about.

It's also important to remember that the point of strength training in those days was to build *strength*. Even the lifters who were most interested in muscle size and aesthetics learned to lift heavy iron.

Finally, the bodybuilders back then, even the champions, had day jobs. Nobody had the luxury of training 6 days a week, with entire workouts devoted to relatively small muscle groups.

In the 1960s, though, all these dynamics changed. Equipment had already begun to improve. The bench press (using actual benches) grew increasingly popular as a muscle-building exercise in the 1940s and '50s. Squat racks became standard equipment in the '50s. And with this equipment came the sport of powerlifting, which featured the bench press, squat, and deadlift. (It also included the barbell biceps curl in its early years, which must've made those contests entertaining to watch.)

Powerlifting provided muscleheads with a midway point between Olympic weightlifting—which included the snatch, clean-and-jerk, and standing shoulder press—and bodybuilding, which had no need for such highly skill-dependent lifts. (The standing shoulder press was eliminated in 1972, leaving the sport of weightlifting with two lifts that virtually nobody in gyms ever does anymore.) The powerlifts were better muscle-building exercises than Olympic lifts, and easier to learn. And, more to the point, workouts could now be designed around exercises that focused on the lower body or the upper body, without a practical need to work all the major muscles in every workout.

All these phenomena preceded the development that ensured a huge and permanent shift in the way bodybuilders trained. Steroid pills were invented in the late 1950s and became wildly popular among athletes of all sorts in the 1960s. They were legal in every sense—doctors could prescribe them to anybody who wanted them, and sports organizations hadn't yet outlawed them. Steroid testing began in the early '70s, but that didn't affect bodybuilders, who were the most obvious and enthusiastic consumers of the drugs. Even when the federal government made steroids illegal in the 1990s, their popularity among bodybuilders continued to grow.

Steroids changed our ideas about training in two important ways: First, they helped lifters recover much faster after workouts. Bodybuilders could now train 2 or 3 hours a day, 6 or 7 days a week, and continue to get bigger. Second, they were equal-opportunity muscle builders. They worked with well- or poorly designed routines, and the lines between the two began to blur.

The famous bodybuilders of the 1960s and '70s were still guys who started out lifting heavy. For example, in *The New Encyclopedia of Modern Bodybuilding*, Arnold Schwarzenegger says that he built his celebrated muscles with max-weight powerlifts, and he laments the fact that bodybuilders had largely abandoned that type of training by the time he retired.

What had worked for Arnold and his generation of musclemen—low-rep sets of heavy powerlifts—was no longer considered necessary by drug-using bodybuilders. You can't argue against the logic: Bodybuilders continued to get bigger, despite a lack of traditional strength and power training. Thus, they *looked* stronger, even if they weren't. If you can get the look you want without doing the work, and the look is all that matters, why would anyone choose to do the work?

You may be asking a similar question about me at this point: Why am I working so hard to emphasize the influence of steroids on pro bodybuilders when I'm writing a book for muscleheads who aren't competitive bodybuilders and don't use drugs?

Simple: The way the mass monsters train filters down to everyone else.

Bodybuilding is probably the only athletic pursuit in which it's assumed that whoever looks the best has the best training program. You wouldn't go to an NBA game and presume that whoever has the most spectacular dunk also has the best workout routine, or look

at baseball stats and declare that whoever hit the most home runs in any given season knows more about training than the guys who didn't hit as many. In just about any sport, in fact, you'd attribute an athlete's achievements first to natural talent, then to that person's work ethic, then to coaching and other opportunities to excel. A successful athlete's workout philosophy would be pretty far down the list.

But, because bodybuilding isn't really a sport, and because its promoters have done everything they can to distance the pursuit of muscle from its athletic origins, most of us are conditioned to think of people with really good physiques as experts on training. If the best conditioning expert in the world was standing next to a 25-year-old bodybuilding champion who wouldn't know how to type "hypertrophy" into a search engine, almost everyone in the room would just assume the guy with the best-looking physique knows the most about how to build muscle. The idea of a natural, genetic predisposition to building muscle quickly and easily hardly exists in modern gym culture, except when lifters lament the fact that they don't have it.

That's why this discussion matters to you. Almost all the advice you've gotten from magazines, personal trainers, friends, and lifting partners has come to those sources from people with great genetics who were using anabolic steroids. Whether drug-free, genetically average lifters can benefit from this methodology is a question that's hardly ever asked. Until now.

UNSPLITTING YOUR WORKOUTS

A typical split routine looks something like this:

DAY	MUSCLE GROUPS WORKED	EXERCISES TYPICALLY SELECTED
MONDAY	CHEST AND BACK	» Bench presses (flat, incline, decline, with barbells and or/ dumbbells and/or machines) » Chest flies (various angles, using dumbbells, cables, and/or a pec-deck machine) » Lat pulldowns (to the front or back) » Rows (bent-over with barbell or dumbbells, or seated with cables or machines)
WEDNESDAY	LEGS AND ABS	» Squats and/or squat variations (front squats, hack squats) » Leg presses » Leg extensions » Stiff-legged deadlifts » Leg curls » Standing and seated calf raises » Crunches, several variations per workout » Hanging leg raises or seated leg tucks
FRIDAY	ARMS AND SHOULDERS	» Biceps curls (standing, seated on a bench, or using a preacher-curl station; with straight or angled barbells, dumbbells, cables, and/or machines) » Triceps extensions (standing, seated, or lying on a bench; using angled barbells, dumbbells, cables, and/or machines) » Shoulder presses (usually seated, with barbells, dumbbells, and/or machines) » Shrugs (using barbells, dumbbells, and/or machines) » Lateral raises (standing or seated, using dumbbells, cables, and/or machines) » Front raises with dumbbells » Reverse flies or bent-over lateral raises (standing or seated, using dumbbells, cables, and/or machines)

I guarantee you this: You can get better results in less time with just three basic, compound exercises per workout. My one firm rule is that you need to do at least one exercise in each of these categories:

» Upper-body pulling

» Upper-body pushing

» Squat or deadlift variation

Here are two simple examples:

EXAMPLE 1

>> Upper-body pulling: chinup

>> Upper-body pushing: dip

>> Deadlift

EXAMPLE 2

>> Upper-body-pulling: row

>> Upper-body pushing: chest press

>> Squat

You can use this template with any system of sets and reps, and pursue any goal: hypertrophy (muscle growth), fat loss, pure strength, athletic performance. I've used it with elite athletes, competitive bodybuilders, clients who were rehabilitating injuries, and everyone in between. In every situation, with every type of client, the results were better than whatever the person was doing before working with me.

(In most cases, the client was doing some kind of body-part split, with a preponderance of isolation exercises for small muscle groups.)

Why does total-body training work better than the alternatives?

YOU STIMULATE MORE TOTAL MUSCLE MASS IN EVERY WORKOUT

This is the key to transforming your body from the way it looks and performs now to what you want it to look like and how you want it to perform. I explained in Chapter 3 why a chinup or chest press will do more for your upper-arm muscles than any type of biceps curl or triceps extension. I could make the same argument for choosing squats over leg presses and leg extensions, and for deadlifts over leg curls. The more muscle you stimulate, the better.

Take a look at the table below to see the muscles used in each exercise category:

EXERCISE CATEGORY	SAMPLE EXERCISES	UPPER-BODY MUSCLES	LOWER-BODY MUSCLES
UPPER-BODY PULLING	CHINUPS/PULLUPS; ROWS; LAT PULLDOWNS	>> Lats, trapezius and rhomboids, rear deltoids, biceps, forearms	
UPPER-BODY PUSHING	CHEST PRESSES, SHOULDER PRESSES, DIPS	>> Pectorals and serratus (on chest presses and dips), trapezius (on shoulder presses), deltoids, triceps	
SQUAT	ALL VARIATIONS OF SQUATS, PLUS LUNGES AND STEPUPS		>> Gluteals, hamstrings, quadriceps, adductors, spinal erectors, calves
DEADLIFT	ALL VARIATIONS OF DEADLIFTS, PLUS CLEANS AND OTHER VARIATIONS ON OLYMPIC LIFTS	>> Trapezius, forearms	>> Gluteals, hamstrings, spinal erectors

In compiling this table, I've left out as many active muscles as I've included. For example, when you do squats and deadlifts, you work not only the lower-body muscles listed in the far right column but also virtually every muscle that's involved in stabilizing your spine, from the ones in your neck to those in your pelvis, including your abdominals.

Furthermore, when you do squats, besides working glutes, hams, quads, and calves, you involve virtually all the supporting muscles in your lower body, from the thin strip on the front of your shins to the thick, powerful muscles on the inside of your thighs. One of the best things about being male is that we don't spend much time thinking about our inner thighs, and even less worrying about our shins. But these are muscles that other people notice, even if they don't realize it. Believe me, if you saw an NFL running back walking along the beach, dressed like everyone else, you could tell in an instant that he's an elite athlete just because he has such well-developed muscles in places where everyone else is thin or flabby. That's what squats do for your physique—they make you look like a player, even if you aren't.

Deadlifts also hit their share of obscure lower-body muscles, with the bonus of working the intricate, layered patchwork of tissues attached to your shoulder blades. The result is a stronger, wider, thicker back—another way to look like an athlete without the hassle of attending the NFL Combine.

YOU PREVENT MUSCLE IMBALANCES AROUND YOUR JOINTS

Workout routines based on body-part splits inevitably emphasize one side of the body over the other. If you have one day for "chest" and another for "shoulders," but just one day for "back," you're probably going to do more pushing than pulling. Then you compound the problem by doing the pushing exercises first in every workout, when you're fresh, and the pulling exercises last, when you're fatigued. Finally, you probably push yourself to use heavier weights with lower reps on pushing exercises, and use relatively lighter weights with higher reps for pulls.

The result is imbalanced strength and stability around your shoulder joints. It exacerbates a problem you might already have from sitting at a desk all day, hunched over a computer. That posture causes the muscles and connective tissues on the front of your torso to get shorter and tighter over time, with the corresponding tissues on the back of your torso getter longer and losing their tensile strength. Even the best exercise routine won't necessarily fix postural problems—you probably need a specialized program for that—but it sure as heck shouldn't reinforce them.

When you push and pull in every workout, with relatively equal intensity on both movements, you help maintain or restore your body's preferred balance. And when you use compound movements to balance your pushing and pulling, you work all your body's muscles the way your body wants to work them: as a coordinated system.

YOU HAVE PLENTY OF OPPORTUNITY TO ADD TARGETED EXERCISES

You can do more than three exercises per workout; you'll see examples throughout *Huge in a Hurry.*

But that doesn't mean you can add exercises willy-nilly and get the same benefits. Every type of stress you put on your muscles and joints presents some risk to those tissues. Additional work above and beyond my guidelines gives your body more fatigue, which means more risk of overtraining and less chance to recover. It's like playing poker with wild cards: The odds change, and random chance becomes more important than skill.

Another type of risk comes when you use machines instead of free weights and cables for the exercises I recommend. But that's such a complex issue that it needs its own section.

WHEN MACHINES ATTACK

I'll concede that it's possible to train your entire body without free weights. I've seen bodybuilders who rarely if ever touch a barbell, using machines for almost all their heavy-duty compound movements. The workouts certainly take longer, but that's not an issue for them. The machines prevent their bodies from working in natural, coordinated movement patterns, but bodybuilders stopped worrying about functional strength two generations ago.

So why am I so down on machines?

Because I think they subject your body to considerable and unnecessary injury risk.

Everything you do in the gym is slightly unnatural. A deadlift—pulling a barbell up off the floor—isn't exactly the same as lifting a heavy appliance. A squat with a barbell on your shoulders doesn't precisely replicate anything you do in sports or real life. And if you tried to imagine situations in which your body needed maximum strength for pushing and pulling, you'd probably choose a tug of war for pulling; pushing would likely involve a car with an empty tank and a gas station just over the horizon. Those are total-body exercises, and there's nothing we can do in commercial gyms that comes close.

So free-weight and cable exercises are already a compromise. Cable rows and chest presses aren't a whole lot like real-life pulling and pushing. (You'll notice that I make a distinction between cable systems and other types of machines. A bar that's attached to a cable allows your body to select its own trajectory, making these exercises more like working with free weights and less like fixed-arm machines.) They present some risk to your joints and connective tissues. But you compound that risk when you use machines instead of barbells, dumbbells, or cable stations.

Let's say you do your bench presses on the Smith machine (the barbell-on-rails device you find in every gym) instead of using a conventional barbell. It *looks* like the same exercise, but it's less intimidating, since the rails give the bar a fixed path and take away the risk of unpredictable movement. (I'm being generous here when I say people use the Smith because of safety issues. The bar only weighs 15 pounds, versus 45 pounds for the Olympic barbell we use for bench presses. A guy can throw two 45-pound plates on each side and look like he's benching 225 when in reality it's just 195.)

But while you decrease the risk of an accident, the irony is that you increase the risk of an injury. Your shoulders aren't meant to move objects in a fixed plane. Barbells and dumbbells rarely move straight up and down during a bench press. The typical trajectory is J-shaped, meaning the bar moves back toward your head slightly during the lift. That's the natural movement pattern. Furthermore, the pattern is more pronounced for novices than for advanced lifters. Elite bench pressers learn to push the bar straight up to shorten the range of motion. Inexperienced lifters are most likely to have a pronounced J-shaped pattern. They're also the most likely to use a Smith machine, which means they're the most likely to force their shoulder joints to do something unnatural and potentially dangerous.

When you change that natural pattern, you change everything. Smaller muscles in your shoulders and torso no longer need to go into action to keep the bar stabilized, creating imbalances. The ball-and-socket shoulder joint is forced into an artificial movement pattern, which could put unusual and cumulative strain on the connective tissues holding it in place.

Something similar happens when you do a rowing exercise on a machine, instead of using free weights or cables. When you rest your chest against a pad, instead of standing for a bent-over row or sitting upright for a cable row, you deactivate all the muscles in your shoulders and torso that would ordinarily work hard to keep you from falling over.

It's even worse for lower-body exercises. Using the Smith machine for squats forces your back, hips, and knees into an unnaturally straight up-and-down movement pattern, putting unnecessary stress on the connective tissues in those areas. Over time, any number of overuse injuries could result. The leg press takes your back and torso out of the movement altogether. You make your legs stronger without developing proportional strength in the muscles that support your legs in high-powered actions like running and jumping.

This is my strongest argument against machines: Any time you develop isolated strength, you throw your body out of balance. The muscles that exist to stabilize joints and support bigger muscles during maximum-force-generating movements will not be as strong as they need to be. The more imbalances you create, and the more severe the imbalances become, the greater your risk of injury.

Again, I've always found this kind of ironic, since machines became popular in part because misguided researchers believed that free-weight exercises are dangerous. (I say "in part" because marketing played the biggest role. Health-club entrepreneurs quickly figured out that their prospective customers were less intimidated by machines and found chrome more appealing than iron.) The squat, in particular, has been falsely cited since the 1960s as a major cause of knee injuries. The leg press was seen as the more enlightened alternative.

Are all machines bad? One device I find useful is the assistance machine for chinups and dips. The exercise is basically the same for your shoulder joints; you just get a little help until you're strong enough to do those exercises without assistance.

IF BODYBUILDERS ARE WRONG, WHY ARE THEY BIGGER THAN EVERYONE ELSE?

I've already mentioned steroids, genetics, and the fact that bodybuilders don't need to worry about what their bodies can and can't do. Their only concerns are size, symmetry, and body-fat percentage. Which is fine for them. I like

bodybuilders, and I've worked with several over the years. Besides, I'd be the last person to tell anyone what to do with his own body.

But even if you take steroids out of the equation, a natural bodybuilder still needs to do specialized, muscle-isolating exercises.

The exercises I focus on in *Huge in a Hurry* build muscle size and strength in a balanced, proportional way. My programs should be perfect for athletes and most gym rats. They'll even get a drug-free bodybuilder most of the way there. But if you're serious about bodybuilding, you need proportions that are dramatic and eye-catching. In other words, you need *unnatural* development in certain areas. You especially need every bit of muscle tissue you can build in your upper torso.

And if you have weak genetics in any particular muscle group—the dreaded "lagging body part"—you need to take more extreme measures to make those muscles look like they belong on the same body with the ones that grow easily. A lot of guys who're naturally beefy in the shoulders and arms, for example, have relatively small calves. Bodybuilders with thickly muscled legs often have relatively narrow shoulders.

As I said, a balanced workout based entirely on compound lifts isn't enough for these guys. That's where the technique I describe in the next chapter—high-frequency training—comes into play.

CHAPTER 5

HIGH-FREQUENCY TRAINING

'm sure a lot of people will tell you they had life-altering experiences in Las Vegas. It's not like the moniker "Sin City" came out of a Chamber of Commerce focus group. Many more will deny they've had such moments there, even though the evidence might suggest they did.

The Vegas moment that changed my career in 2001 had nothing to do with sex, gambling, gluttony, or any of the usual temptations—although, if all I told you about were the steak dinner and the two densely muscled men, you might get that impression.

I'd started training clients in 1996, and I was proud of the fact that I'd been busy as all hell since then. Downtime was rare, and I tried to enjoy it as much as I could. At the top of my vacation to-do list was a Cirque du Soleil show called *Mystère* that my clients and friends in the strength-and-conditioning business had been raving about. (In the movie *Knocked Up*, two of the main characters go to see *Mystère* during an acid trip. Personally, I suggest seeing it drug-free.)

I knew when I took my seat in the theater at the Treasure Island casino that I was going to see an entertaining show, with astonishing displays of physical prowess, athleticism, and beauty. To that end, I'd prepared myself with a winning streak at the blackjack tables, a protein infusion from a slab of medium-rare beef at a high-end steakhouse on the Strip (more on that in a moment), and as many glances at beautiful women as I could manage without looking like a dipweed. Plus, there was the extra oxygen that casinos are rumored to pump into the air.

Even with all those attitude-enhancing factors going for me, I wasn't prepared to rethink my entire view of training. But that's what I did when the Alexis Brothers took the stage. When I describe them as "densely muscled men," I'm just scratching the surface. Either of these guys— their real names are Paolo and Marco Lorador—could've won any bodybuilding contest in the pre-steroid era without breaking a sweat. They would've scared off everyone else just by showing up. But it's what they could *do* with those muscles that took my breath away. One of them hoisted the other over his head and held him there with one hand. One lay on his stomach and performed a leg curl with his brother doing a handstand on his feet. They did dozens more, with each stunt shifting my concept of human potential more than the one that preceded it.

Which brings me back to the steak dinner. While waiting for a table, I got into a conversation with the bartender and mentioned that I was going to see *Mystère*. He told me that Paolo and Marco lived next door to him and worked on their routine in their backyard almost every day. By then my table was ready, so I paid for my drink, thanked him for the conversation, and didn't think any more about it. (I was hungry, after all.)

At that time in my career, as I said, I'd been keeping very busy training clients. (I was also in graduate school at the University of Arizona.) If you'd asked me, I would've told you I was pretty good at what I did. I worked with people from all walks of life and with as wide a range of goals and challenges as any trainer I knew. I was never shy about violating conventional training methods if I thought it would help my clients get better results. So I used heavier weights with lower reps with clients who were used to doing the opposite. I sometimes had clients who were used to body-part splits switch to total-body workouts.

But I wasn't really as innovative as I'd imagined. I still used split routines as often as not—mostly upper- and lower-body splits, but some clients did body-part splits straight out of the bodybuilding playbook. And when it came to training frequency, I was as conventional as anybody. Most of my clients worked out three times a week, and even with split routines nobody did more than four sessions in 7 days. I believed, as everybody did then and almost everyone does now, that muscles needed at least 48 hours to recover from a workout, and that more advanced lifters needed to give their muscles 72 hours before they could risk hitting them again. If they didn't, the muscles wouldn't recover fully, and clients wouldn't get the results they wanted.

Seeing the Alexis Brothers, and remembering what the bartender had told me about their practice schedule, made me rethink that.

First is an obvious point: For Paolo and Marco and their fellow Cirque du Soleil performers, every performance is a full-body workout. Nothing they did isolated any muscle group, or required upper- or lower-body strength in the absence of strength from the other half.

But you already know that I prefer total-body workouts, even if I wasn't a complete convert back in 2001.

Now for a less obvious point: The brothers didn't restrict their performances to Monday, Wednesday, and Friday, resting their muscles for 48 hours in between. According to their Web site (alexisbrothers.com), they work 5 consecutive nights each week, with 2 performances a night. That's 10 full-body workouts in 5 days, on top of the almost-daily practice the bartender described. They also train with weights, which is obvious from looking at them and confirmed by clicking the "About Us" link on their site.

How does any of this affect you? Good question (assuming you asked it). You can probably think of at least three reasons not to change our entire concept of training frequency because of two ripped dudes in Las Vegas:

>> The brothers are genetic freaks. They might be the only two people on earth who possess their combination of strength, coordination, muscular endurance, and the ability to recover quickly from workouts and performances.

>> They're professional performers. It's their job to train and recover from training. They don't have to sit in front of computers all day, like many of us.

>> Who even wants to exercise that often?

Believe me, I took all these questions and arguments into account. And I kept coming back to this: According to conventional wisdom, what the brothers were doing should have been impossible, regardless of their genetics or how much they were being paid. The most basic concept in the field of strength and conditioning tells us that muscles have to be challenged and then allowed to recover. Violate the first part and you get no results. Violate the second part and your body breaks down. But here were two guys who clearly pushed their bodies in their workouts and performances, clearly didn't have much time to recover, and just as clearly weren't breaking down.

I asked myself a tough question: Was I short-changing my clients? Would they get better results by training more frequently? If so, how frequently, and how much of the body could be trained that way?

NOT-SO-FREQUENTLY ASKED QUESTIONS ABOUT FREQUENCY

In 2000, the year before my epiphany in the desert, University of Alabama scientists published a study in the *Journal of Strength and Conditioning Research* that I hadn't paid any particular attention to at the time. They designed a total-body workout program with three sets of each exercise. Half the study participants did the entire workout once a week. The other half worked out three times a week, doing one set of each exercise each time. In 12 weeks, they all did the same *volume* of exercise. The only variable was frequency. One group did 12 workouts, while the other did three times that many. Just about any expert, quoting from any textbook, would've told you that the results should've been more or less the same.

They weren't.

The group doing more workouts gained 38 percent more strength, on average. They also gained more muscle and lost more fat, although those changes didn't rise to the level of statistical significance. If they had, this would have been one of the most talked about studies of the year. The three-times-a-week group—five men and four women—gained an average of 10 pounds of muscle while decreasing their body fat by a full percentage point.

Because of the small number of people involved in the study, I don't want to make too much of it, except to note that the strength changes *were* statistically significant. That is, the strength increases were consistent enough for all the lifters in the study that it's safe to draw conclusions from the results. And those results suggest that lifting three times a week increases your strength more, all else being equal.

This information shouldn't change your worldview in any dramatic way. You knew before you picked up this book that you couldn't get huge by training once a week. More to the point of this chapter, it doesn't say anything about working out *more* than three times a week.

So let's put this discussion into a practical context that all muscleheads can appreciate.

Let's say you're already doing three total-body workouts a week, but you have some stubborn muscles that just won't grow as fast as the others. To keep it simple, let's say it's

your upper arms that lag behind everything else. (I only had a 95 percent chance of calling that one correctly.) And to keep it *really* simple, let's say your goal is to add an inch to your upper-arm circumference.

If you read bodybuilding magazines regularly, you've probably seen one of those articles promising you can add an inch with just 1 or 2 crazy-ass days of lifting. You've been around long enough to know that's insane. You know it can't be done in a week, much less a day. Muscle growth doesn't happen fast for anybody, and the longer you've been lifting, the more time it takes to make measurable gains. So if I said you could do it in 4 weeks, you'd think I was crazy, but you might still be curious enough to hear me out.

First, though, let's recast the question and make sure we're all thinking about it the same way.

A typical lifter with some experience is probably doing a body-part split similar to the one I showed in Chapter 4. So, for this example, we'll say you're working your chest and back on Monday and your shoulders and arms on Friday. That means you hit your upper-arm muscles two times a week—once with compound exercises such as rows and bench presses, once with isolation exercises such as curls and extensions (with one compound lift, the shoulder press, which works your triceps). Over 6 weeks, you'd work those muscles 12 times.

Could you put an inch on your arms with

this system in the next 4 weeks? Well, considering you've been doing it for a long time and haven't seen the growth you want, I'd say no, you can't.

But what if I had you work your upper arms six times a week, instead of twice? We'll keep the logistics simple: You'd do three total-body training sessions a week wherever you currently work out (gym, home, prison), and three specialized workouts at home with some basic free weights and a bench. Now we're talking about 24 workouts in 4 weeks, instead of 8 workouts. It's clearly different from what you're currently doing, but do you think it would work?

Back in 2001, following my mind-expanding Vegas experience, I was eager to find out. I had 15 clients, a mix of men and women, several of whom weren't remotely interested in building bigger muscles. But I had two male clients who looked like perfect subjects for case studies. One wanted to put an inch on his arms; the other wanted bigger calves.

The high-frequency program I designed looked something like this:

Total-body workouts: Monday, Wednesday, Friday, a.m.

Specialized high-frequency workouts: Monday, Wednesday, Friday, p.m.

I varied it a bit from week to week, but that's the basic idea. And it worked even better than I'd hoped. The first client put just over an inch on his arms. The second added three-quarters of an inch to his calves.

This doesn't prove that high-frequency training (which I'll abbreviate as HFT from now on) works better than what we do now, even if it worked pretty damned well for my two clients. But I was sure of one thing: It didn't backfire on my clients and me, and it was worth pursuing.

TRUSTING A THEORY, IGNORING THE EVIDENCE

By the time I started experimenting with HFT, I was 25 and had been working out since I was 14. I'd studied biology and exercise science for 7 years in college and grad school. And, as I mentioned, I'd been training clients for 6 years. All that time, the trends in both science and practice were going away from HFT. The question of how *little* training was needed to make gains was more often explored than the question of how much training a human body could use to its advantage.

There were practical reasons for taking research this direction, since dedicated exercisers were breaking down with overuse injuries and the nonathletic population was reluctant to exercise at all. Still, as a trainer, I knew that my income and reputation depended on the results I got for my clients. If someone wanted to work out more often and I had reason to believe it might help and probably wouldn't hurt, why shouldn't I try it?

There was one example from bodybuilding that I could look to for inspiration. In his *New Encyclopedia of Modern Bodybuilding*, Arnold Schwarzenegger writes that he turned to his own version of HFT two different times. When he realized that his (relatively) puny calves were going to be a problem for him when he competed against the world's best bodybuilders, he started training them 6 days a week, 30 to 45 minutes a day. He even tried walking differently, rising all the way up on his toes, as if he were doing calf raises every time he walked across the street.

You always need a bit of skepticism when considering bodybuilding legends. Schwarzenegger is among the most genetically gifted musclemen ever, and by his own admission he was taking steroids. There were also rumors that he'd gotten calf implants and made up the story of excessive training to explain the areas' sudden growth. And if his calves had stayed the same size and shape as he got older and cut back on his training, the surgery story might be a credible theory. But they didn't, and it's not. You can almost never be sure what's real and what's not in bodybuilding, but I think we can trust the source on this one.

A less-well-known Schwarzenegger story concerns his best-known muscles. According to his book, his left biceps used to be smaller than his right. He targeted the problem: "I noticed that whenever I was asked to show my biceps, I would automatically flex the right arm. So I consciously made an effort to flex my left arm as much or more than my right. Eventually I was able to make my left biceps the equal of my right."

Again, I have no way to verify or refute the story. I just think it's interesting that when he had a problem with muscles lagging behind, his instincts as a bodybuilder told him to train them more frequently. And it worked for him, according to his own accounts.

I also had some personal experience with HFT that I'd never before thought relevant to the way I trained my clients.

When I was an undergrad at Western Illinois University in Macomb, I worked at a campus apartment complex. The students who lived there didn't have much respect for the furniture . . . or for education, for that matter, although that's a different book. My job was to lug out the ruined mattresses, incinerated sofas, crushed kitchen tables, and whatever else they'd managed to mangle in their pursuit of whatever it was they were pursuing. (Like I said, it sure as hell wasn't education.) Then I'd have to lug in the new stuff.

I despised the work as much as I despised the idiots who made sure I had so much of it. I'd lug flimsy mattresses and unwieldy couches up and down narrow stairwells all afternoon on Monday, and on Tuesday morning I had to go back in and do the same crummy work again, only this time with my forearms, biceps, shoulders, and upper back screaming with post-exertion soreness.

At that time, in the mid-1990s, just about every professor I encountered in the classroom and all the gym rats I knew from the weight room believed that muscle soreness was a big stop sign for a lifter. It meant your muscles hadn't yet recovered from the previous workout.

This belief grew out of something called the "one-factor" theory of recovery. The idea was that a workout drained your body of materials that had to be replenished. So if you ran a long distance, your legs would be drained of glycogen (the form of carbohydrate your body uses for energy), and recovery would involve restoring it. Your body would then adapt to the training challenge by storing more of the substance than it had originally, a process called *supercompensation*.

As applied to strength training, the one-factor theory suggested that a workout would break down the protein in the affected muscles, and in the process of recovery, your body would supercompensate by giving your muscles more protein than they'd had before the workout.

The graph below shows how this works.

You'll note that supercompensation doesn't last very long before you return to your normal levels of whatever it is you've drained from your muscles. Thus, according to the one-factor theory, there's a relatively small window in which you get maximum benefit from your most recent workout. Do your next workout

SUPERCOMPENSATION CHART

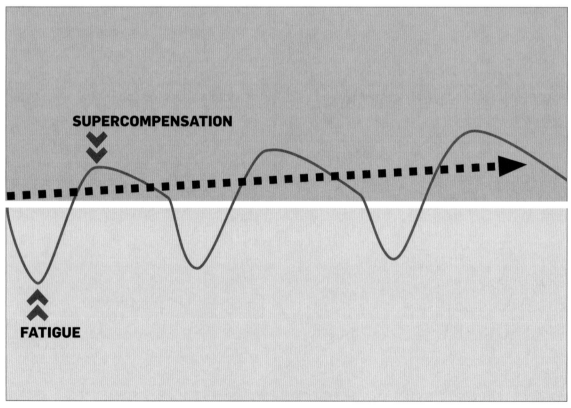

PROPER RECOVERY

too soon, and your muscles will still be depleted. Do it too late, and you miss the chance to work out with the enhanced energy or strength or muscle mass you got from supercompensation.

Knowing all this, I feared that my campus job was ruining my muscles along with my opinion of my fellow students. I didn't have the luxury of waiting for supercompensation to take place before I had to go in and break down my muscles all over again.

But my muscles didn't break down. In fact, my forearms, biceps, and shoulders grew more in my first month of manual labor than they had in the previous year of serious, uninterrupted strength training.

ALL WE REALLY KNOW IS HOW MUCH WE *DON'T* KNOW

I should note here that scientists had already moved away from the one-factor theory as it applied to muscle building. Russian sports scientist Vladimir Zatsiorsky sums it up nicely in *Science and Practice of Strength Training*: "In general, the theory of supercompensation is too simple to be correct." The book was published in 1995, the same time I was trying to avoid piles of student vomit as I hauled furniture up and down apartment stairwells. But I hadn't yet read it, and I was still taking on faith what everyone believed about workouts and recovery.

Currently, we don't really know how many

factors are involved in the muscle-building process, or how much each matters. There's more than one factor, of course—everyone agrees on that—but, when studying the issue, there's no all-encompassing model that works for everybody. I focus most on the nervous system, but I know that everything comes into play. Energy stores need to be replenished, muscle protein is constantly breaking down and being replaced, and hormone levels fluctuate. And no matter how sophisticated your approach to all those variables, you also have to consider how you actually perform as a result of your training. If you're not getting bigger and stronger, then you have to decide whether the problem is too much exercise or too little. (And I haven't even begun to discuss nutrition, the subject of Chapters 22 and 23.)

The simplest and most useful perspective is to assume that your muscles will adapt—for better or for worse—to any training stimulus that doesn't break down your body. For example, if a runner trains his body to run long distances without breaking down, his body will adapt by making his muscle fibers smaller and better able to perform lots of low-intensity repetitions at a steady pace. Which, of course, is the opposite of what *you're* after. If you do my HFT program while eating enough food and getting plenty of rest to ensure recovery after your workouts, your body will adapt by giving you what you want: bigger, stronger muscles.

CHAPTER 6

EIGHT KEYS TO SUCCESSFUL WORKOUTS

know from long experience that some guys reading this book have a certain type of question: "Do I have to do your workouts exactly the way you wrote them? Can I substitute *this* for *that?*" A lot of guys just like to tinker with workouts. I understand, believe me. But there are good substitutions and bad substitutions. Some keep you on track for the results you'd get if you did my workouts to the letter, and some derail you by compromising the intensity of the programs. Change some parameters and you make the workouts too easy; change others and you make them so difficult that you can't recover sufficiently from one workout to the next.

With that in mind, I want to explain to you the most important considerations affecting my program design. And yes, they are listed in order of importance.

1. CHOOSE THE RIGHT EXERCISES

When I started training, I was 14 and lived in a small town with no gym. My only equipment was an Olympic barbell and some weight plates, unless you count the rafters in the garage, which I used for pullups. No bench, no squat rack. Every exercise had to start with the bar on the floor, which is why my workouts were built around deadlifts, standing shoulder presses, and the self-taught version of the power clean that I used to get the bar to my shoulders for the presses.

By no coincidence, I gained muscle and strength much faster than anyone I knew.

It's funny to think about, but if you'd given me the option of working out in a gym with every machine that existed back then, I would've taken you up on the offer without hesitation. And I would've missed out on the best muscle-building exercises on Earth.

Gyms today, as I noted earlier, are designed to promote the least effective exercises. You might not find a squat rack, or even a place to put a bar on the floor for deadlifts, but you can do curls just about anywhere. You'll find curl machines, cable stations with special bars for curls, preacher-curl stations, and a row of adjustable benches in front of the dumbbell rack, at least half of which are being used by people doing curls at any given time. In fact, in some gyms, it's hard to find a place to do *standing* curls with free weights. Worse, if a gym has a squat rack, you'll often find guys using it for barbell curls, since there's no other spot to do them without people walking into you. I sometimes get the impression that the entire health-club industry is involved in a massive conspiracy to make strength training as ineffective as possible.

Make this your rallying cry: Fight for your right to do compound exercises. Don't let the forces of flab pressure you into choosing single-joint exercises. And if you want to do single-joint exercises, at least do them on your own two feet.

The more muscles an exercise requires, including the ones you use to maintain balance and coordination, the more you'll get out of it.

2. TRAIN ALL YOUR MUSCLES IN EVERY WORKOUT

I gave you the full argument in favor of total-body training in Chapter 4, so I won't repeat myself here. The rules are simple: For my program to work, you must do a compound pushing exercise and a compound pulling exercise, combined with a squat or deadlift variation, in every workout. You can use free weights, body weight, or a cable machine. Your goal is to work as much of your body's total muscle mass as possible each training session, and thus transform your body as quickly and safely as possible.

3. DECIDE ON A PROGRESSION PLAN, AND STICK WITH IT

Everything we want from strength training, the sum total of exercise science and practice, culminates in a single principle: If you want to change your body, you must force it to do something it's not used to doing. It doesn't matter what you want to change. Whether you want it to be stronger, faster, bigger, or leaner, you have to present your body with a new stimulus, a unique challenge that can only be met with the physiological transformation you desire.

That's the simple part. The complications grow from there. If you've been lifting for a while, you've probably found your comfort zone: exercises, techniques, and program configurations that you enjoy and that your body performs pretty well. Chances are, you made your best gains with these workout parameters, which is how you got comfortable with them in the first place. But now your body has made all the adaptations possible with your current system, and you have to decide what comes next—what your body hasn't yet done, and which of those unique stimuli best suits your abilities and goals.

Even then, you have to put your new strategy into the form of a progression plan, allowing you to get from where you are to where you want to be without getting hurt or burned out. I know just about everybody reading this will have a combination of goals: bigger muscles, stronger muscles, less fat. But when I designed the workouts in this book, I did so with the idea that one goal would be paramount in each program. So, while you'll certainly get stronger and probably get leaner in the Get Big program, I used a progressive plan that would put the most emphasis on muscle growth.

Here are the main progression plans you'll find in the *Huge in a Hurry* workouts.

GET BIG

To gain muscle as fast as possible, you want to increase your training volume over time. The traditional way is to add reps and sets to your workouts. I don't do that in *Huge in a Hurry*—the repetitions per exercise remain constant. But because you increase the amount of weight you use for the same number of reps as you get stronger, you end up lifting more total weight from week to week.

GET STRONG

Anybody could tell you to put more weight on the bar. The key is adding it gradually and consistently. You want to avoid big jumps in load that cause you to peak before you've made all the gains you could have achieved with more gradual, consistent improvement. I recommend increasing the load by 2 percent or 5 pounds, whichever is more, on each set of each exercise each time you repeat a workout.

GET LEAN

Your metabolism is the best tool you have to attack your body's fat. To speed it up, you need to give your body a more intense training stimulus that results in a faster metabolism as you recover from the workout. One sure way

WHAT ABOUT CARDIO?

When fitness geeks like me talk about running or other types of endurance exercise, we call it "energy-systems training." If you're doing sprints, you're working your anaerobic energy systems. If you're jogging, swimming, or riding a bike for a specified distance or amount of time—an hour-long run at lunchtime, for example—you're training your aerobic energy system.

You don't need to do any energy-systems work in most of my programs in *Huge in a Hurry*. The exception is the "Get Lean" program in Chapter 14, which includes some sprint intervals after the weight workouts. You can add intervals to most of the other workouts if you want, although it's strictly optional. Just don't add them—or any other nonprescribed training—to the "Get Even Bigger" workouts shown in Chapter 11.

If you want the extra work, do up to 20 minutes of high-intensity intervals, three times each week, either after your workouts or on separate days. I prefer 45 seconds of walking, followed by 15 seconds of sprinting. (I go into more detail, and show a progression plan, in Chapter 14.) Running outside or on a track is ideal, but you can also use a treadmill, bike, or elliptical machine in a gym.

I don't recommend any traditional endurance exercise when you're trying to build strength and muscle size.

to do that is to perform the same amount of work in less time each time you repeat a workout. Just cut your rest time between sets by 5 seconds. If you keep the load constant, it'll feel like more work, since you're allowing less recovery between sets.

4. NEVER SACRIFICE FORM FOR SPEED

I've talked a lot about lifting as fast as possible. And I've mentioned that the actual speed of a lift depends on the load: The heavier the weight, the slower you'll lift it, no matter how fast you're *trying* to lift.

I think all of us are cautious about form when we're using weights close to our max. We'll always have idiots among us—I've seen enough of them on YouTube to realize there's an inexhaustible supply of people who not only lift heavy weights with spine-buckling form but record their stupidity on digital video.

The rest of us make sure we know how to lift, before we push our limits. And then the weights themselves help prevent mistakes. Here's what I mean: If your one-repetition maximum (the most weight you can lift once) on the deadlift is 320 pounds, and I tell you to lift it as fast as you can, the actual speed of your lift won't be any different than if I'd told you to lift at your normal speed. There's really only one way to pull a max weight off the floor.

But if I told you to put 160 on the bar and lift it as fast as you can, all kinds of things might go wrong. You can probably guess why, based on what you've read so far. You aren't used to recruiting so many muscle fibers when you lift a weight that's only 50 percent of your maximum. As soon as the bar starts moving, your muscles are in uncharted territory, and chances are something will happen that you aren't expecting.

Another example: The standing cable row is one of my favorite pulling exercises. The cable-row station isn't designed for standing, so there aren't any supports to help you keep your balance. (That's why I like it so much.) Picture yourself standing up, your feet straddling the bench that everyone else sits on for the traditional version of the exercise, and pulling the bar to your chest. How do you keep from falling forward? By keeping your body rigid from head to toe. The only moving parts are your shoulders and arms. Even when you lift slowly, it takes some effort to keep your feet planted firmly on the ground so that you stay upright.

Now picture yourself pulling the bar to your chest as fast as possible. It's not hard to imagine losing your balance, is it? Trust me: In real life, almost everyone struggles to remain standing—which is exactly why it's a great exercise to do fast.

You want to challenge your balance and coordination. You'll activate more of your stabilizing muscles, especially those in your core and lower body. Some of them have to work with slow lifts, too, but not as many, and not as hard.

What you don't want is to allow those stabilizing muscles to throw off your form. There's no point in doing an exercise faster if it turns into a different exercise, powered by different muscles. On the standing cable row, the faster you pull, the more your hips try to move to help with the lift. But those muscles are much bigger and stronger than the ones you're targeting. If they help, it shortens the range of motion for your upper-back, shoulder, and arm muscles, diminishing their workload. It also decreases the challenge to the stabilizing muscles in your core, since they no longer have to hold your hips and torso in one position. The solution is obvious: Don't let your hips overpower your upper body on the exercise.

5. COUNT REPETITIONS, AND LET THE SETS TAKE CARE OF THEMSELVES

Bill Starr, a great lifter and one of the first professional strength coaches in the United States, popularized the "5 × 5" combination of sets and reps in a book called *The Strongest Shall Survive*. He recommended 5 sets of 5 reps of 3 core exercises: the power clean, bench press, and squat. The book was targeted to football players and coaches (Starr was the first strength coach of the Baltimore Colts), but 5 × 5 was a hit with strength and power athletes of all sorts, as well as with muscleheads like me.

Another popular workout configuration is 3 × 8. As I said in the Introduction, I first got attention with online articles recommending that lifters flip around popular recommendations and do more sets with fewer reps. So 3 × 8 would become 8 × 3.

The great thing about all these configurations is that each one works for anybody who hasn't done it before. The guy who starts out lifting the conventional way—3 × 10—will realize that he makes better gains with 3 × 8. If he moves on to 5 × 5, he'll do even better. And many lifters, including me, have made our best gains in size and strength with 8 × 3.

But ask yourself: What's the one thing that all three configurations share?

When you do the math, you get to about the same place: 24 or 25 reps per exercise.

I'm not suggesting that two dozen is a magic number. But I don't think it's a coincidence that doing 24 or 25 reps per exercise works for a large cross-section of lifters. As long as we stay in the middle range (3 × 8, 5 × 5, 8 × 3) and avoid the extremes (1 × 24, 24 × 1), lifters seem to hit a "sweet spot" of volume and intensity. That is, we use weights heavy enough to build strength, and lift them enough times to add size, without doing so much work that recovery becomes problematic.

That's why I've moved away from prescribing specific combinations of sets and reps. Instead, I give a target number of reps per exercise, which varies according to your goals:

GET BIG

Most muscleheads who are trying to gain pure size—like, say, readers of a book called *Huge in a Hurry*—are eating an excess of calories. As the poet said, "Eat big to get big." So if you're looking to move up a weight class, I recommend more volume: 35 reps per exercise. This makes workouts longer and more fatiguing, but you balance that out with the extra food you're eating. Thus, you're able to recover from one workout to the next. The extra lifting combined with extra calories gives you more of a stimulus for creating new muscle tissue, along with more food to use for that goal.

GET STRONG

You have to focus on lifting weights that are close to your max, which fatigues your nervous system. That's why I go down to 15 reps per exercise. If most of your sets are triples (3 reps), doubles, and singles, getting to 15 can be so exhausting you barely have the energy to finish your postworkout protein shake.

GET LEAN

This is the type of client I see most often—the person who doesn't want to gain weight but wants to look better. That is, he's trying to build bigger muscles while losing fat. He might also want to get stronger. (Most of the mixed-martial-arts athletes I work with fall into this category—the whole point is to get stronger and faster in their current weight class.)

If this describes you, chances are you're keeping a close watch on your diet. Even if you aren't cutting calories, you're not increasing them. That means you have to be careful that the volume of your workouts doesn't exceed your ability to recover from them. For you, the aforementioned sweet spot of 25 reps per exercise should be just right: plenty of stimulus, but little risk of overtraining.

6. LIFT ENOUGH WEIGHT

I mentioned that you should avoid working at the extremes when it comes to total reps—1 set of 24, or 24 sets of 1—but I didn't say why, and I think it's an important question. Let's consider the first possibility: 1 set of 24 reps. To achieve any gains at all, you need to work with at least 60 percent of your one-rep maximum (1RM) in that exercise. So if your 1RM in the bench press is 200 pounds, 120 pounds is the bare minimum you could use with any hope of building muscle. A typical lifter would be able to do 20 to 22 reps with 60 percent of his max. So to get to 24 in one set of bench presses, you'd probably have to use less than 120 pounds.

That's at a normal lifting speed. If you're trying to lift faster than normal, you'd have to use even less. That would make the weight too light to allow you to bring your biggest motor units into play.

If you went the other direction—24 × 1, on all 3 exercises in your workout—you'd do a total of 72 sets. That would take 2 or 3 hours

to do. Believe me, if you have that much time to train, there are much better ways to use it.

So, how do you know how much to use? I've tried all kinds of complicated formulas, but we can keep it simple by thinking in terms of these four categories of load:

Light: a weight you could lift 20 to 22 times

Medium: a weight you could lift 10 to 12 times

Heavy: a weight you could lift 4 to 6 times

Superheavy: a weight you could lift 2 or 3 times

One more note about reps: When I say "24 per exercise," I'm not including anything you do in your warmup sets. All these reps are within "work" sets—the ones you do with weights heavy enough to build muscle and increase strength. For the sake of simplicity and efficiency, and to avoid arguments about sharing equipment in crowded gyms, I recommend doing all your reps with the same weight in each workout.

7. WORK A DIFFERENT ANGLE IN EACH WORKOUT

Stand with your hands on the fronts of your thighs. Now lift them straight up overhead. No, it's not a mobility exercise. It's just a reminder that you can do pushing and pulling exercises anywhere within that 180-degree range of motion.

For pulling exercises, you have a range that goes from chinups at one end to power cleans at the other, with all kinds of rows and pull-downs in between, for a total of five angles:

>>Traditional lat pulldowns, a more-or-less straight vertical pull downward

>>Lat pulldowns with your torso leaning back

>>Traditional seated cable rows, with a horizontal pull

>>Standing cable rows, which I described earlier

>>Power cleans, a vertical pull upward

For pushes, you can go from overhead presses to dips, with incline, flat, and decline bench presses along the trajectory.

These variations become crucial when we're talking about three total-body workouts a week. As you'll see in the workout chapters, you'll never push or pull at the same angle twice in the same week. The goal is to give your upper-body muscles a variety of challenges (you don't need me to tell you that dips, flat bench presses, and shoulder presses hit your pectorals and deltoids in different ways) and prevent the excessive stress on your joints that could occur if all or most of your pushes or pulls hit the same movement patterns.

This concept also applies to the lower body—the squats and deadlifts—although it's a little harder to picture. The key point is to consider what joints are moving most or working hardest in each exercise. Most lower-body exercises can be classified as either hip- or knee-dominant. A deadlift is a hip-dominant exercise, since that's where almost all the

movement takes place; your knees have a small range of motion. A front squat, on the other hand, is knee-dominant. (Some trainers say "quad dominant" instead.) Your hips have a pretty big range of motion, and the muscles that move your hips—glutes and hamstrings—get a workout. But the exercise is harder for your knee joints than it is for your hips, and you'll feel it more in your quads than in your glutes or hamstrings.

Other exercises don't fall as neatly into one category or the other. Most of us would consider lunges knee-dominant, but the range of motion is about the same for the hips. The difference, again, is that it's harder for your knee joints than for your hips. But how do you classify stepups? Many trainers I know would say they're hip-dominant, but try telling that to a guy with bad knees. There may be more of a load on the hips, but the balance component makes it harder on knee joints.

You'll also notice that there are only two possibilities—hip or knee dominance—which means you're going to have to repeat one or the other each week. My advice is to avoid doing two exercises that are clearly hip- or knee-dominant in consecutive workouts, using heavy weights. So, if you do deadlifts on Monday, don't do a different type of deadlift on Wednesday. With exercises that are less obviously hip- or knee-dominant, you'll have to decide for yourself which joints are hardest hit, and schedule them accordingly. If you feel that stepups are toughest on your knees, it doesn't matter whether a trainer says they're a hip-dominant exercise. You'd be in a world of hurt if you did front squats on Monday and stepups on Wednesday. So, you know, don't do that.

Another way to spread the workload around is by changing foot position. If you do a squat with a wide stance, for example, your quadriceps have a less effective line of pull than they do with your feet shoulder-width apart. Your inner-thigh muscles—hip adductors—take on the work your quads can't do. For some lifters, the wide-stance squat is easier on the knees, making it a useful alternative.

A wider or narrower stance also changes the emphasis of hip-dominant exercises. Your back is more upright when you do a sumo-style deadlift, which requires an extremely wide stance, than if you do it the traditional way. That means less work for your lower-back muscles and more for your hip adductors. Conversely, if you do a stiff-legged deadlift with a narrow stance, you increase the range of motion for your hip joints, making all the muscles on the back of your body work harder, including those that protect your lower back.

8. DON'T COMPRESS YOUR SPINE IN EVERY WORKOUT

Most powerlifters who've been in the game for more than a decade are shorter than when they started. I don't mean a *little* shorter; they lose several inches. It's easy to figure out the reason: A steady routine of heavy squats and deadlifts will compress the spinal column, specifically the jelly-doughnut-like discs between your vertebrae. Many powerlifters are forced to retire with back injuries, to no one's surprise. The less space there is between discs, the harder it is for your nerves to transmit electrical signals to your muscles. If you've ever put a kink into a garden hose, you get the idea. Water still gets through, but not as much, and not as fast.

If heavy squats and deadlifts are crucial to the results you want but also compress your spine, how can you make gains now without injuries you'll pay for later? I recommend two strategies.

DON'T LIFT HEAVY IN EVERY WORKOUT

You know that fast contractions allow you to recruit big motor units without using max weights. (If you don't know that by now, you must've skipped every chapter before this one.) So, even if one of your goals is to improve your strength, you can reach that goal with two heavy workouts a week, and use the third workout for faster lifts with lighter weights. That'll take some burden off your spine.

DON'T DO EVERY EXERCISE ON TWO LEGS

At least one workout each week should include single-leg versions of the squat and deadlift. You'll get two important benefits:

>> These exercises recruit a lot of stabilizer muscles that might be understimulated by traditional squats and deadlifts.

>> They unload your spine, since you're forced to use less weight. A guy who can deadlift 300 pounds might use 50-pound dumbbells when doing a single-leg deadlift. If he maxes out with 275 on the squat, he'd have all he could handle with a 25-pound weight plate on a single-leg squat.

Each of those exercises gives muscles plenty of work, with hardly any load on your spine. I've tried them with professional athletes and serious competitive powerlifters, and I've seen how it works for them. Sometimes we'll go a week to 10 days doing nothing but single-leg exercises. Invariably, they get stronger when they return to their normal exercises with heavy loads, thanks to the restoration of the normal spaces between their vertebrae and the improvement in nerve transmissions.

If it works for them, it should work for you.

CHAPTER 7

WARMING UP AND COOLING DOWN

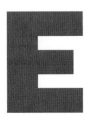veryone who exercises knows that it's good to have flexibility. Until recently, most experts would have agreed that everyone should stretch more than they do, since flexibility is crucial to health and performance. If you heard about "mobility," it was probably in the context of an injury or disability—a doctor trying to restore mobility to an injured leg, for example.

Lately, though, the more forward-thinking strength and conditioning specialists have drawn a sharp distinction between flexibility and mobility. Flexibility can be good, but it's sometimes not—people with too much flexibility, usually women, can set themselves up for injuries because their joints aren't protectively stiff where they need to be. And stretching can be useful in some situations, but in others it's probably a bad idea. Mobility, on the other hand, is increasingly seen as the gold standard for skeletal health and injury-free performance.

Before we get into that, let's define the terms.

Flexibility is your passive range of motion. If you went to a physical therapist, and he wanted to assess your lower-body flexibility, he'd have you lie on your back on a table. He'd lift each leg as high as possible, showing the muscles' ability to lengthen, as well as whether there's a difference in passive flexibility from one leg to the other. He might do the same with your ankles and knees.

Mobility is your active range of motion. If you were to pull your own leg up until you felt the stretch in your hamstrings, you'd be testing mobility, rather than flexibility.

Is one better than the other? No. Flexibility and mobility are both important and should be trained if either is lacking. They just need to be trained at different times, using different techniques.

Mobility exercises should come before strength training, and flexibility exercises should come after. A good workout revs up your nervous system and produces a high level of tension in your muscles. After the workout, you want to release that muscle tension so you can begin the recovery process. That can't happen until your nervous system slows down. (This is why so many of us feel pain in the neck or upper back when we're stressed. Stress excites the nervous system, which stiffens muscles.) Flexibility exercises help with both goals: Used properly, they can slow down your nerves and relax your muscles.

But before your workout, the last thing you want is relaxed muscles and a decelerated nervous system. You'll weaken the signals your brain is sending to your muscles, reducing the amount of force you can generate. The result, over time, can be smaller, weaker muscles.

Mobility training, done right, turns on the switches that allow peak performance. If you've ever watched Olympic swimmers right before they dive into the water for a race,

you'll notice that they do big, fast arm circles to prepare their shoulders. Deliberately and actively moving the muscles through a full range of motion stimulates the motor nerves that control the muscles, allowing the nerves to recruit more motor units, and to recruit them faster. The movements also help the joints produce a lubricant called synovial fluid that reduces friction. That not only enhances performance immediately by allowing the shoulders to move faster, it also has the potential to reduce injury risk over time.

Flexibility and mobility training combine to give you three big benefits:

>> You'll be able to use a full range of motion in your exercises.

>> You'll potentially reduce your risk for joint injuries, since you'll have fewer areas that are chronically stiff and restricted over time. Not every problem can be fixed with pre- and postworkout drills, but at least you'll know where the problems are, and whether they're getting better on their own or need professional intervention.

>> You'll unbind your muscles, giving them more room to grow.

None of which is to say that mobility exercises, by themselves, are all you need to do to warm up before a workout, especially if you're going to be lifting heavy weights as fast as you can. Even with perfect form, you

EXTRA CREDIT

You can do these drills on days you don't lift. They'll work best if you start with the mobility exercises and move from them into the flexibility training. But you can also do the flexibility exercises—the stretches—by themselves if you want. The only rule: Don't do them first thing in the morning or immediately after sitting for long periods.

When you sleep, your spinal disks fill with fluid and are more prone to rupture. A half-hour of verticality should get you out of the danger zone.

Sitting, of course, leaves some tissues shorter and stiffer than they should be, setting you up for injury if you do stretches without loosening up a bit first. It takes only a few minutes of walking around to get your body ready for flexibility exercises.

need to prepare your muscles and joints for specific lifts.

This chapter tackles its three subjects in order of how you'll do them:

>> preworkout mobility exercises

>> warmup techniques for specific lifts

>> postworkout flexibility exercises

MOBILITY EXERCISES

Do these at the start of each workout. The entire routine should take just 5 to 10 minutes.

EXERCISE	REPS
ARM CIRCLES	5*
LEG CIRCLES TO FRONT	5***
FOOT CIRCLES	5***
PUSHUP WITH T ROTATION	5*
CAMEL/CAT	5
SINGLE-LEG DEADLIFT	5**
SIDE LUNGE WITH OVERHEAD REACH	5*
OVERHEAD SQUAT	5

* Each direction
** Each limb
*** Each direction, each limb

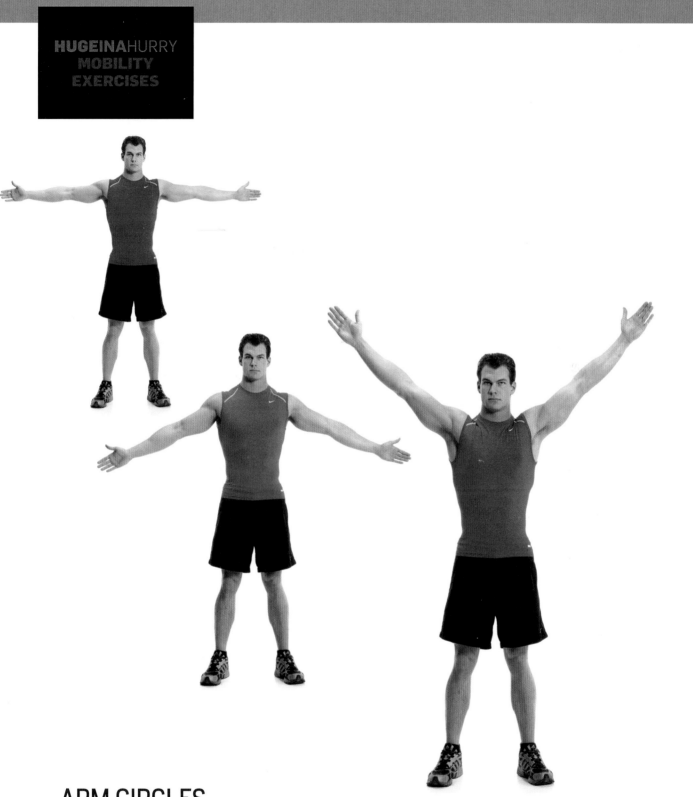

ARM CIRCLES

WHY? Increase mobility of shoulder joints

HOW TO DO THEM: Stand with your arms straight out to your sides, palms forward, thumbs up. Start with small forward circles and progress to big circles by the time you get to the final repetition. Repeat in the opposite direction.

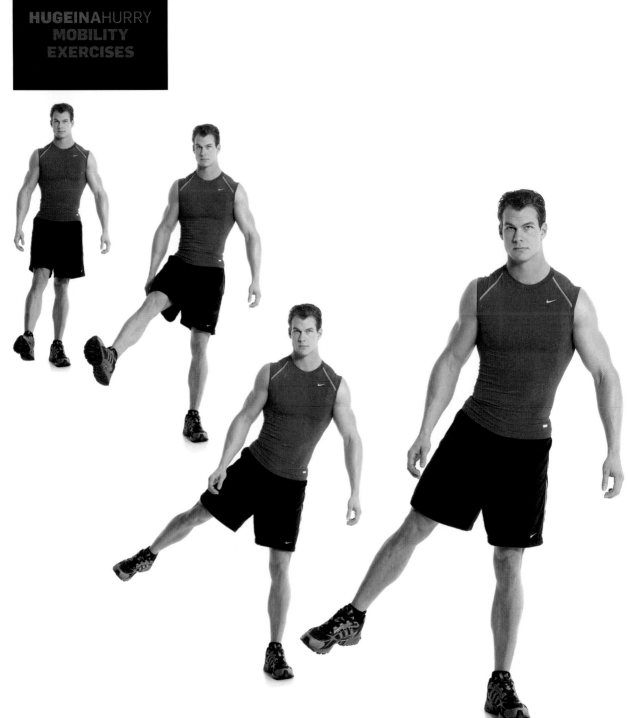

LEG CIRCLES TO FRONT

WHY? Increase mobility of hip joints

HOW TO DO THEM: Stand and lift your right leg about 12 inches out in front of you. Keep the leg straight and foot flexed (don't point your toes, in other words). Do five leg circles clockwise, using the biggest range of motion you can without losing your balance. (It's okay to rest your fingers on a wall to help with balance, but don't use it as a crutch.) Do five more circles counterclockwise, then switch legs and do five in each direction.

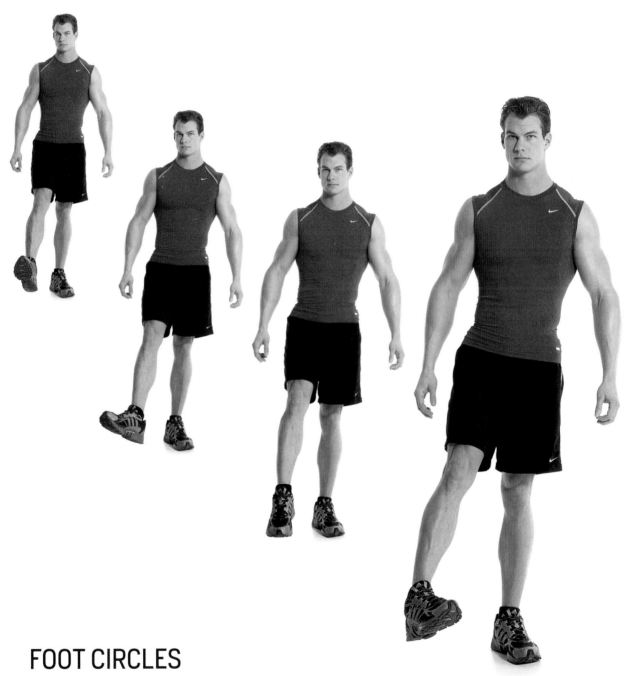

FOOT CIRCLES

WHY? Increase mobility of ankle joints

HOW TO DO THEM: Stand and lift your right foot about 6 inches in front of you with your leg straight. Make five clockwise circles with your right foot, using the biggest range of motion you can. Do five more circles counterclockwise, then switch legs and do five in each direction.

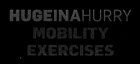

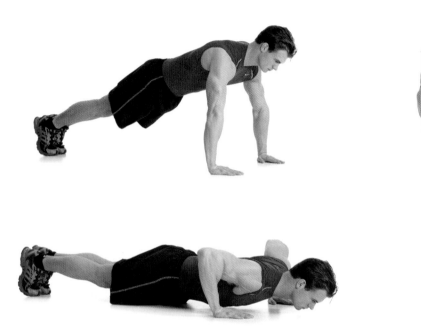

PUSHUP WITH T ROTATION

WHY? Increase mobility of shoulder joints

HOW TO DO IT: Get into a pushup position with your hands directly below your shoulders. Lower your body until your chest touches the floor, then immediately push back up to the starting position. Rotate to the right by twisting your torso and lifting your right arm as high as possible. Turn your head by following your hand with your eyes. Rotate back to the starting position, and then rotate to the left by lifting your left arm as high as possible.

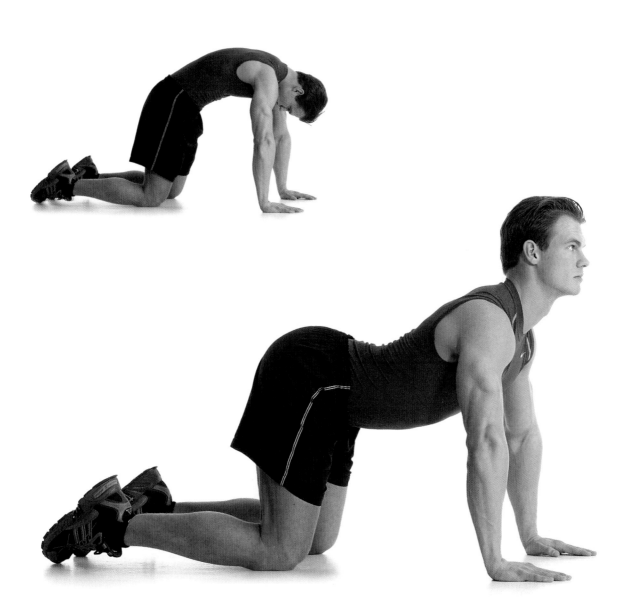

CAMEL/CAT

WHY? Increase core mobility

HOW TO DO IT: Get down on all fours with your hands directly below your shoulders and your knees directly below your hips. Round your back by pushing it upward (camel), then push your abdomen down toward the floor, exaggerating the arch in your back (cat).

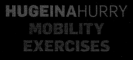

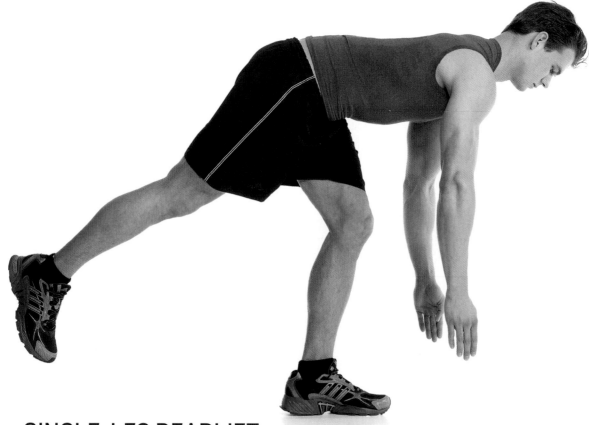

SINGLE-LEG DEADLIFT

WHY? Increase mobility of hips, gluteals, hamstrings, and calves

HOW TO DO IT: Stand with your feet hip-width apart, hands at your sides. Bend your left knee slightly, just enough to lift your right foot off the floor and hold it behind your body. You want your right knee tight, but not locked completely. Push your hips back and shift your torso forward while keeping your back flat. Lower your hands toward the floor until you feel your back start to round. Rise back to the starting position, and finish the set with your left leg. Repeat with your right.

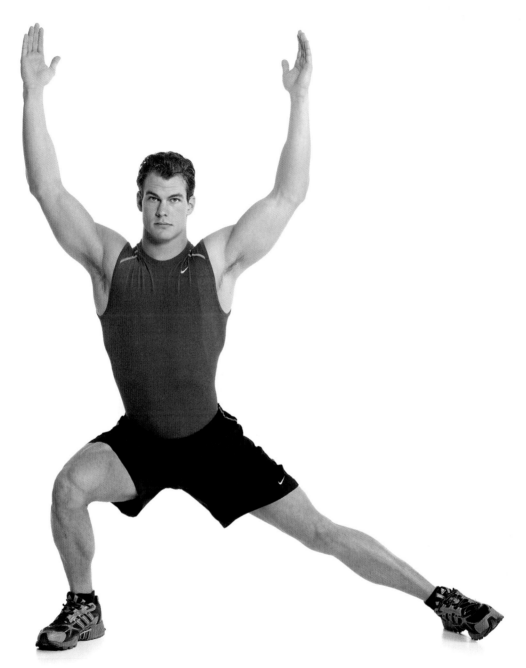

SIDE LUNGE WITH OVERHEAD REACH

WHY? Increase mobility of inner thighs and hips

HOW TO DO IT: Stand with your feet hip-width apart, hands at your sides. Take the longest step you can to your right and drop down into a lunge while reaching toward the ceiling with both arms. Keep your toes pointing forward. Push back to the starting position, lowering your arms. Repeat to your left, and alternate sides until you finish all your reps.

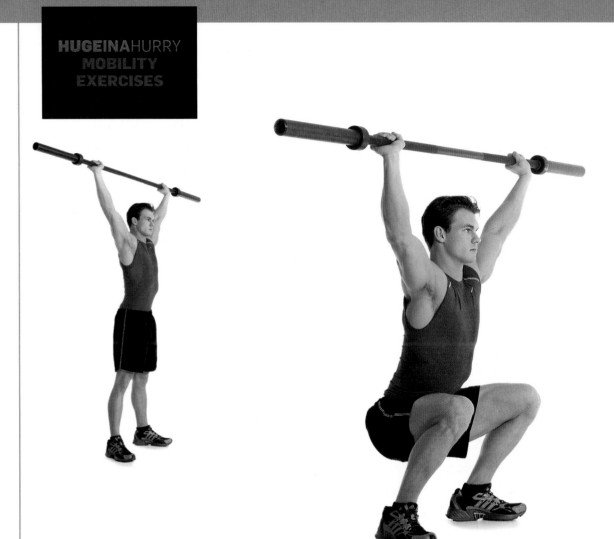

OVERHEAD SQUAT

WHY? Increase mobility of shoulders, thoracic spine (upper back), hips, and ankles

HOW TO DO IT: If you have experience with Olympic lifts, or if you've done this exercise before, you can start with a 45-pound Olympic barbell. Experienced lifters who've never done overhead squats before can use a standard barbell, which weighs 10 pounds. If you are a novice lifter and have no idea what I'm talking about, try this the first time with a broomstick or anything else you can find that's similarly light. No matter how strong you are, don't add any weight to the bar you use.

Grab the bar with a very wide grip and hold it overhead with your feet about shoulder-width apart, toes angled out slightly. Push your hips back while keeping your chest up, and lower yourself into a squat. Keep your elbows locked and the barbell over your head, if not behind it. If you feel the bar moving forward, past your head, stop your descent and return to the starting position.

Also stop your descent if you feel your lower back slipping out of its natural arch in either direction—you don't want your back to round, but you also don't want it to go into an excessive arch. Do all your repetitions with the best range of motion you can with good form, but don't go past the point at which your form breaks down.

If you don't have either problem, descend until your upper thighs are parallel to the floor, or slightly below that if you can, and then return to the starting position and repeat.

WARMUP SETS

At this point, your body is ready to train. But that doesn't mean you're ready to jump right into your work sets, using heavy weights. You'll need to do one or more warmup sets of each exercise before you begin your work sets of that specific exercise. The number of warmup sets you do depends on any number of factors: your age, your experience, your injury history, your comfort level and personal preferences, and whether the exercise is first or last in your workout.

Really, warmup sets are an art, not a science. You're the artist. There's no universal "right" way to prepare for heavy lifts. For one guy it might be four or five warmup sets. Another guy might hate the idea of doing more than one, and he has gotten so used to working with minimal warmup sets that he can do it without any problems. The better you know your body, the better you'll be at preparing it for productive workouts.

This is as good a time as any to call your attention to an aspect of my workouts that differs from most others.

A typical total-body workout will start with squats or deadlifts. We all know the logic: Those exercises use the most muscle and require the most effort and concentration, so it makes sense to do them when you have the most energy. However, they also require the most extensive warmup, perhaps 5 to 10 minutes more than you'd need to warm up for pulling or pushing exercises.

That's why I have upper-body exercises first in most of my *Huge in a Hurry* workouts. It takes less time to warm up for them, and by the time you're finished with work sets of pulls and pushes, you'll be able to do heavy squats or deadlifts with fewer warmup sets.

Here are a few suggestions for how to approach exercise-specific warmups.

CONSIDER THE LOAD

In Chapter 6, I gave you four general categories of weights you'll use in my workouts:

» Light (20 to 22 reps)

» Medium (10 to 12 reps)

» Heavy (4 to 6 reps)

» Superheavy (2 or 3 reps)

I don't think anyone reading this book would consider doing warmup sets for "light" weights. A lot of you wouldn't want to be seen with a weight you could lift more than 20 times, even if you were only using it to warm up for "heavy" or "superheavy" sets. But what do you do when the program calls for "medium" work sets? There's no right or wrong answer; I'd estimate that half my clients would do a warmup set, and half wouldn't.

When the program calls for heavy or superheavy weights, I think everyone needs to do 2 or 3 warmup sets. Let's say you're doing deadlifts and plan to use 250 pounds for your work sets. An easy way to warm up would be to use the weights you have to put on the bar anyway. So, you'd start with 135 pounds—the bar with a 45-pound plate on each end—and progress like this:

>> 135 pounds, 3 or 4 reps

>> 185 pounds, 2 or 3 reps

>> 225 pounds, 1 or 2 reps

Now you're ready to add the final weights and do your work sets with 250. I'm not suggesting everyone should warm up this way, just that it's simple and time-efficient.

CONSIDER YOUR AGE

Let's say you're 40, you were a serious athlete in high school, and you've been lifting consistently for more than 20 years, while playing recreational sports off and on in your twenties and thirties. You are in good shape and always have been, but your knees have taken a hell of a beating over the years. For you, a good warmup is the difference between feeling great for the next week . . . or limping around like someone twice your age.

Your lower-body exercise is front squats, and you're going to do work sets with 225 pounds. (Like I said, you're in good shape.) But you probably take a lot longer to get to that weight than someone younger would. In fact, your first warmup set might be with an empty barbell:

>> 45 pounds, 3 reps

>> 95 pounds, 3 reps

>> 135 pounds, 3 reps

>> 185 pounds, 2 reps

An equally strong lifter who's 20 years younger might skip those first two steps and jump right into warmups with 135. Even that might be a concession to a coach or training partner; I've seen plenty of young lifters whose idea of a warmup was a couple of deep breaths before lifting near-max weights. I don't recommend the no-warmup strategy, but in some circumstances, as I'll explain next, even that can work.

CONSIDER YOUR REASONS FOR TRAINING

Some of my clients have been members of elite military or police units. At first I trained them the same way I'd train any other athletes, with plenty of warmup sets. But then one Special Forces soldier explained the finer points of his job: Sometimes, he said, he has to go from deep sleep to a full-on uphill sprint carrying 40 pounds of gear. Once or twice he got to wherever he was going before he even realized he was awake.

I wasn't doing him any favors by training him in the gym with extensive warmups. Anything his body could do, it had to be able to do without warning. From then on, we went right into heavy work with little or no specific preparation.

Most of us have less urgent reasons for

training, to the great relief of our wives and girlfriends. My point is to keep in mind that whatever you do in the weight room—including your approach to warming up—will have some effect on how you perform in other parts of your life.

CONSIDER THE ORDER OF EXERCISES

Ideally, you'll do my workouts as a circuit—a typical one might include chinups, dips, and deadlifts, in that order. I can't say with complete veracity or confidence that any exercise is "safe." But I can say that upper-body pulling exercises seem to pose the least risk, which is why most of my workouts start with one of those.

You may find that you don't need to warm up for the second and third exercises in the circuit. Let's say you do two warmup sets before your first work set of chinups. (You'll probably use the lat pulldown machine for this.) That might be enough to prepare your shoulder joints for the first work set of dips. And after you've done a set of chinups and a set of dips, you might feel as if you're ready for a work set of deadlifts without additional warmup sets.

Is that an ideal way to do that circuit?

If you're using medium weights, sure. With heavy weights, you probably want to do two warmup sets for each exercise before you jump into work sets for that exercise. And with superheavy weights, I think you'll do best with two or three warmup sets of each exercise before you do your work sets of that exercise.

I know many of you won't do the workouts in circuits. If you're working out in a crowded gym, it's out of the question—as soon as you walk away from a station, it might be 10 or 15 minutes before you can use it again. But even if it's possible, some of you won't want to work out that way. Which, of course, is fine: It's your workout, even if you're using my programs. In that case, you probably want to include at least one warmup set for the second and third exercises if you're using heavy weights. For superheavy loads, I recommend three warmup sets for the first exercise and at least two for the others.

Unless, that is, you're considering a career in Delta Force. . . .

FLEXIBILITY TRAINING

I recommend these stretches immediately following each training session. Hold each position for 15 seconds.

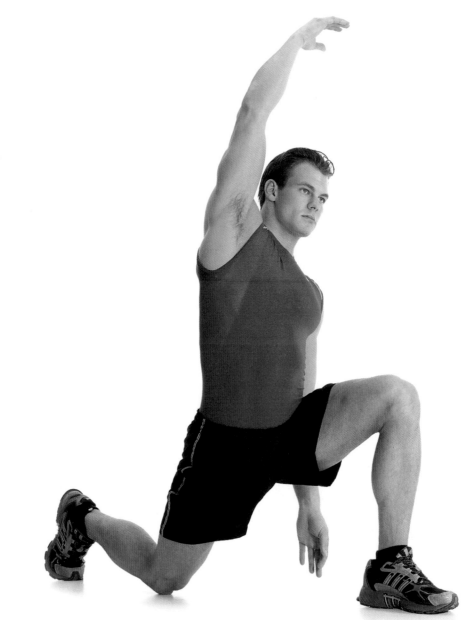

HIP FLEXOR STRETCH

Kneel on your right knee, with your torso upright, your left foot flat on the floor, and your left knee bent about 90 degrees. (It's like the bottom position of a lunge, only with your right knee on the floor instead of just above it.) Lean back, pushing your hips forward and pulling your chest back, as you reach up and over your head with your right arm. Hold that position, feeling the stretch in the right side of your pelvis. Repeat on the other side.

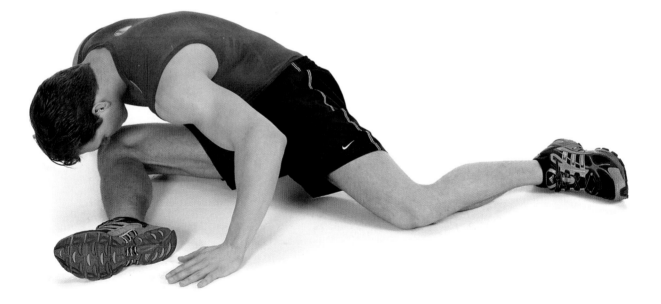

OUTER THIGH STRETCH

Sit on the floor in what we used to call "Indian style." (It's like the lotus position in yoga, except the outer edges of your feet are on the floor.) Pull your left leg back and to the side so your left foot is behind you, with your left knee slightly bent. Now lean forward from your hips and try to touch your nose to your right calf. Hold as you feel the stretch in your right outer thigh. Repeat on the opposite side.

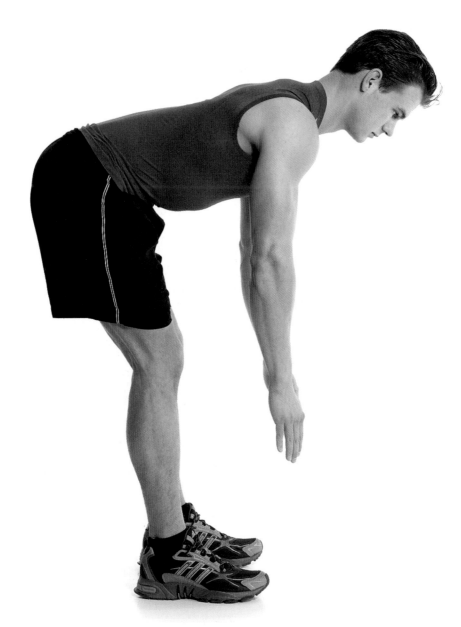

GLUTEALS, HAMSTRINGS, AND CALVES (GASTROCNEMIUS) STRETCH

Stand with your feet together and your knees nearly straight, but not locked. Push your hips back while keeping your lower back in its natural arch, and reach toward the floor. You want to go as far as you can without your lower back losing its arch. Hold that position.

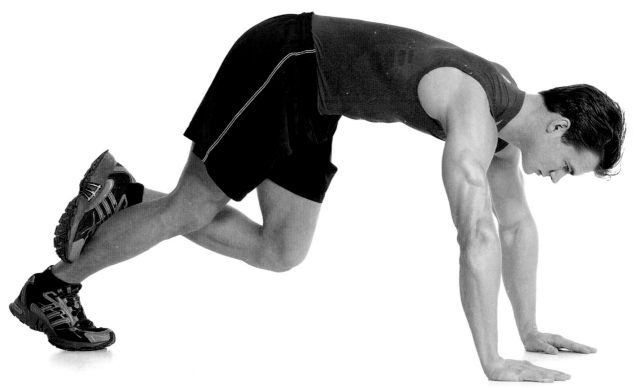

CALVES (SOLEUS) STRETCH

Stand, bend forward from the hips, and place your hands on the floor, keeping your hips up. Lift your left foot off the floor, and place it behind your right calf. Bend your right knee slightly, and feel the stretch in the soleus of your right leg. (The soleus is the flat calf muscle beneath the diamond-shaped gastrocnemius.) Hold, then repeat on the opposite side.

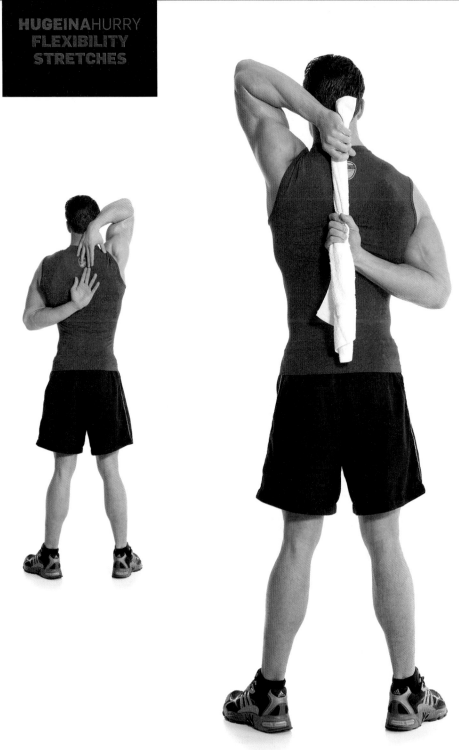

FRONT SHOULDER STRETCH

Lift your right arm up and over your right shoulder and place your hand between your shoulder blades, palm down. Place your left hand behind your lower back, palm turned out, and reach up to touch the fingers of your right hand. Hold, then repeat with your arms reversed. If you can't touch your fingers, you can use a towel—hold one end in your top hand, and grasp it as high as you can with your bottom hand.

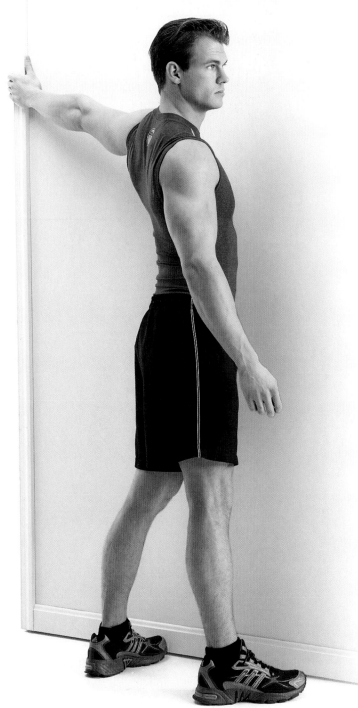

CHEST STRETCH

Stand facing a wall. Reach your left arm out to the side, parallel to the floor, with your left palm against the wall. Twist your body to the right as far as possible and hold. Repeat on the opposite side.

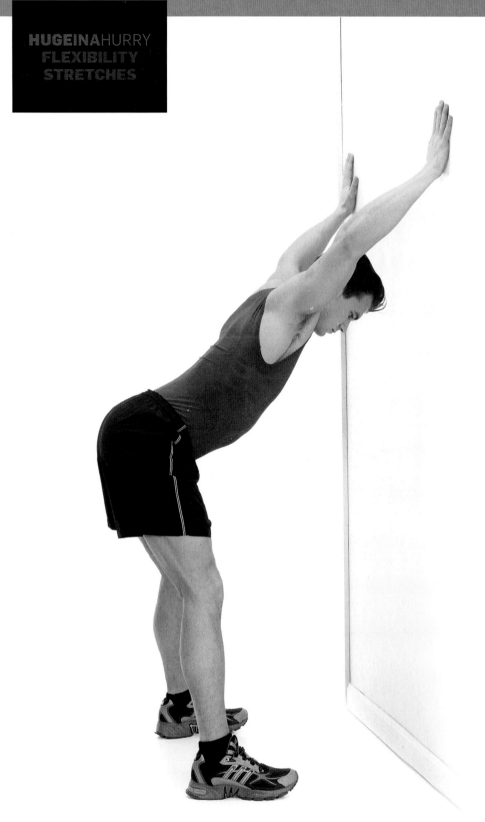

LAT STRETCH

Stand facing a wall with your arms extended overhead, shoulder-width apart, and your palms
against the wall. Push your hips back, lower your chest toward the floor, and hold.

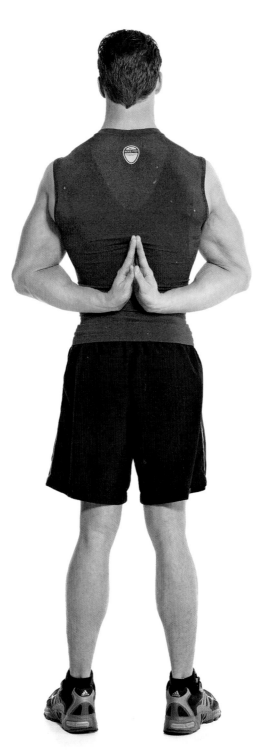

WRIST FLEXORS STRETCH

This stretch is sometimes called "reverse prayer," which helps you visualize the position: Press your palms together behind your back, fingertips pointed up, and hold.

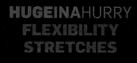

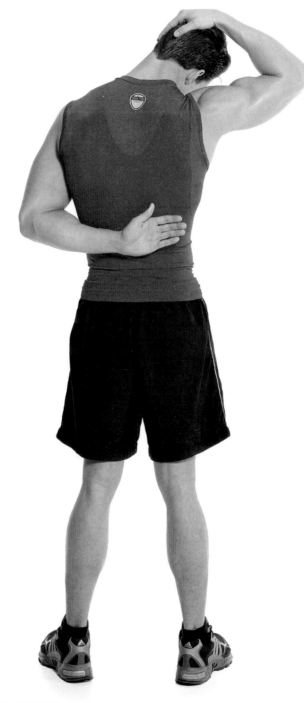

UPPER TRAPS STRETCH

Stand and place your left arm behind your lower back, your palm turned out. With your right hand, grasp the lower-left part of your head. *Gently* pull your head diagonally, toward your right hip, and hold. Repeat on the opposite side.

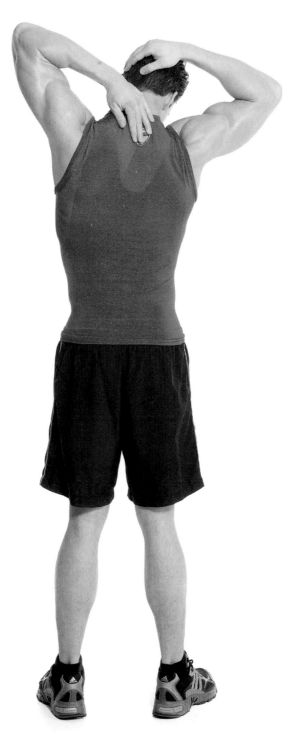

LEVATOR SCAPULAE STRETCH

Lift your left arm up and over your left shoulder so your left hand rests palm-down on your upper back. Grab the left-rear side of your head with your right hand and *gently* pull your head diagonally toward your right hip. Hold, then repeat on the opposite side.

CHAPTER 8

HOW TO USE THE PROGRAMS

n Part 3, you'll see exactly how to do the workouts I've been talking about for the previous seven chapters. I know you can't wait to get to them, so I'll try to keep these instructions as brief as possible while still giving you the information you need to succeed.

THE BASICS

You know from previous chapters that I'm going to give you a specific number of repetitions to do for each exercise, rather than a combination of sets and reps. Your goal is to do as many as you can per set with good form, while lifting as fast as possible. When a repetition is slower than the first one you did in that set, it becomes the last rep in that set.

As we've discussed, the weight you use will fall into one of these four categories:

Light: a weight you could lift 20 to 22 times

Medium: a weight you could lift 10 to 12 times

Heavy: a weight you could lift 4 to 6 times

Superheavy: a weight you could lift 2 or 3 times

Don't worry about memorizing, since I'll remind you of the range on each workout chart. It'll look like this:

Load: heavy (4–6 RM)

"RM" stands for "repetition maximum," which means exactly what you think: the most reps you can do with a given weight on your first work set, when you're fresh.

That's a crucial point, so I'll repeat it: *Select your weight based on what you can do in your first set.* The other sets will take care of themselves. You don't need to hold back on your first set so you can do the same number of reps on subsequent sets. It doesn't matter if you do fewer reps per set as you go along.

But how do you know how much weight to use on that first set? That is a great question, and contrary to what I just said about being as brief as possible, it requires a detailed answer.

HOW TO CHOOSE THE RIGHT WEIGHT

On the one hand, my system is simple to use, since the idea is to do every set of every exercise in each workout with the same weight. But what if you don't use the correct weight on the first set? And if you've never done that particular exercise in that particular rep range, how do you even guess how much to start out with?

The answer is "trial and error." The following strategies should help you get it right sooner rather than later.

USE YOUR WARMUP TO ESTIMATE THE CORRECT LOAD

Remember the standing cable row I described in Chapter 7? Chances are, you've never done it before, nor have you ever seen anyone else doing it. You have absolutely no way to know how much weight you should use for your first set. Even if I wanted to help you out by suggesting a starting weight, I couldn't, since I don't know what kind of cable system you'll be using. Forty pounds on one machine might feel like 60 on another.

That's where your warmup comes in handy. Start with what looks like a ridiculously light weight, and try a few reps, focusing on your balance and form. Go up a plate or two, and try that. You should know within two or three reps whether it's the right weight for the category. If it's not, add another plate or two. As soon as you find a weight that feels right, rest for a minute, and then use that weight for your first work set. If you selected correctly, you should be able to use that weight for all your sets.

ADJUST THE WEIGHT UP OR DOWN FOR YOUR SECOND SET

So you've selected a weight that you think qualifies as "heavy"—one you can lift four to six times on your first set. But you shoot past your sixth rep and get seven without slowing down or changing your form, and you know you could keep going for another rep or two, or maybe even three. Here's what you do:

>> Stop at seven reps. I don't want you to stop at six if you haven't slowed down, since that puts the wrong idea into your head. You'll start focusing on reps instead of rep speed. But it's easy enough to quit at seven.

>> For your second set, add 2 percent or 5 pounds, whichever is more, and take the designated amount of rest. If you still blow past six reps, stop after seven, and add another 2 percent or 5 pounds.

>> If that doesn't work, and you get past six again, do the same adjustment for your final set. Stop when you hit your 25th total rep, and plan to use more weight the next time you do that workout.

If the weight is too heavy, and you can't get four reps on your first set without slowing down, make the adjustment in reverse: subtract 2 percent or 5 pounds, whichever is more. If that's still too much, subtract again, and continue until you get it right.

On some exercises—particularly, squats and deadlifts—there's a chance you'll miss by a lot more than 2 percent or 5 pounds. If it's clear you need to add or subtract more than what I recommend, use your own judgment. I just want you to avoid having to make reverse adjustments on subsequent sets, overshooting in one direction and then undershooting in the other.

MANAGING YOUR REPETITIONS

Let's say you've gotten it exactly right on your first set. The workout calls for 25 total reps with a "heavy" load, and you get four, five, or six reps with the weight you've selected. Now what?

Different lifters recover at different speeds, so nobody can predict what will happen on subsequent sets. If your nervous system is efficient at recruiting the largest motor units, your second set will probably be around four reps. If it isn't efficient—it needs a set or two before you can tap into your largest motor units—you might be able to get seven reps on your second set before the speed slows down. That's fine. The key is to get the first set right.

Which brings me to another important point: After the first set, you might not get four reps with a heavy load before your speed slows down. That's fine, too.

Let's look at two potential outcomes, based on the lifter's experience. A veteran musclehead might reach 25 reps this way:

Set 1: 5 reps

Set 2: 5 reps

Set 3: 4 reps

Set 4: 4 reps

Set 5: 4 reps

Set 6: 3 reps

Conversely, a novice lifter's workout chart might look like this:

Set 1: 6 reps

Set 2: 7 reps

Set 3: 6 reps

Set 4: 6 reps

The experienced lifter has more ability to recruit his largest motor units. That's why he might be working with three times as much weight as the beginner on any given exercise. Those big motor units can't recover as fast as smaller motor units, which is why the vet's first set with a heavy or superheavy weight will generally be his best set on that exercise.

Meanwhile, the entry-level lifter is using smaller motor units. His inability to tap into the biggest ones limits the amount of weight he can lift, but the motor units he *can* recruit recover faster. That's why his performance tends to improve on his second set, and why it doesn't fall very far on subsequent sets.

PROGRESSION

The programs in *Huge in a Hurry* have similar structures: Most take 16 weeks. The programs include three 4-week phases. Each phase has three workouts—A, B, and C. Ideally, you'll do three workouts a week, with at least 1 day off in between (Monday, Wednesday, and Friday, for example), and complete the phase in 4 weeks. If you can't do three workouts every week, make sure you do workouts A, B, and C four times each, in that order, before you move on.

Each phase is followed by a week of workouts (usually designated as "unloading") designed to help you with recovery and boost your benefits. You won't work out at all the 16th and final week of each phase.

Nothing in this book will work if you don't push yourself to improve your performance from one week to the next. Different programs emphasize different types of progression, such as higher volume for hypertrophy, heavier weights for strength, and shorter rest periods for fat loss. But the most important progression is the amount of weight on the bar. As soon as you can exceed the designated number of repetitions you perform on your first set of each exercise, add 2 percent or 5 pounds, whichever is more. You should be able to do this on almost every exercise from one week to the next.

CIRCUITS AND SUPERSETS

In a perfect world, I'd design virtually all of my workouts as circuits—doing a set of every exercise in the routine before repeating an exercise. You'd end up with about 3 minutes to recover from one set of an exercise to the next set of that exercise. In my experience, that's the most effective and time-efficient way to train.

The world, alas, is imperfect. If you work out in a commercial gym, you can't take up three stations for the duration of a workout. Even if you work out at home, you might not have enough equipment to set up for three different exercises at the same time.

So, reluctantly, I prescribe straight sets for most of the workouts in this book. If, however, you have the luxury of performing any of the workouts as a circuit, I recommend it. Or, at least, try it for a workout to see if you like it. Or alternate circuits and straight sets each time you repeat a workout.

If a workout includes the chinup, dip, and deadlift, with 60 seconds of rest between sets, a circuit would look like this:

>> Chinups

>> Rest 60 seconds

>> Dips

>> Rest 60 seconds

>> Deadlifts

>> Rest 60 seconds

>> Repeat the circuit

Another option, which is more realistic for many lifters, is to alternate between the two upper-body exercises, and then finish the workout with straight sets of the lower-body exercise. As with the circuits I just described, you'd take the designated amount of rest after each set of each exercise.

One potential problem: You do more reps per set with one exercise, which means you reach the target reps with that exercise before you finish the others.

Let's say your workout starts with chinups and dips, and you decide you're going to super-set those two exercises. It calls for a "heavy"

load, a weight you could lift four to six times while fresh. You know you can do a lot of dips with your body weight, so you wear a dipping belt with a 10-pound weight attached. The problem is that you're not yet very good at doing chinups with your body weight. You do just three or four chinups per set, compared with five or six dips. You hit your target reps on dips with four chinups left to perform.

The solution is simple enough: Just continue with the chinups as straight sets until you finish all your reps, resting for the designated time after each set. In most cases, it takes only one set to make up the difference.

ORPHAN REPS

Here's a question that will come up the first time you do these workouts: What do you do with leftover reps? If the target is 25 reps, and after five sets you've completed 24, what happens to the leftover rep? You're going to hate my answer.

Take the specified amount of rest, and then do the final repetition as its own set.

See, I knew you'd hate the answer.

But you don't have to like the solution to appreciate the logic behind it. If you don't do the final rep, your workout doesn't have the requisite volume. If you do more reps in that final set, the volume exceeds the parameters, which can affect your recovery and your performance in future workouts.

The same answer applies to two corollary questions:

>> What happens if I hit the target reps when I'm in the middle of a set, and I know I can do two or three more?

>> If I get to within one rep of the target and my speed starts to slow down, is it okay to grind out that last repetition, even though it's noticeably slower than the others?

In the first scenario, yes, I really do want you to stop the set even though you're leaving one or more reps in the tank. In the second, no, I don't want you to grind out that last rep.

Those are the official answers. But, to be honest, I know you're going to follow your own instincts. That's what experienced lifters are supposed to do. You learn by experimenting and you come to trust your own judgment.

However, in my experience, too many inexperienced or moderately experienced lifters trust instincts they don't yet have. They start improvising with workouts designed by people like me before they've given them a chance to work.

So, I'm not saying the programs won't work unless you do them exactly as written. And I'm certainly not the kind of control freak who blows a head gasket if anyone questions my philosophy of program design. As former nightclub bouncers go, I'm surprisingly easygoing.

All I ask is this: Try it my way first, before you start improvising. You'll at least understand how I meant for it to work.

SAMPLE TRAINING LOG

PROGRAM/STAGE:

WORKOUT:

REPETITION RANGE:

EXERCISE	WEIGHT	REPETITIONS PERFORMED IN EACH SET							
		SET 1	SET 2	SET 3	SET 4	SET 5	SET 6	SET 7	SET 8
UPPER-BODY PULL									
UPPER-BODY PUSH									
SQUAT OR DEADLIFT VARIATION									
ACCESSORY EXERCISE									

NOTES:

PUTTING TOGETHER
A LONG-TERM PROGRAM

I've trained just about every type of athlete, from fighters to figure competitors, and just about every type of nonathlete, from young to old and thin to thick. What I don't know is how to classify you personally. I can guess that you're a male, under 40, who bought this book to learn how to put on a lot of muscle mass in as little time as possible. (Who else would buy a book called *Men's Health Huge in a Hurry*?)

But I can't possibly make assumptions about your genetics, your experience, your skill as a lifter, your comfort level with unfamiliar lifts and techniques, or any of the dozens of variables that determine the best way for you to use my workouts.

If you've read the Contents, you know that the chapter following this one is called Get Ready, and you can probably guess that it includes an introductory workout, designed to prepare you for the ones that follow.

Likewise, I'm sure you've figured out that the chapter called Get Big focuses on muscle hypertrophy, and that the subsequent chapter, Get Even Bigger, includes an advanced hypertrophy program. (Actually, it has two advanced programs; you'll learn why when you get there.)

Then there's Get Strong (a strength program) and Get Even Stronger (an advanced strength program). I wrap up with Get Lean, and I won't insult your intelligence by explaining what that title means.

You're free to use these workouts in any order you want, with just two rules:

>> Everyone should do the 3-week prep workouts in Get Ready. It doesn't matter whether you've been training for 20 minutes or 20 years. You will not get the results you want from the other programs if you skip this step. You need this step to train your body to do the workouts that follow.

>> Always do the basic workouts (Get Big or Get Strong) before tackling the advanced programs (Get Even Bigger or Get Even Stronger).

Other than that, you're free to start off with Get Big, Get Strong, or Get Lean. I think most readers will get the best results by doing the hypertrophy workouts before the strength programs, but the most advanced lifters can certainly go straight from Get Ready to Get Strong.

The fat-loss programs in Get Lean employ Olympic lifts, which certainly involve a learning curve. That's why I think most readers will be better off doing the hypertrophy or strength workouts before tackling fat loss. But an experienced lifter could start there, and then move on to Get Big or Get Strong.

Here are some suggested paths for lifters at different levels.

LESS THAN 2 YEARS
OF SOLID TRAINING EXPERIENCE

1. Get Ready

2. Get Big

3. Get Strong

4. Get Lean

5. Get Even Bigger (optional)

6. Get Even Stronger (optional)

**2 TO 5 YEARS
OF SOLID TRAINING EXPERIENCE**

1. Get Ready

2. Get Big

3. Get Even Bigger (optional)

4. Get Strong

5. Get Even Stronger (optional)

6. Get Lean

**MORE THAN 5 YEARS
OF SOLID TRAINING EXPERIENCE**

1. Get Ready

2. Get Strong

3. Get Even Stronger

4. Get Lean

5. Get Big

6. Get Even Bigger (optional)

Again, these aren't the only ways to do these programs, and I don't want to talk anyone out of trying anything, as long as you use common sense and follow the two inviolable rules: Do Get Ready first, and do the basic programs before the advanced ones in the same category. If you need to lose a lot of fat, it's best to start with Get Lean. The leaner you are, the less likely it is that you'll add fat when you put on muscle.

Now, finally, it's time to lift.

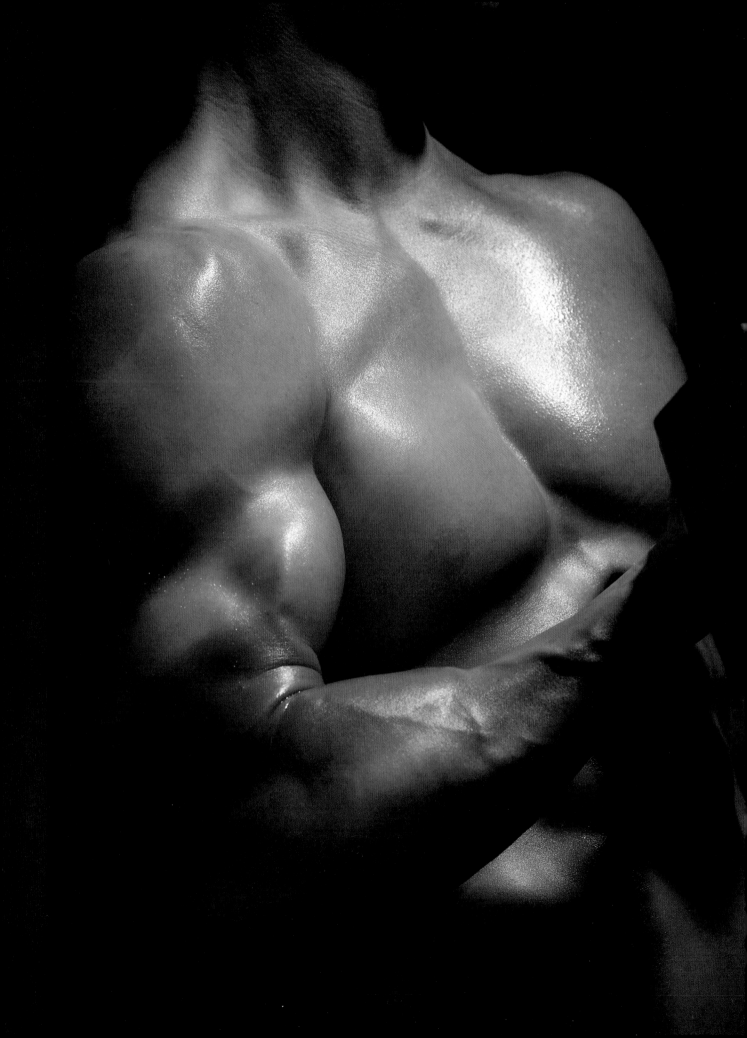

PART 3: THE PLANS

CHAPTER 9

GET READY

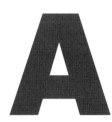

Are you ready for a little cognitive dissonance? Here it comes: Throughout this book, I've been pushing the idea of lifting with maximal speed with enough volume and weight to get the results you want, while maintaining perfect form. That's too much to master all at once, which is why I want you to start with this break-in program. You'll do three total-body workouts a week for 3 weeks, with the goal of getting used to my workout parameters.

It's that whole "walk before you run" thing.

And yes, I want everyone to do this program. It doesn't matter whether you're a beginner, intermediate, or advanced lifter. In fact, I don't even want you to think in those terms right now. Even if you've been training for 20 years, a lot of this will be new to you.

Your goal in these first 3 weeks is to focus on the speed of your lifts in conjunction with your form.

All of the parameters will remain constant except for the load you use for each exercise. The reason the load won't remain constant is because for the first few weeks, you'll probably miscalculate the weight that corresponds with the prescribed rep range. Each week you'll probably be able to add at least 5 pounds since your nervous system and muscles will quickly adapt.

This 3-week phase serves two essential purposes. First, it teaches you to focus on speed and total reps per exercise instead of a target number of sets and reps. So instead of doing five sets of 5, you'll perform as many sets as it takes to get to 25 total reps and stop each set when the last rep is noticeably slower than the first rep. Second, it prepares you for the core programs that are outlined in the following chapters.

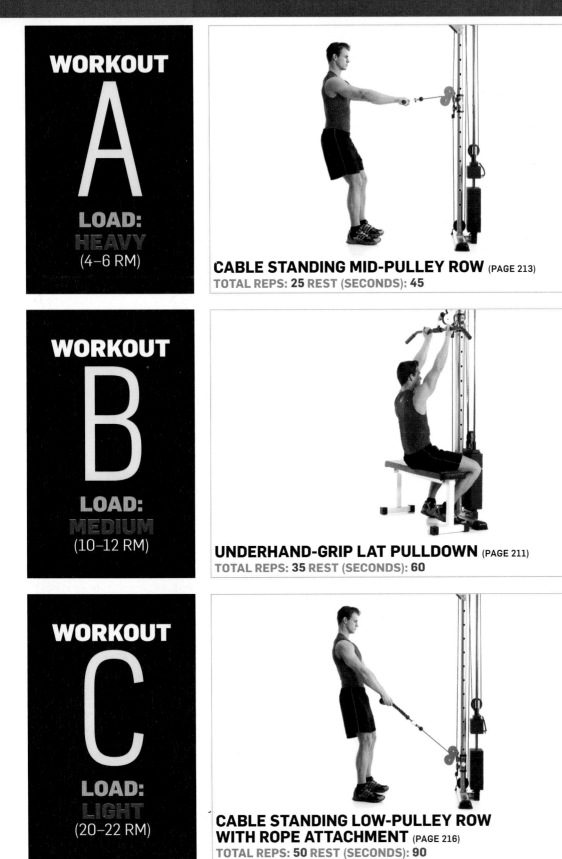

WORKOUT A

LOAD: HEAVY (4–6 RM)

CABLE STANDING MID-PULLEY ROW (PAGE 213)
TOTAL REPS: 25 REST (SECONDS): 45

WORKOUT B

LOAD: MEDIUM (10–12 RM)

UNDERHAND-GRIP LAT PULLDOWN (PAGE 211)
TOTAL REPS: 35 REST (SECONDS): 60

WORKOUT C

LOAD: LIGHT (20–22 RM)

CABLE STANDING LOW-PULLEY ROW WITH ROPE ATTACHMENT (PAGE 216)
TOTAL REPS: 50 REST (SECONDS): 90

Start with your weaker side first, then immediately do the same number of reps with your stronger limb. Rest after working both sides.

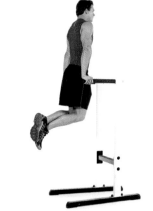

DIP OR DUMBBELL DECLINE BENCH
PRESS WITH NEUTRAL GRIP (PAGES 223 AND 227)
TOTAL REPS: 25 REST (SECONDS): 45

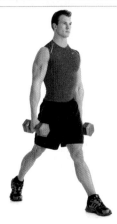

DUMBBELL SPLIT SQUAT* (PAGE 247)
TOTAL REPS: 25 REST BETWEEN SETS (SECONDS): 45

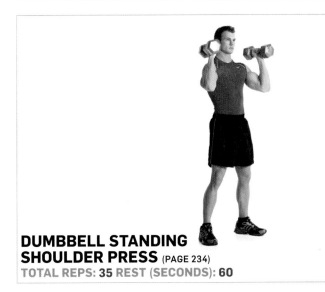

DUMBBELL STANDING
SHOULDER PRESS (PAGE 234)
TOTAL REPS: 35 REST (SECONDS): 60

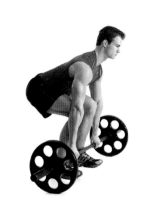

DEADLIFT (PAGE 254)
TOTAL REPS: 35 REST (SECONDS): 60

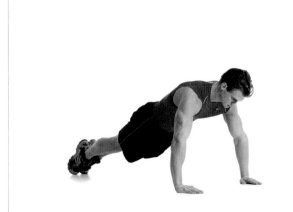

PUSHUP (PAGE 231)
TOTAL REPS: 50 REST (SECONDS): 90

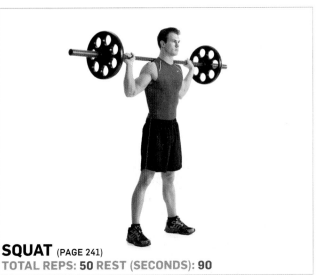

SQUAT (PAGE 241)
TOTAL REPS: 50 REST (SECONDS): 90

CHAPTER 10

GET BIG

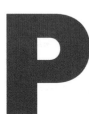icture two Olympic athletes. The first is a weightlifter. As you expect, he has huge thighs, and if you watch him perform snatches and cleans in competition, you understand why. Those lifts force him to drop into a full squat, ass to calves, with hundreds of pounds held overhead or on the front of his shoulders. Then he has to stand up from that position. You imagine his thigh muscles grow just thinking about doing something so obviously extreme and difficult.

The second is a cyclist. He also has large, well-developed thigh muscles—not nearly as big as the weightlifter's, but still showing obvious signs of training-induced muscle growth. And yet, the demands of his sport don't in any way resemble Olympic weightlifting. He probably does some strength training, but it's unlikely to involve all-out, max-effort lifts. Almost all his training is on the bike, with a focus on endurance. So how did his thighs get so big?

Short answer: Because all of your muscle fibers, from the smallest to the largest, have the potential to grow.

But if we leave the comparison where it stands, we negate everything I've written so far about the importance of tapping into your biggest and most powerful motor units. Right?

Not really. Let's consider two important qualifiers that I haven't yet mentioned:

›› The cyclist only has this kind of development in one muscle group: his quadriceps. He might also have reasonably well-developed calves, but if you just looked at him from the waist up, you'd never guess that he's an elite athlete. On the other hand, if the weightlifter walked into a room, he'd look like a guy who lifts weights. Even if you didn't know why he lifted, you'd guess in an instant that he's a serious athlete of some sort.

>> The weightlifter achieved a high level of overall muscularity in a fraction of the time the cyclist spent building his thighs—perhaps 10 hours a week of lifting, versus several times that riding.

My goal when I designed this 16-week muscle-building program was to include all five of the key considerations for muscle growth—three that I've covered in detail elsewhere in this book, and the two I just noted:

>> Recruit all your motor units.

>> Induce enough fatigue for them to grow.

>> Give them plenty of food (you'll find the details in Chapter 23).

>> Hit all the major muscles with a variety of movement patterns.

>> Do all this in the most time-efficient way possible.

Results? I think you can expect to add 10 pounds of muscle in this 16-week program. Some of you who haven't been training will do much better and add a pound each week, while others will remain in single-digit muscle growth. But I'm confident that everyone will notice an impressive difference after 4 months.

WORKOUT A

LOAD: HEAVY

(4–6 RM)

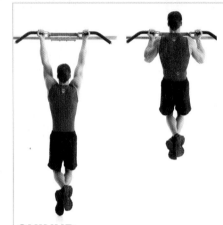

CHINUP (PAGE 207)
TOTAL REPS: **25** REST BETWEEN SETS (SECONDS): **60**

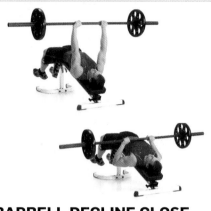

BARBELL DECLINE CLOSE-GRIP BENCH PRESS (PAGE 226)
TOTAL REPS: **25** REST BETWEEN SETS (SECONDS): **60**

WORKOUT B

LOAD: MEDIUM

(10–12 RM)

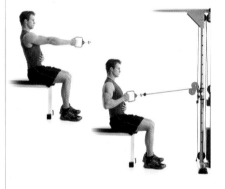

CABLE SEATED ONE-ARM ROW WITH NEUTRAL GRIP*
(PAGE 217)
TOTAL REPS: **40** REST (SECONDS): **75**

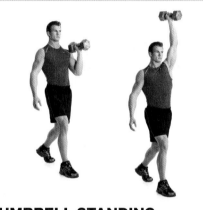

DUMBBELL STANDING ONE-ARM SHOULDER PRESS*
(PAGE 235)
TOTAL REPS: **40** REST (SECONDS): **75**

WORKOUT C

LOAD: LIGHT

(20–22RM)

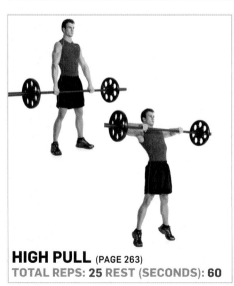

HIGH PULL (PAGE 263)
TOTAL REPS: **25** REST (SECONDS): **60**

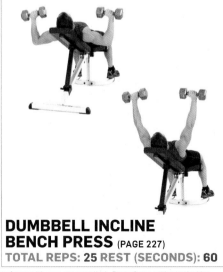

DUMBBELL INCLINE BENCH PRESS (PAGE 227)
TOTAL REPS: **25** REST (SECONDS): **60**

Start with your weaker side first, then immediately do the same number of reps with your stronger limb. Rest after working both sides.

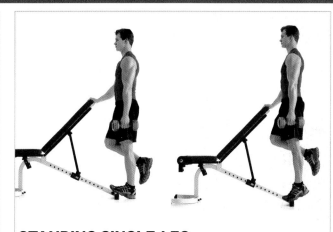

DEADLIFT (PAGE 254)
TOTAL REPS: **25** REST BETWEEN SETS (SECONDS): **60**

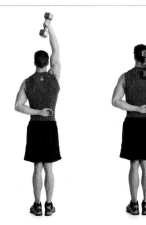

**STANDING SINGLE-LEG
CALF RAISE*** (PAGE 280)
TOTAL REPS: **25** REST BETWEEN SETS (SECONDS): **45**

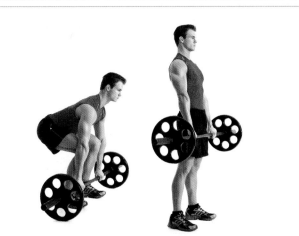

BULGARIAN SPLIT SQUAT (PAGE 248)
TOTAL REPS: **40** REST (SECONDS): **75**

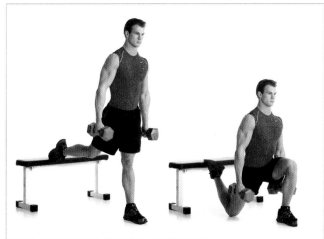

**DUMBBELL STANDING ONE-ARM
TRICEPS EXTENSION*** (PAGE 285)
TOTAL REPS: **40** REST (SECONDS): **60**

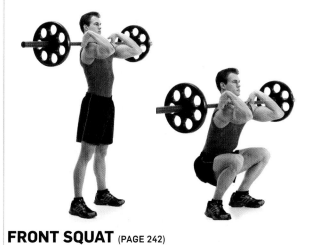

FRONT SQUAT (PAGE 242)
TOTAL REPS: **25** REST (SECONDS): **60**

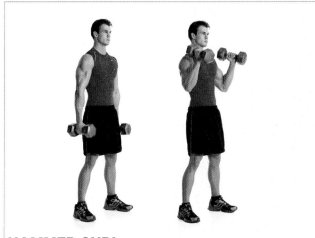

HAMMER CURL (PAGE 284)
TOTAL REPS: **25** REST (SECONDS): **45**

WORKOUT A

LOAD: LIGHT

(20–22 RM)

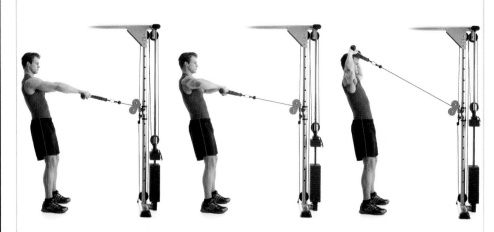

CABLE STANDING MID-PULLEY FACE PULL (PAGE 214)
TOTAL REPS: **50** REST (SECONDS): **75**

WORKOUT B

LOAD: MEDIUM

(10–12 RM)

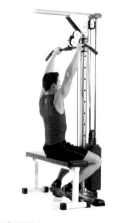
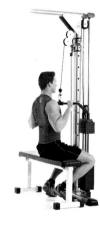

LAT PULLDOWN (PAGE 210)
TOTAL REPS: **30** REST (SECONDS): **60**

WORKOUT C

LOAD: MEDIUM

(10–12 RM)

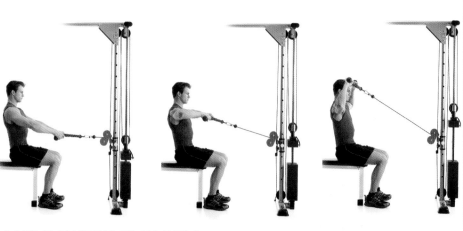

CABLE SEATED FACE PULL (PAGE 217)
TOTAL REPS: **30** REST (SECONDS): **60**

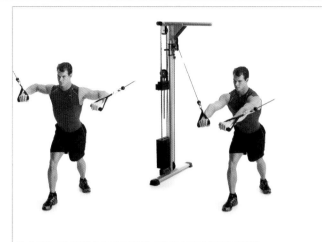

CABLE STANDING CHEST PRESS (PAGE 229)
TOTAL REPS: 50 REST (SECONDS): 75

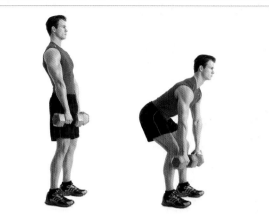

DUMBBELL ROMANIAN DEADLIFT
(PAGE 256)
TOTAL REPS: 50 REST (SECONDS): 75

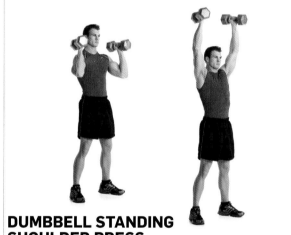

DUMBBELL STANDING
SHOULDER PRESS (PAGE 234)
TOTAL REPS: 30 REST (SECONDS): 60

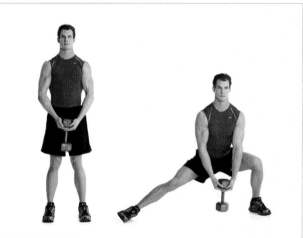

SIDE LUNGE (PAGE 249)
TOTAL REPS: 30* REST (SECONDS): 60
*With each leg

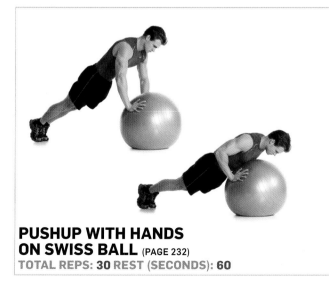

PUSHUP WITH HANDS
ON SWISS BALL (PAGE 232)
TOTAL REPS: 30 REST (SECONDS): 60

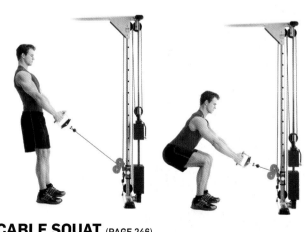

CABLE SQUAT (PAGE 246)
TOTAL REPS: 30 REST (SECONDS): 60

WORKOUT A

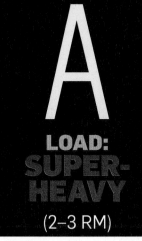

LOAD: SUPER-HEAVY
(2–3 RM)

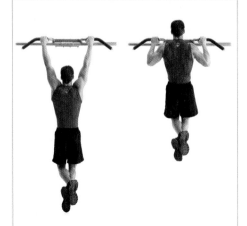

PULLUP (PAGE 207)
TOTAL REPS: 15 REST (SECONDS): 45

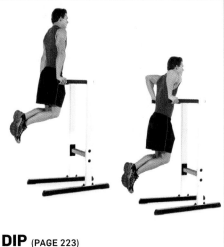

DIP (PAGE 223)
TOTAL REPS: 15 REST (SECONDS): 45

WORKOUT B

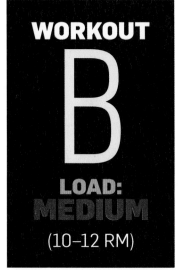

LOAD: MEDIUM
(10–12 RM)

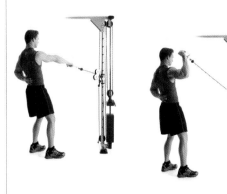

CABLE STANDING ONE-ARM MID-PULLEY ROW, PALM UP*
(PAGE 214)
TOTAL REPS: 40 REST (SECONDS): 75

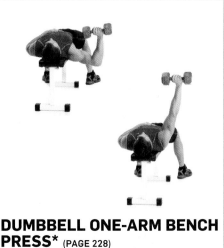

DUMBBELL ONE-ARM BENCH PRESS* (PAGE 228)
TOTAL REPS: 40 REST (SECONDS): 75

WORKOUT C

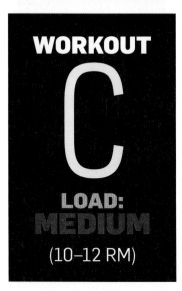

LOAD: MEDIUM
(10–12 RM)

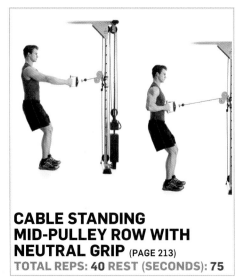

CABLE STANDING MID-PULLEY ROW WITH NEUTRAL GRIP (PAGE 213)
TOTAL REPS: 40 REST (SECONDS): 75

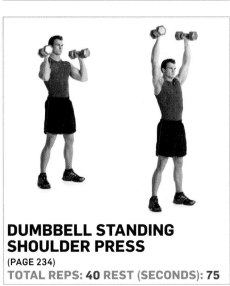

DUMBBELL STANDING SHOULDER PRESS
(PAGE 234)
TOTAL REPS: 40 REST (SECONDS): 75

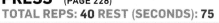

Start with your weaker side first, then immediately do the same number of reps with your stronger limb. Rest after working both sides.

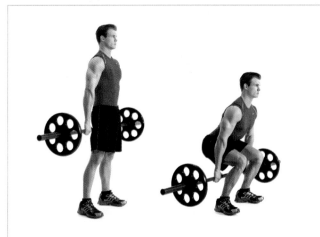

HACK SQUAT (PAGE 245)
TOTAL REPS: **15** REST (SECONDS): **45**

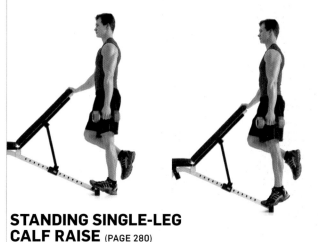

STANDING SINGLE-LEG CALF RAISE (PAGE 280)
TOTAL REPS: **15** REST (SECONDS): **30**

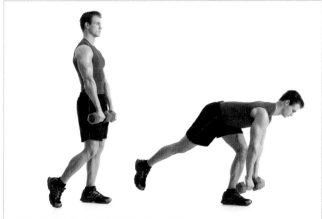

DUMBBELL SINGLE-LEG DEADLIFT* (PAGE 257)
TOTAL REPS: **40** REST (SECONDS): **75**

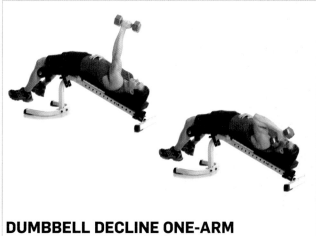

DUMBBELL DECLINE ONE-ARM TRICEPS EXTENSION* (PAGE 287)
TOTAL REPS: **40** REST (SECONDS): **60**

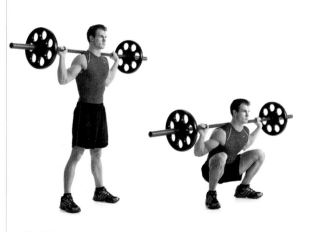

SQUAT (PAGE 241)
TOTAL REPS: **40** REST (SECONDS): **75**

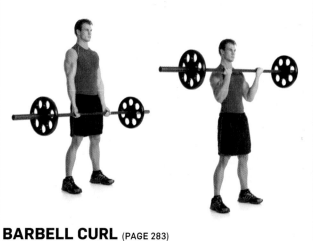

BARBELL CURL (PAGE 283)
TOTAL REPS: **40** REST (SECONDS): **60**

WORKOUT A

LOAD: LIGHT

(20–22 RM)

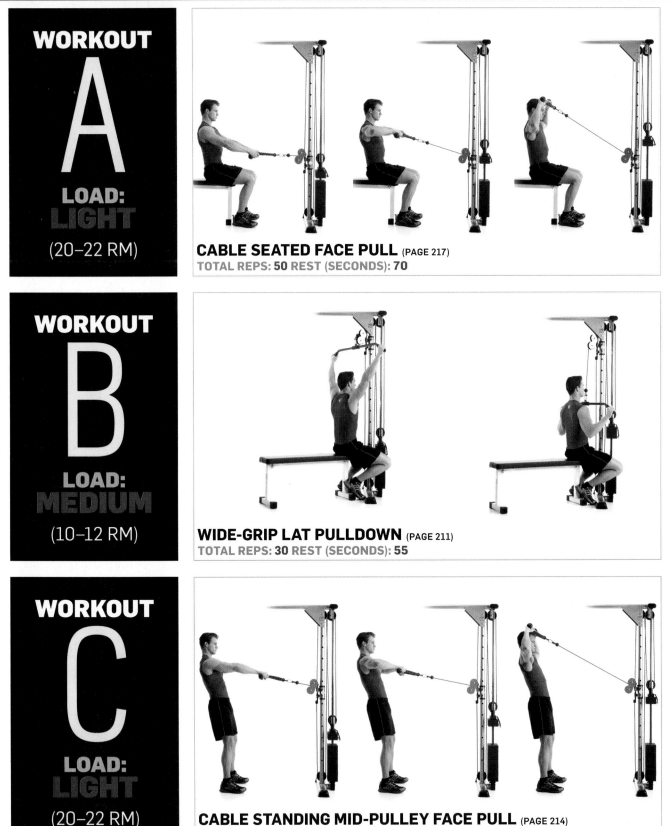

CABLE SEATED FACE PULL (PAGE 217)
TOTAL REPS: **50** REST (SECONDS): **70**

WORKOUT B

LOAD: MEDIUM

(10–12 RM)

WIDE-GRIP LAT PULLDOWN (PAGE 211)
TOTAL REPS: **30** REST (SECONDS): **55**

WORKOUT C

LOAD: LIGHT

(20–22 RM)

CABLE STANDING MID-PULLEY FACE PULL (PAGE 214)
TOTAL REPS: **50** REST (SECONDS): **70**

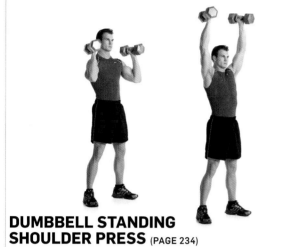

**DUMBBELL STANDING
SHOULDER PRESS** (PAGE 234)
TOTAL REPS: 50 REST (SECONDS): 70

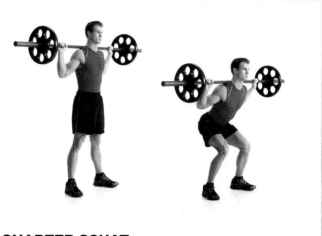

QUARTER SQUAT (PAGE 241)
TOTAL REPS: 50 REST (SECONDS): 70

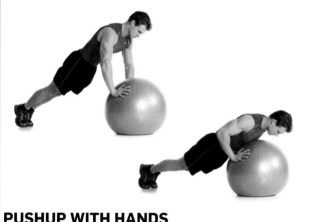

**PUSHUP WITH HANDS
ON SWISS BALL** (PAGE 232)
TOTAL REPS: 30 REST (SECONDS): 55

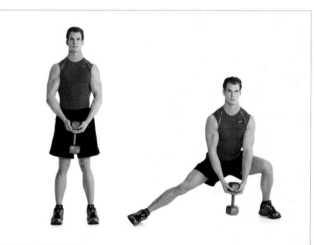

SIDE LUNGE (PAGE 249)
TOTAL REPS: 30* REST (SECONDS): 55
*With each leg

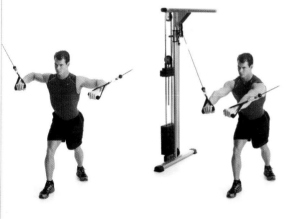

CABLE STANDING CHEST PRESS (PAGE 229)
TOTAL REPS: 50 REST (SECONDS): 70

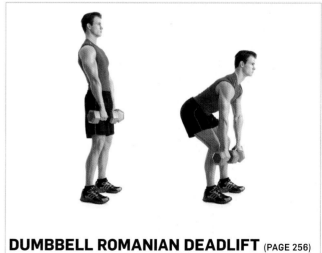

DUMBBELL ROMANIAN DEADLIFT (PAGE 256)
TOTAL REPS: 50 REST (SECONDS): 70

WORKOUT A

LOAD: SUPER-HEAVY

(2–3 RM)

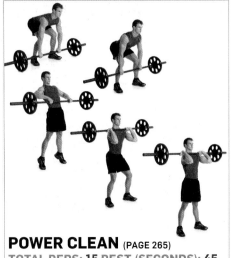

POWER CLEAN (PAGE 265)

TOTAL REPS: **15** REST (SECONDS): **45**

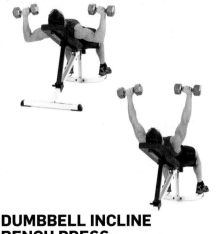

DUMBBELL INCLINE BENCH PRESS (PAGE 227)

TOTAL REPS: **15** REST (SECONDS): **45**

WORKOUT B

LOAD: MEDIUM

(10–12 RM)

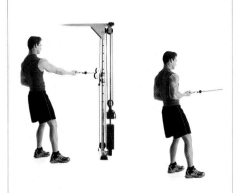

CABLE STANDING ONE-ARM MID-PULLEY ROW, PALM UP*

(PAGE 214)

TOTAL REPS: **40** REST (SECONDS): **75**

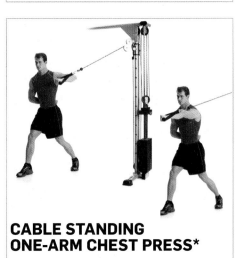

CABLE STANDING ONE-ARM CHEST PRESS*

(PAGE 230)

TOTAL REPS: **40** REST (SECONDS): **75**

WORKOUT C

LOAD: HEAVY

(4–6 RM)

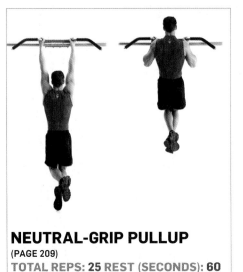

NEUTRAL-GRIP PULLUP

(PAGE 209)

TOTAL REPS: **25** REST (SECONDS): **60**

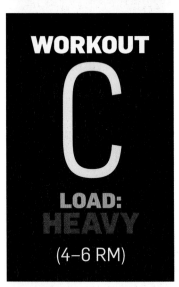

DIP (PAGE 223)

TOTAL REPS: **25** REST (SECONDS): **60**

Start with your weaker side first, then immediately do the same number of reps with your stronger limb. Rest after working both sides.

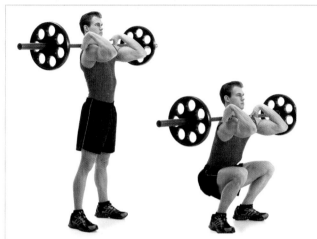

FRONT SQUAT (PAGE 242)
TOTAL REPS: **15** REST (SECONDS): **45**

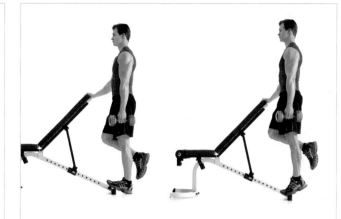

STANDING SINGLE-LEG CALF RAISE* (PAGE 280)
TOTAL REPS: **15** REST (SECONDS): **30**

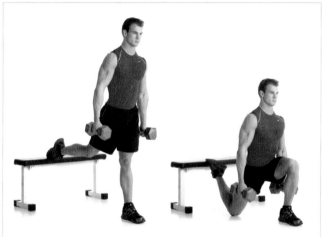

BULGARIAN SPLIT SQUAT* (PAGE 248)
TOTAL REPS: **40** REST (SECONDS): **75**

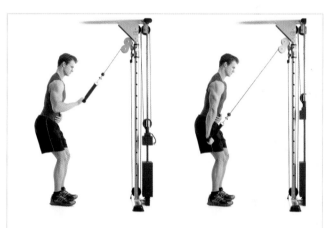

CABLE ONE-ARM TRICEPS PUSHDOWN* (PAGE 287)
TOTAL REPS: **40** REST (SECONDS): **60**

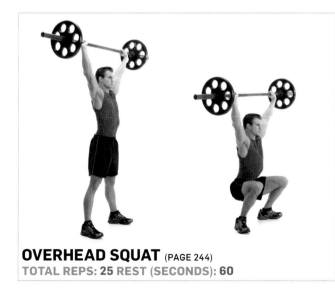

OVERHEAD SQUAT (PAGE 244)
TOTAL REPS: **25** REST (SECONDS): **60**

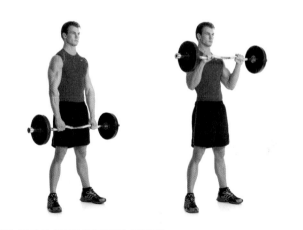

EZ-BAR REVERSE CURL (PAGE 284)
TOTAL REPS: **25** REST (SECONDS): **45**

WORKOUT A

LOAD: LIGHT
(20–22 RM)

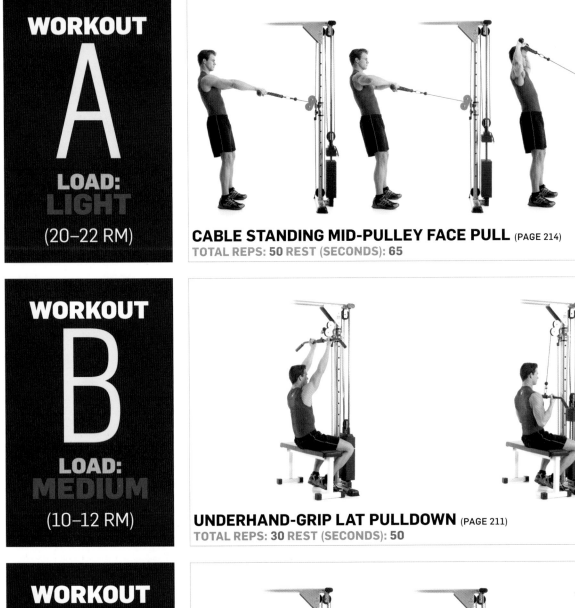

CABLE STANDING MID-PULLEY FACE PULL (PAGE 214)
TOTAL REPS: **50** REST (SECONDS): **65**

WORKOUT B

LOAD: MEDIUM
(10–12 RM)

UNDERHAND-GRIP LAT PULLDOWN (PAGE 211)
TOTAL REPS: **30** REST (SECONDS): **50**

WORKOUT C

LOAD: LIGHT
(20–22 RM)

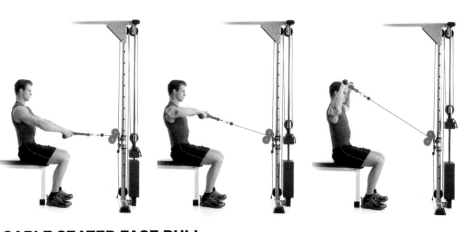

CABLE SEATED FACE PULL (PAGE 217)
TOTAL REPS: **50** REST (SECONDS): **65**

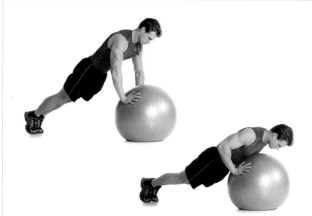

PUSHUP WITH HANDS ON SWISS BALL (PAGE 232)
TOTAL REPS: 50 REST (SECONDS): 65

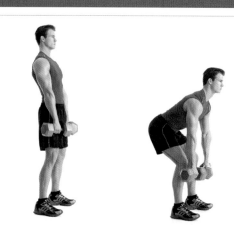

DUMBBELL ROMANIAN DEADLIFT (PAGE 256)
TOTAL REPS: 50 REST (SECONDS): 65

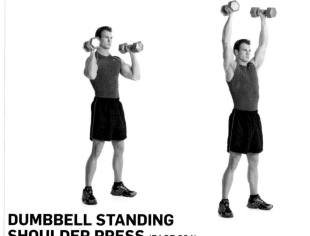

DUMBBELL STANDING SHOULDER PRESS (PAGE 234)
TOTAL REPS: 30 REST (SECONDS): 50

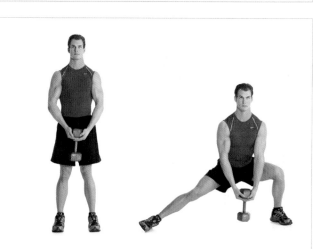

SIDE LUNGE (PAGE 249)
TOTAL REPS: 30* REST (SECONDS): 50

*With each leg

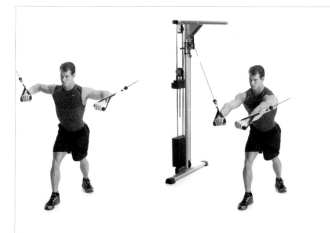

CABLE STANDING CHEST PRESS (PAGE 229)
TOTAL REPS: 50 REST (SECONDS): 65

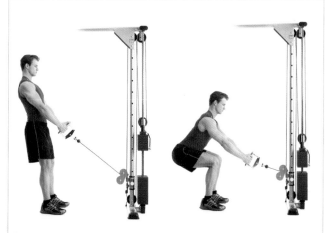

CABLE SQUAT (PAGE 246)
TOTAL REPS: 50 REST (SECONDS): 65

CHAPTER 11

GET EVEN BIGGER

I f you asked me which of my workout systems builds muscle the fastest, I'd say "high-frequency training" without any doubt or hesitation. But if you asked which is the toughest to do and trickiest to get right, I'd give you the same answer.

I talked about the surprising power of HFT in Chapter 5, but I didn't go into the fine print beyond acknowledging that few lifters have the time or desire to work out six or more times a week—three total-body workouts like those you just saw in Get Big (Chapter 10) and will see in Get Strong (Chapter 12), plus two, three, or four additional workouts.

In this chapter, I'll give you two sample HFT programs. The first one focuses on your biceps and triceps, and I wouldn't be surprised if it turned out to be the most talked about workout in this entire book. As I noted in Chapter 5, one of my clients added an inch to the circumference of his upper arms with my first version of this program. Another client added considerable size to his calves in just 6 weeks with HFT. I can't imagine anyone doing these workouts without achieving significant, measurable, and visible results.

The second is a total-body HFT program, and let me warn you, it's a monster. The arm workouts won't be easy for anyone reading this, but the total-body program is in another league. If training programs were animals, HFT for Arms would be a pit bull—a tough sumbitch by any standard—while Total-Body HFT is Sasquatch. The end results are as unique as a fingerprint. Some guys put on lots of muscle, while others add less but burn off so much fat that they *look* as if they've added more muscle. The one constant is that your body should look very different after you complete the total-body HFT program.

You can try my sample HFT programs or design your own, as long as you understand the rules.

GUIDELINES FOR HFT

Provide the proper nutritional support. You can't build measurable muscle mass on a calorie-restricted diet. That goes double for HFT programs. Without enough food, it just won't work. (You'll learn how to figure out what's "enough" in Chapter 23.)

Avoid the most fatiguing exercises. Compound exercises challenge hundreds of different muscles at once, which is why they build size and strength so quickly and dependably, and why I use them almost exclusively in my workout programs. They're also a lot more demanding than isolation exercises, breaking down more muscle tissue and requiring more time for recovery.

So if you're going to add extra workouts for specific muscle groups, you should build those workouts around single-joint exercises when possible. When your choice of useful isolation exercises is limited, opt for multi-joint exercises that hit the muscles you want to build without taking a big toll on the rest of your body.

For example, there aren't many good exercises for your chest and lats in which the action is restricted to your shoulder joints—you have flies for your chest and pullovers for your lats. Most of the other good exercises involve movement at your elbow joints. You have to include variations on pushups and rows to hit the muscles you're targeting. But as

you'll see later in this chapter, you can do versions of those exercises that limit the stress you put on the rest of your body.

Protect your joints. If you want to build your biceps and triceps—as you will in HFT for Arms—you'll end up putting a lot of stress on your elbow joints. In my experience, triceps extensions are more problematic than biceps curls. That's why HFT for Arms uses a mix of single-joint and compound exercises for your triceps.

Use different exercises throughout the week. This one is kind of cautionary, and kind of commonsense. Few of you will want to do the same exercises over and over again in the same week, so you'd probably mix up your exercises even if I didn't say you had to. Boredom is a powerful precursor to creativity.

There's also a physiological reason to use a variety of movement patterns: Your joints don't like doing the same exercises at the same angle multiple times a day.

Consider your biceps. The best, most direct way to work the muscle is to do a chinup or curl with an underhand grip. I mean, in the entire history of strength training, has it ever taken more than a week for an entry-level meathead to figure this out? And yet, because it's so simple and straightforward, there are relatively few working parts involved. It's easy to put more strain on the ligaments and tendons of your elbow joints than they can handle.

The easiest fix is to use a variety of hand positions—neutral (palms facing each other) and overhand (palms down) as well as the traditional palms-up grip.

You can also start the movement from a different angle. For example, if you lie on your back on an incline bench, with your arms hanging straight down from your shoulders, you begin a curl with your biceps in a stretched position. You don't want to do incline-bench curls too often, since you'd create at least as many problems as you're trying to solve. But if you use these variations judiciously, you end up with stronger, healthier joints.

Work one or two muscle groups at a time. You can't prioritize everything at once. So while HFT is a powerful way to build one or two lagging muscle groups, it probably wouldn't work if you tried to use it for more than two body parts at the same time. It could work for chest and back, but if you tried to build your chest, back, and arms with HFT, I think you'd quickly overtrain those muscles without achieving the gains possible by focusing on one or the other.

If you feel a need to prioritize more than one or two muscle groups at a time, you should probably give Total-Body HFT a shot. I wasn't kidding when I described it as a monster, but it is designed to build overall muscle mass faster than you could with my other programs.

Incorporate an unloading week. The Get Big and Get Strong programs in this book show you how to unload your muscles every fifth week. Rather than taking the entire week off from training, you scale back the weights you use and allow your body to catch up on its recovery.

I used the same system with HFT for Arms—three prescribed unloading workouts after the 4-week programs.

Total-Body HFT is unique in that you'll stop after 3 weeks of HFT workouts, and then do a single unloading workout the fourth week.

Resume HFT after the unloading week, if you want. If, after finishing the unloading workouts, you want to continue with HFT for those same muscles, you don't have to build back up to seven workouts a week. You can pick up where you left off, using the workouts from the third and fourth weeks. Or you can scale back to two or three HFT workouts—it's your choice.

Consider taking a weeklong break from training. After you finish the unloading workouts in Week 5, you'll probably benefit from taking an entire week off before resuming HFT or moving on to another training program. I won't say it's a requirement or a mandate, but it will certainly help your connective tissues recover more completely from the challenge of working the same muscles and joints seven times a week.

HFT FOR ARMS

I designed this program as a follow-up to Get Big. (You can also use it after Get Strong.)

Make sure you take a full week off following the conclusion of either program before you attempt HFT for Arms.

You'll do three total-body workouts a week, plus two, three, or four additional workouts that focus on your upper-arm muscles.

After 4 weeks, you'll do three unloading workouts. After that, you can resume HFT for Arms, as I said earlier, or take an entire week off from training.

The biggest rule is that you have to do these workouts exactly as I designed them, especially when it comes to the specified days and times of day. It doesn't matter whether Day 1 is Monday or another day of the week; you just have to arrange your schedule in 7-day blocks from that starting point. On days when you do two workouts, make sure you put at least 6 hours in between the day's a.m. and p.m. training sessions. That gives you enough time to restore enough of the energy supplies in your muscles to get you through the second workout.

However, you *don't* have to use the exact same exercises I have on these charts. You've already done the 3-week Get Ready program, plus 16 weeks of Get Big. If you're getting tired of my exercise choices, you should know my system well enough to substitute some of your favorites. You can replace barbell exercises with dumbbells, free weights with cables, cable exercises with free weights. . . . Just follow the *program* the way I've written it, using your judgment to make one-for-one substitutions when you want or need to.

DAY 1

WORKOUT A1 ^{AM}

LOAD: **HEAVY** (4–6 RM)

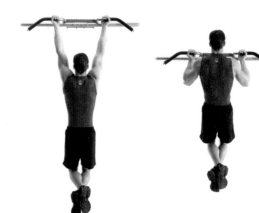

CHINUP (PAGE 207)
TOTAL REPS: 20 REST BETWEEN SETS (SECONDS): 60

WORKOUT B1 ^{PM}

LOAD: **HEAVY** (4–6 RM)

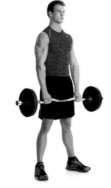 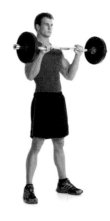

EZ-BAR REVERSE CURL (PAGE 284)
TOTAL REPS: 20 REST (SECONDS): 45

DAY 2 = OFF

DAY 3

WORKOUT C1 ^{AM}

LOAD: **MEDIUM** (10–12 RM)

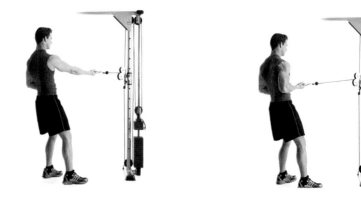

CABLE STANDING ONE-ARM MID-PULLEY ROW, PALM UP* (PAGE 214)
TOTAL REPS: 35 REST (SECONDS): 75

Start with your weaker side first, then immediately do the same number of reps with your stronger limb. Rest after working both sides.

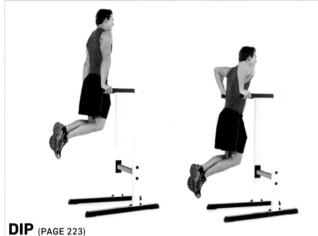

DIP (PAGE 223)
TOTAL REPS: **20** REST BETWEEN SETS (SECONDS): **60**

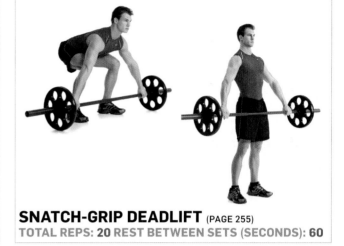

SNATCH-GRIP DEADLIFT (PAGE 255)
TOTAL REPS: **20** REST BETWEEN SETS (SECONDS): **60**

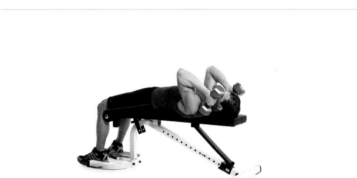

DUMBBELL LYING TRICEPS EXTENSION (PAGE 286)
TOTAL REPS: **20** REST (SECONDS): **45**

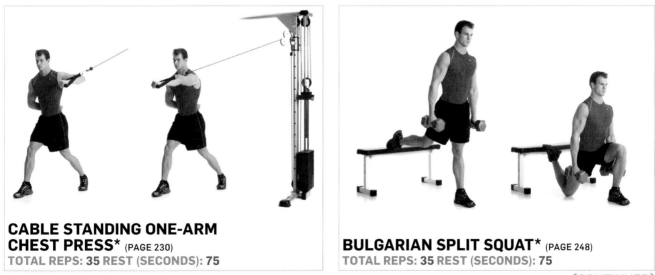

**CABLE STANDING ONE-ARM
CHEST PRESS*** (PAGE 230)
TOTAL REPS: **35** REST (SECONDS): **75**

BULGARIAN SPLIT SQUAT* (PAGE 248)
TOTAL REPS: **35** REST (SECONDS): **75**

(CONTINUED)

DAY 3

WORKOUT

D1 PM

LOAD:
MEDIUM
(10–12 RM)

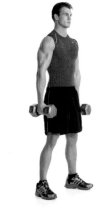

HAMMER CURL (PAGE 284)
TOTAL REPS: 30 REST (SECONDS): 60

DAY 4 = OFF

DAY 5

WORKOUT

E1 AM OR PM

LOAD:
MEDIUM
[10-12 RM]

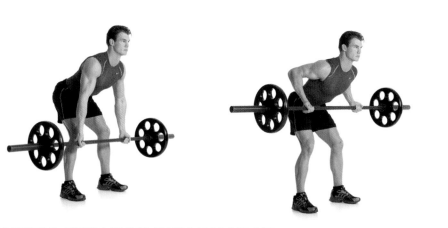

BARBELL BENT-OVER ROW, PALMS UP (PAGE 218)
TOTAL REPS: 20 REST (SECONDS): 60

DAYS 6 AND 7 = OFF

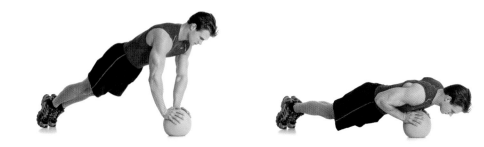

PUSHUP WITH HANDS ON MEDICINE BALL (PAGE 233)
TOTAL REPS: **30** REST (SECONDS): **60**

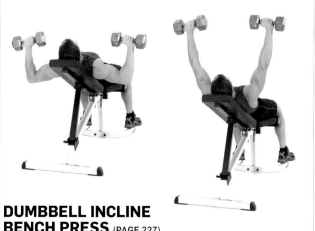

**DUMBBELL INCLINE
BENCH PRESS** (PAGE 227)
TOTAL REPS: **20** REST (SECONDS): **60**

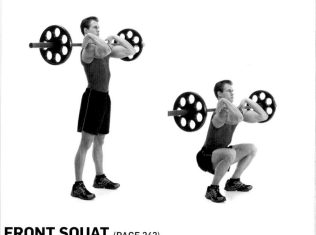

FRONT SQUAT (PAGE 242)
TOTAL REPS: **20** REST (SECONDS): **60**

DAY 1

WORKOUT A2 AM
LOAD: HEAVY
(4–6 RM)

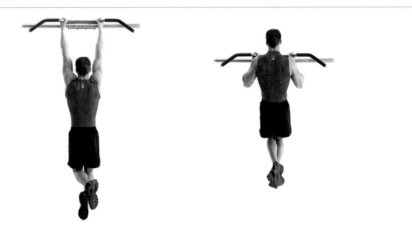

NEUTRAL-GRIP PULLUP (PAGE 209)
TOTAL REPS: 20 REST (SECONDS): 60

WORKOUT B2 PM
LOAD: HEAVY
(4–6 RM)

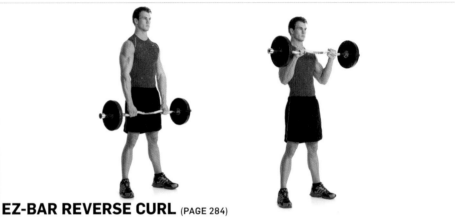

EZ-BAR REVERSE CURL (PAGE 284)
TOTAL REPS: 20 REST (SECONDS): 45

DAY 2 = OFF

DAY 3

WORKOUT C2 AM
LOAD: MEDIUM
(10–12 RM)

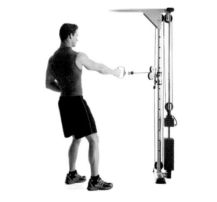
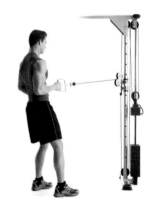

CABLE STANDING ONE-ARM MID-PULLEY ROW, ELBOW IN*
(PAGE 213)
TOTAL REPS: 35 REST (SECONDS): 75

Start with your weaker side first, then immediately do the same number of reps with your stronger limb. Rest after working both sides.

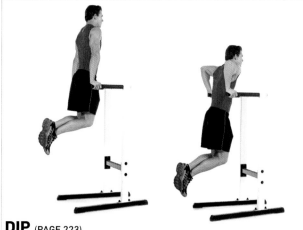

DIP (PAGE 223)
TOTAL REPS: **20** REST (SECONDS): **60**

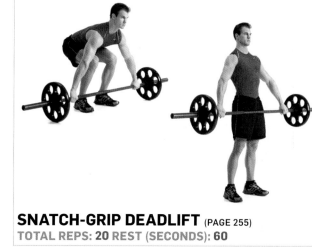

SNATCH-GRIP DEADLIFT (PAGE 255)
TOTAL REPS: **20** REST (SECONDS): **60**

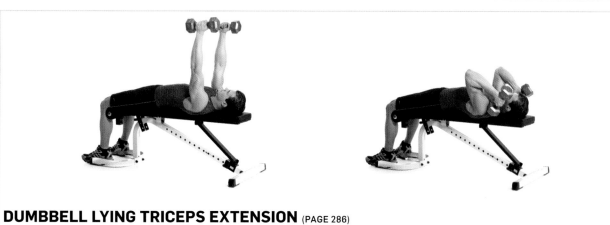

DUMBBELL LYING TRICEPS EXTENSION (PAGE 286)
TOTAL REPS: **20** REST (SECONDS): **45**

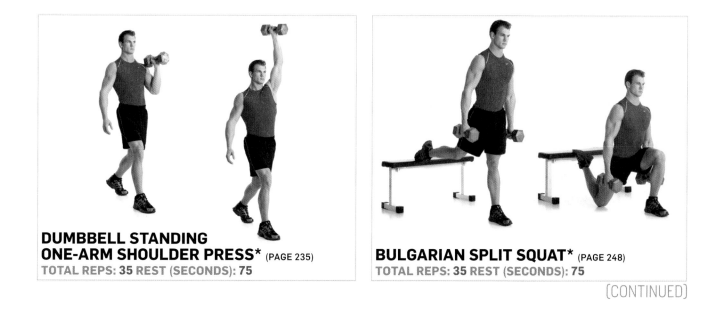

**DUMBBELL STANDING
ONE-ARM SHOULDER PRESS*** (PAGE 235)
TOTAL REPS: **35** REST (SECONDS): **75**

BULGARIAN SPLIT SQUAT* (PAGE 248)
TOTAL REPS: **35** REST (SECONDS): **75**

(CONTINUED)

DAY 3, CONT.

WORKOUT D2 PM
LOAD: MEDIUM
(10–12 RM)

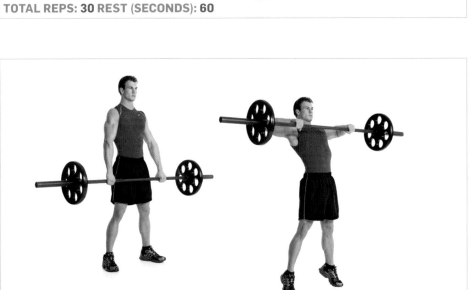

HAMMER CURL (PAGE 284)
TOTAL REPS: **30** REST (SECONDS): **60**

DAY 4 = OFF

DAY 5

WORKOUT E2 AM
LOAD: HEAVY
(4–6 RM)

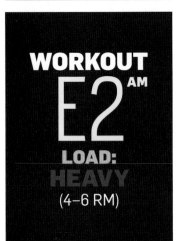

HIGH PULL (PAGE 263)
TOTAL REPS: **20** REST (SECONDS): **60**

WORKOUT F2 PM
LOAD: HEAVY
(4–6 RM)

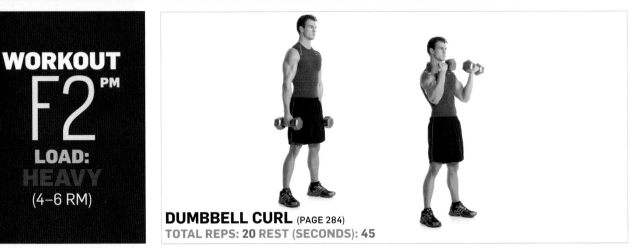

DUMBBELL CURL (PAGE 284)
TOTAL REPS: **20** REST (SECONDS): **45**

DAYS 6 AND 7 = OFF

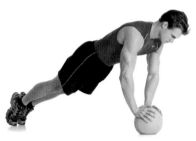

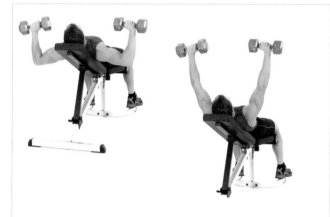

PUSHUP WITH HANDS ON MEDICINE BALL (PAGE 233)
TOTAL REPS: **30** REST (SECONDS): **60**

DUMBBELL INCLINE BENCH PRESS
(PAGE 227)
TOTAL REPS: **20** REST (SECONDS): **60**

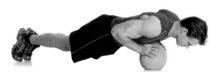

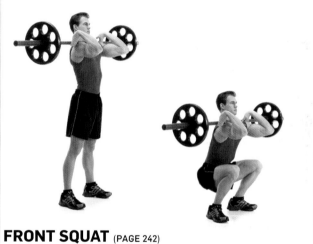

FRONT SQUAT (PAGE 242)
TOTAL REPS: **20** REST (SECONDS): **60**

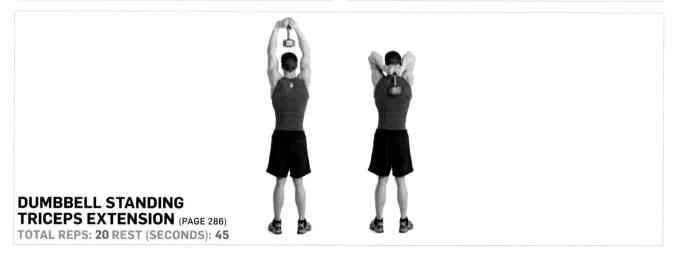

**DUMBBELL STANDING
TRICEPS EXTENSION** (PAGE 286)
TOTAL REPS: **20** REST (SECONDS): **45**

DAY 1

WORKOUT A3 AM

LOAD: HEAVY

(4–6 RM)

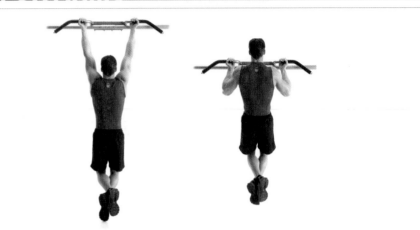

CHINUP (PAGE 207)
TOTAL REPS: 20 REST (SECONDS): 60

WORKOUT B3 PM

LOAD: MEDIUM

(10–12 RM)

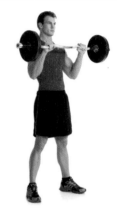

EZ-BAR REVERSE CURL (PAGE 284)
TOTAL REPS: 30 REST (SECONDS): 60

DAY 2 = OFF

DAY 3

WORKOUT C3 AM

LOAD: MEDIUM

(10–12 RM)

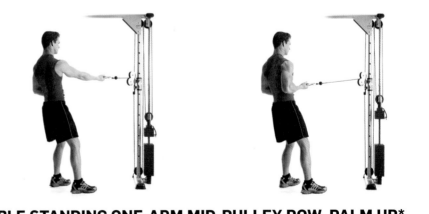

CABLE STANDING ONE-ARM MID-PULLEY ROW, PALM UP*
(PAGE 214)
TOTAL REPS: 35 REST (SECONDS): 75

Start with your weaker side first, then immediately do the same number of reps with your stronger limb. Rest after working both sides.

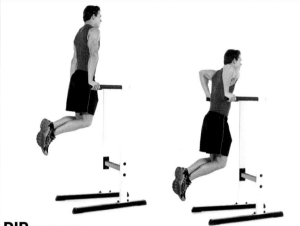

DIP (PAGE 223)
TOTAL REPS: 20 REST (SECONDS): 60

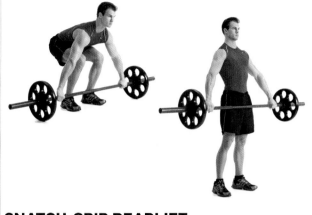

SNATCH-GRIP DEADLIFT (PAGE 255)
TOTAL REPS: 20 REST (SECONDS): 60

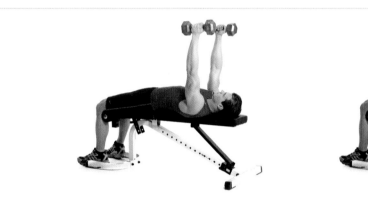

DUMBBELL LYING TRICEPS EXTENSION (PAGE 286)
TOTAL REPS: 30 REST (SECONDS): 60

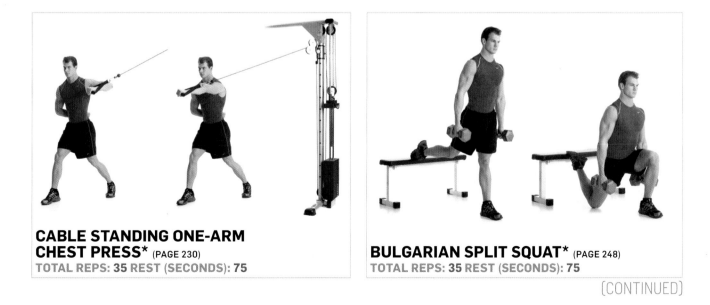

CABLE STANDING ONE-ARM CHEST PRESS* (PAGE 230)
TOTAL REPS: 35 REST (SECONDS): 75

BULGARIAN SPLIT SQUAT* (PAGE 248)
TOTAL REPS: 35 REST (SECONDS): 75

(CONTINUED)

DAY 3, CONT.

WORKOUT D3 PM
LOAD: HEAVY
(4–6 RM)

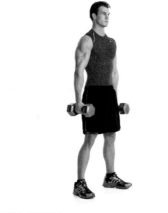

HAMMER CURL (PAGE 284)
TOTAL REPS: 20 REST (SECONDS): 45

DAY 4 = OFF

DAY 5

WORKOUT E3 AM
LOAD: HEAVY
(4–6 RM)

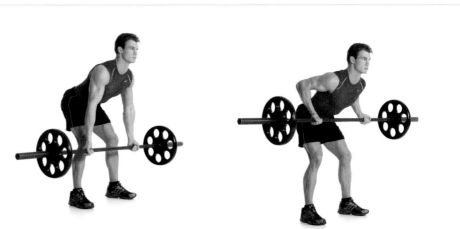

BARBELL BENT-OVER ROW, PALMS UP (PAGE 218)
TOTAL REPS: 20 REST (SECONDS): 60

WORKOUT F3 PM
LOAD: MEDIUM
(10–12 RM)

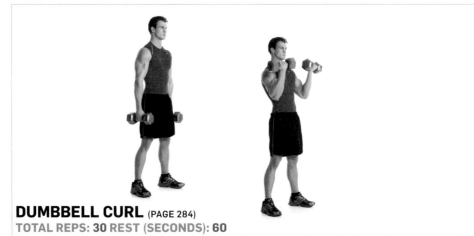

DUMBBELL CURL (PAGE 284)
TOTAL REPS: 30 REST (SECONDS): 60

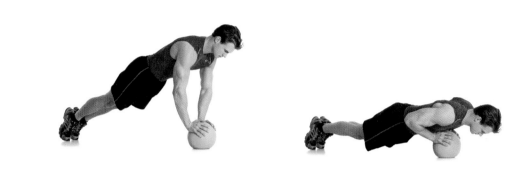

PUSHUP WITH HANDS ON MEDICINE BALL (PAGE 233)
TOTAL REPS: 20 REST (SECONDS): 45

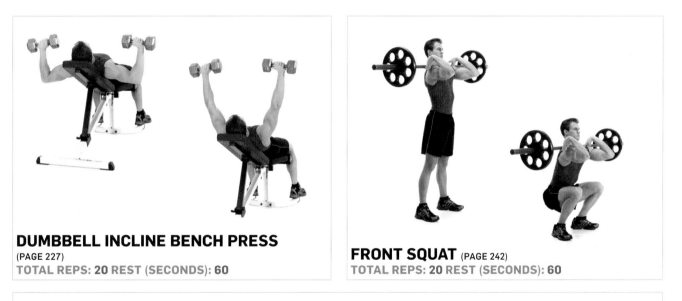

DUMBBELL INCLINE BENCH PRESS
(PAGE 227)
TOTAL REPS: 20 REST (SECONDS): 60

FRONT SQUAT (PAGE 242)
TOTAL REPS: 20 REST (SECONDS): 60

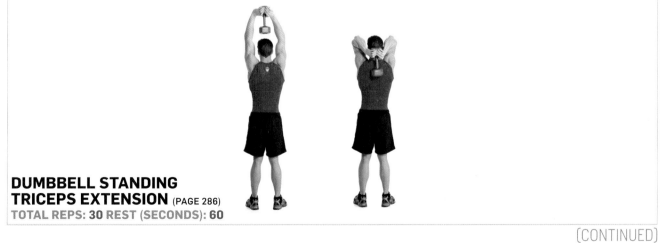

DUMBBELL STANDING
TRICEPS EXTENSION (PAGE 286)
TOTAL REPS: 30 REST (SECONDS): 60

(CONTINUED)

DAY 6

WORKOUT G3 AM OR PM

LOAD: HEAVY
(4–6 RM)

DAY 7 = OFF

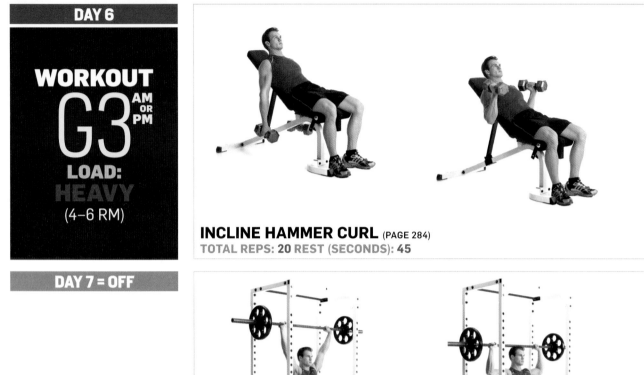

INCLINE HAMMER CURL (PAGE 284)
TOTAL REPS: **20** REST (SECONDS): **45**

BARBELL SEATED PARTIAL SHOULDER PRESS (PAGE 236)
TOTAL REPS: **20** REST (SECONDS): **45**

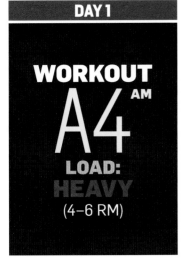

DAY 1

WORKOUT

A4 AM

LOAD:
HEAVY
(4–6 RM)

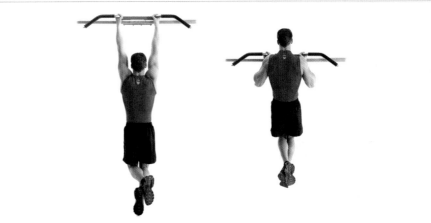

NEUTRAL-GRIP PULLUP (PAGE 209)
TOTAL REPS: 20 REST (SECONDS): 60

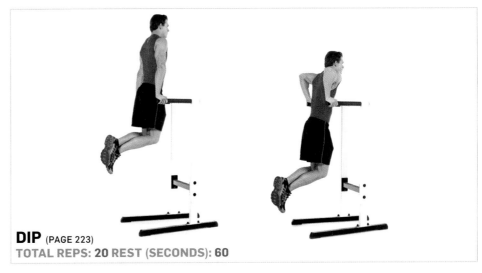

DIP (PAGE 223)
TOTAL REPS: 20 REST (SECONDS): 60

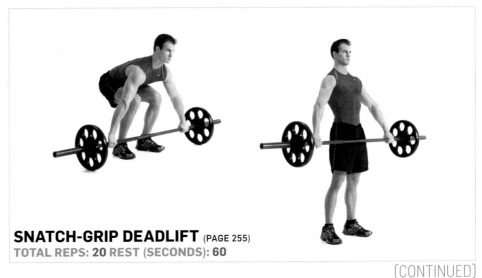

SNATCH-GRIP DEADLIFT (PAGE 255)
TOTAL REPS: 20 REST (SECONDS): 60

(CONTINUED)

DAY 1, CONT.

WORKOUT B4 PM

LOAD: MEDIUM
(10–12 RM)

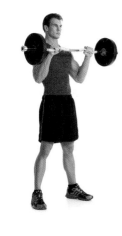
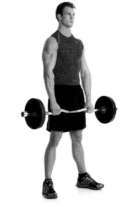

EZ-BAR REVERSE CURL (PAGE 284)
TOTAL REPS: 30 REST (SECONDS): 60

DAY 2 = OFF

DAY 3

WORKOUT C4 AM

LOAD: MEDIUM
(10–12 RM)

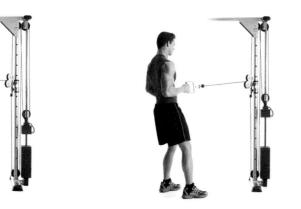

CABLE STANDING ONE-ARM MID-PULLEY ROW, ELBOW IN*
(PAGE 213)
TOTAL REPS: 30 REST (SECONDS): 75

WORKOUT D4 PM

LOAD: HEAVY
(4–6 RM)

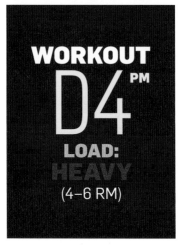
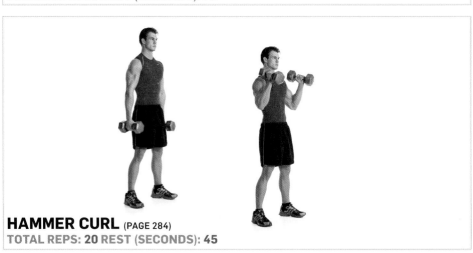

HAMMER CURL (PAGE 284)
TOTAL REPS: 20 REST (SECONDS): 45

Start with your weaker side first, then immediately do the same number of reps with your stronger limb. Rest after working both sides.

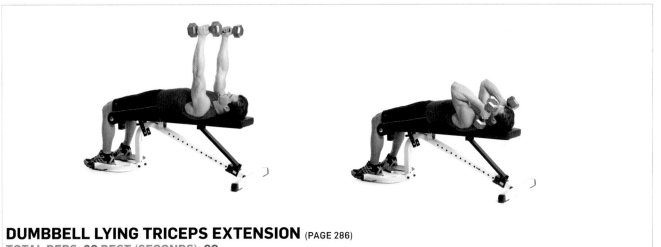

DUMBBELL LYING TRICEPS EXTENSION (PAGE 286)
TOTAL REPS: **30** REST (SECONDS): **60**

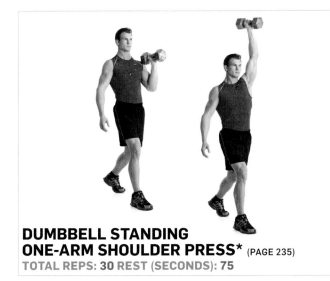

**DUMBBELL STANDING
ONE-ARM SHOULDER PRESS*** (PAGE 235)
TOTAL REPS: **30** REST (SECONDS): **75**

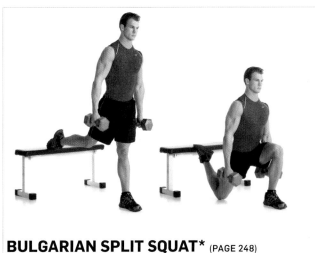

BULGARIAN SPLIT SQUAT* (PAGE 248)
TOTAL REPS: **30** REST (SECONDS): **75**

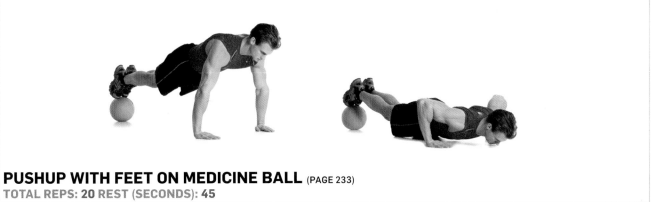

PUSHUP WITH FEET ON MEDICINE BALL (PAGE 233)
TOTAL REPS: **20** REST (SECONDS): **45**

(CONTINUED)

DAY 4 = OFF

DAY 5

WORKOUT E4

LOAD: HEAVY

(4–6 RM)

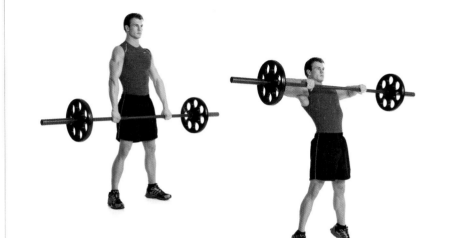

HIGH PULL (PAGE 263)
TOTAL REPS: 20 REST (SECONDS): 60

WORKOUT F4

LOAD: MEDIUM

(10–12 RM)

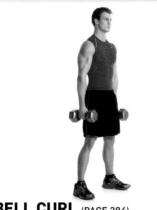
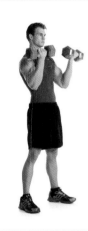

DUMBBELL CURL (PAGE 284)
TOTAL REPS: 30 REST (SECONDS): 60

DAY 6

WORKOUT G4

LOAD: HEAVY

(4–6 RM)

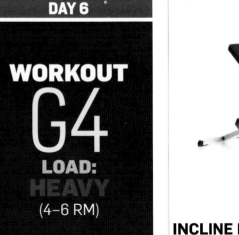
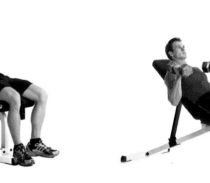

INCLINE HAMMER CURL (PAGE 284)
TOTAL REPS: 20 REST (SECONDS): 45

DAY 7 = OFF

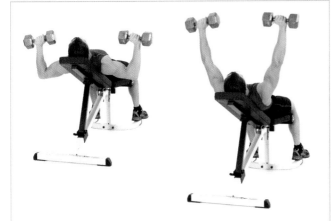

DUMBBELL INCLINE BENCH PRESS
(PAGE 227)
TOTAL REPS: 20 REST (SECONDS): 60

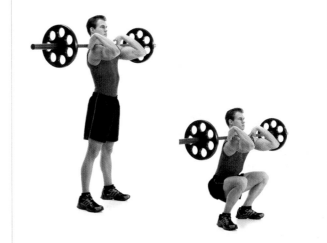

FRONT SQUAT (PAGE 242)
TOTAL REPS: 20 REST (SECONDS): 60

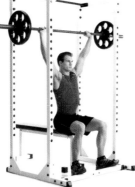

DUMBBELL STANDING
TRICEPS EXTENSION (PAGE 286)
TOTAL REPS: 30 REST (SECONDS): 60

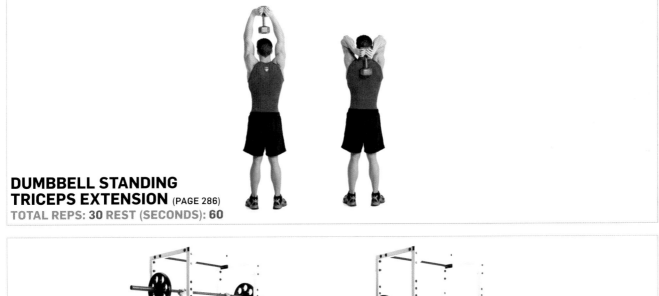

BARBELL SEATED PARTIAL SHOULDER PRESS (PAGE 236)
TOTAL REPS: 20 REST (SECONDS): 45

DAY 1

WORKOUT A5

LOAD: LIGHT
(20–22 RM)

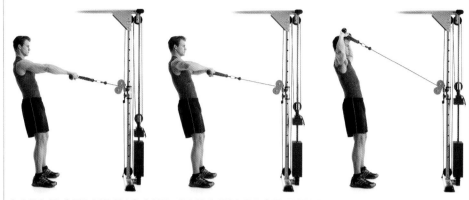

CABLE STANDING MID-PULLEY FACE PULL (PAGE 214)
TOTAL REPS: 50 REST (SECONDS): 75

DAY 2 = OFF

DAY 3

WORKOUT B5

LOAD: MEDIUM
(10–12 RM)

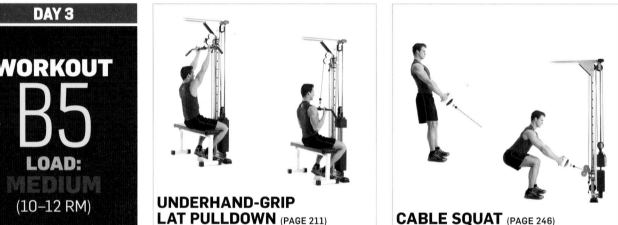

UNDERHAND-GRIP LAT PULLDOWN (PAGE 211)
TOTAL REPS: 30 REST (SECONDS): 60

CABLE SQUAT (PAGE 246)
TOTAL REPS: 30 REST (SECONDS): 60

DAY 4 = OFF

DAY 5

WORKOUT C5

LOAD: MEDIUM
(10–12 RM)

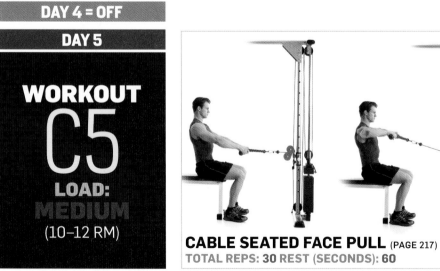

CABLE SEATED FACE PULL (PAGE 217)
TOTAL REPS: 30 REST (SECONDS): 60

DAYS 6 AND 7 = OFF

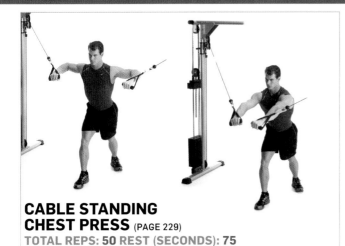

CABLE STANDING CHEST PRESS (PAGE 229)
TOTAL REPS: 50 REST (SECONDS): 75

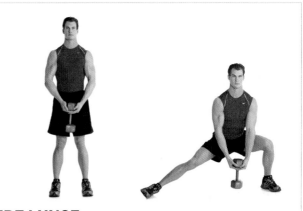

DUMBBELL ROMANIAN DEADLIFT
(PAGE 256)
TOTAL REPS: 50 REST (SECONDS): 75

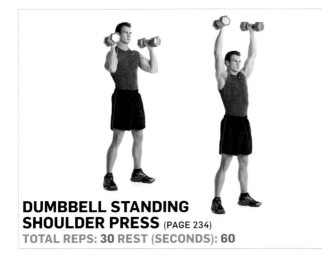

DUMBBELL STANDING SHOULDER PRESS (PAGE 234)
TOTAL REPS: 30 REST (SECONDS): 60

SIDE LUNGE (PAGE 249)
TOTAL REPS: 30* REST (SECONDS): 60

*With each leg

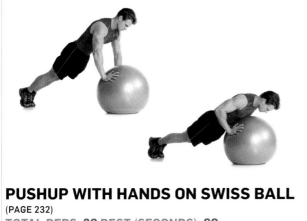

PUSHUP WITH HANDS ON SWISS BALL
(PAGE 232)
TOTAL REPS: 30 REST (SECONDS): 60

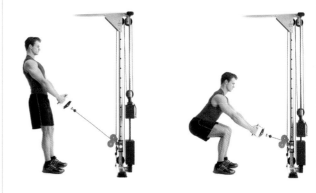

CABLE SQUAT (PAGE 246)
TOTAL REPS: 30 REST (SECONDS): 60

HFT FOR OTHER MUSCLE GROUPS

I don't recommend going directly from one HFT program to another, but I also have no plans to travel out to wherever you live to prevent you from doing it. It's my book, but it's your life and your physique.

If you decide to do another HFT program at some point, I recommend using the HFT for Arms template. You can keep it really simple by doing the three total-body workouts as written, and plugging in your own exercises for whatever muscle groups you want to emphasize. You'll do two HFT workouts the first week, three the second, and four per week in the third and fourth weeks. Do three unloading workouts the fifth week—the ones I created or your own— and consider taking the sixth week off before moving on to your next training program.

Some possibilities for HFT emphasis, and exercises you can use:

FOREARMS

>> Barbell wrist curl (page 288)

>> Dumbbell wrist curl (page 289)

>> EZ-bar reverse wrist curl (page 289)

>> Dumbbell reverse wrist curl (page 289)

DELTOIDS

>> Lateral raise (page 292)

>> Lateral raise with thumbs up (page 293)

>> Lateral raise with pinkies up (page 293)

>> Lean-away lateral raise (page 293)

>> L-raise (page 294)

CHEST

>> Dumbbell decline fly (page 290)

>> Pushup with clap (page 233)

>> Pushup with hands on Swiss ball (page 232)

>> Pushup with wide hand position, feet elevated (page 232)

LATS

>> Dumbbell decline pullover (page 291)

>> Dumbbell decline one-arm pullover (page 291)

>> Dumbbell one-arm bent-over row (page 219)

>> Dumbbell one-arm bent-over row with palm up (page 219)

>> Barbell rollout (page 272)

GLUTES/HAMSTRINGS

>> Cable hip/knee extension (page 295)

>> Single-leg bridge (page 296)

>> Hip abduction with band (page 297)

>> Dumbbell single-leg deadlift (page 257)

>> Swiss-ball leg curl (page 298)

>> Dumbbell Romanian deadlift (page 256)

>> Single-leg good morning (page 259)

QUADRICEPS

>> Single-leg squat (page 251)

>> High stepup (page 299)

>> Reverse lunge (page 250)

>> Stepup on decline bench (page 299)

CALVES

>> Standing single-leg calf raise (page 280)

>> Seated single-leg calf raise (page 280)

>> Single-leg donkey calf raise (page 281)

>> Single-leg hop (page 282)

When you pair up two muscle groups (chest and lats; hamstrings and quadriceps; biceps and triceps), do one exercise for each in your HFT workouts. Otherwise, do two exercises for the targeted muscle or muscle group.

TOTAL-BODY HFT

I already sounded the alarms about this program at the beginning of the chapter, so I won't repeat them here. (Except to remind you of the importance of proper nutrition; food is your friend.) Some key differences between this program and HFT for individual muscle groups:

>> You'll perform six total-body workouts each week for 3 weeks—two a day, followed by at least 1 full day with no workouts.

>> You'll do a single unloading workout the fourth week (as in, one workout in a 7-day period).

>> Don't even think about embellishing these programs with extra exercises for your favorite muscles. Stick with the simplest total-body workouts: upper-body pull, upper-body push, squat or deadlift. Don't do anything else—no curls, no calf raises, no calisthenics, no tantric yoga.

>> You can't use this system with intervals, steady-state cardio, or any type of sport-specific training and live to tell about it.

>> Naps are damned near mandatory. Massages will help, too, if you can find a willing masseuse in your price range.

>> If you want to repeat Total-Body HFT after you've finished the 4-week program, wait at least 2 months. Three times a year (March, August, and November, for example) is the absolute limit.

DAY 1

WORKOUT A AM

LOAD: HEAVY
(4–6 RM)

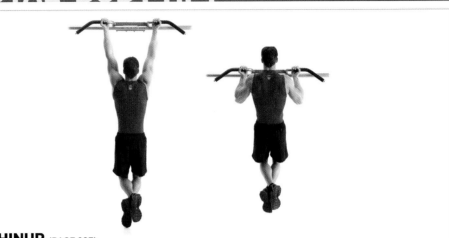

CHINUP (PAGE 207)
TOTAL REPS: 20 REST (SECONDS): 60

WORKOUT B PM

LOAD: MEDIUM
(10–12 RM)

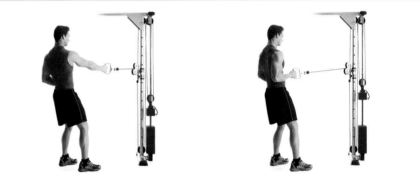

CABLE STANDING ONE-ARM MID-PULLEY ROW, ELBOW IN*
(PAGE 213)
TOTAL REPS: 30 REST (SECONDS): 75

DAY 2 = OFF

DAY 3

WORKOUT C AM

LOAD: HEAVY
(4–6 RM)

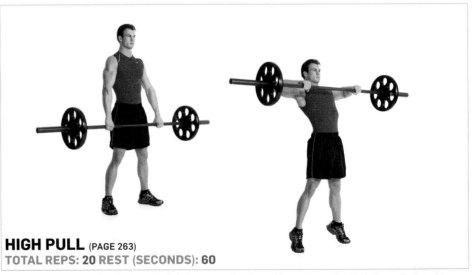

HIGH PULL (PAGE 263)
TOTAL REPS: 20 REST (SECONDS): 60

Start with your weaker side first, then immediately do the same number of reps with your stronger limb. Rest after working both sides.

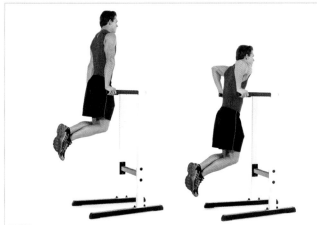

DIP (PAGE 223)
TOTAL REPS: **20** REST (SECONDS): **60**

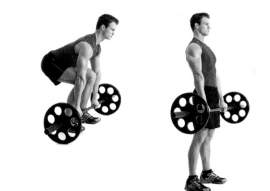

DEADLIFT (PAGE 254)
TOTAL REPS: **20** REST (SECONDS): **60**

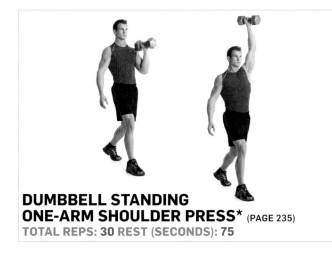

**DUMBBELL STANDING
ONE-ARM SHOULDER PRESS*** (PAGE 235)
TOTAL REPS: **30** REST (SECONDS): **75**

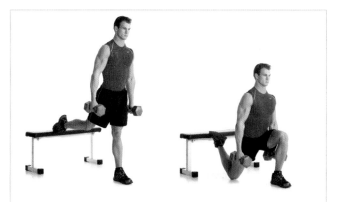

BULGARIAN SPLIT SQUAT* (PAGE 248)
TOTAL REPS: **30** REST (SECONDS): **75**

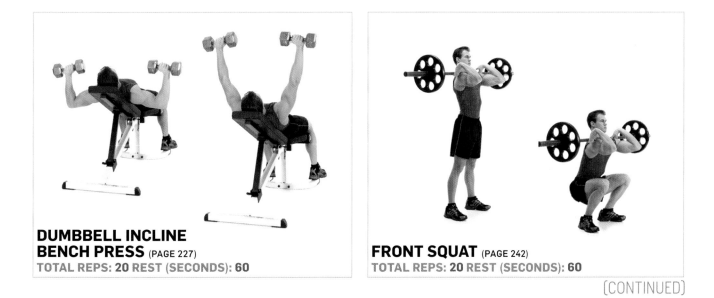

**DUMBBELL INCLINE
BENCH PRESS** (PAGE 227)
TOTAL REPS: **20** REST (SECONDS): **60**

FRONT SQUAT (PAGE 242)
TOTAL REPS: **20** REST (SECONDS): **60**

(CONTINUED)

DAY 3, CONT.

WORKOUT D PM
LOAD: MEDIUM
(10–12 RM)

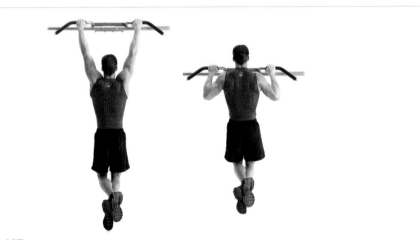

ONE-ARM LAT PULLDOWN* (PAGE 211)
TOTAL REPS: **30** REST (SECONDS): **75**

DAY 4 = OFF

DAY 5

WORKOUT E AM
LOAD: HEAVY
(4–6 RM)

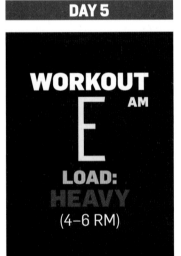

PULLUP (PAGE 207)
TOTAL REPS: **20** REST (SECONDS): **60**

WORKOUT F PM
LOAD: MEDIUM
(10–12 RM)

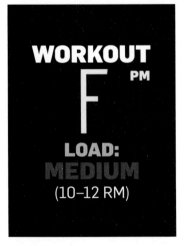

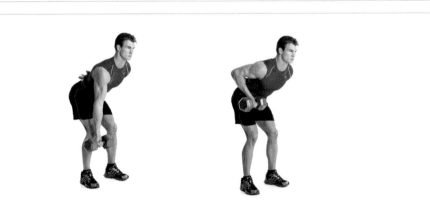

DUMBBELL ONE-ARM BENT-OVER ROW, PALM UP* (PAGE 219)
TOTAL REPS: **30** REST (SECONDS): **75**

*Start with your weaker side first, then immediately do the same number of reps with your stronger limb. Rest after working both sides.

DAYS 6 AND 7 = OFF

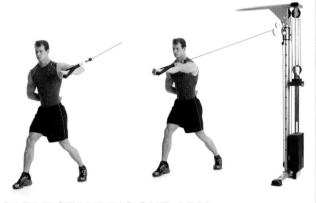

CABLE STANDING ONE-ARM CHEST PRESS* (PAGE 230)
TOTAL REPS: 30 REST (SECONDS): 75

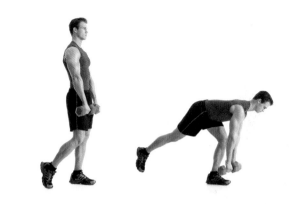

DUMBBELL SINGLE-LEG DEADLIFT* (PAGE 257)
TOTAL REPS: 30 REST (SECONDS): 75

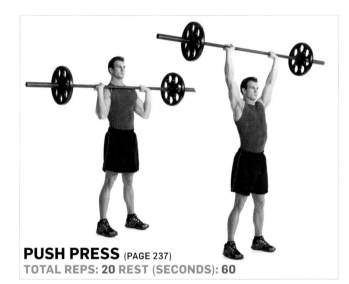

PUSH PRESS (PAGE 237)
TOTAL REPS: 20 REST (SECONDS): 60

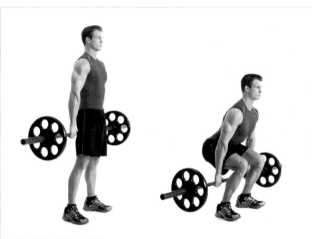

HACK SQUAT (PAGE 245)
TOTAL REPS: 20 REST (SECONDS): 60

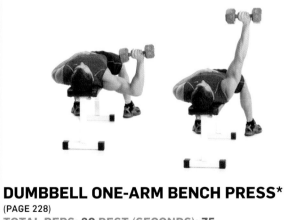

DUMBBELL ONE-ARM BENCH PRESS* (PAGE 228)
TOTAL REPS: 30 REST (SECONDS): 75

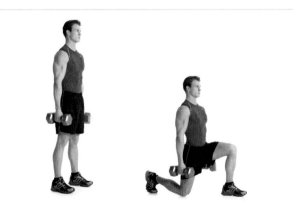

REVERSE LUNGE* (PAGE 250)
TOTAL REPS: 30 REST (SECONDS): 75

(CONTINUED)

147

WORKOUT
A
LOAD:
LIGHT
(20–22 RM)

PERFORM THIS WORKOUT ONCE, AT LEAST 4 DAYS AFTER YOU COMPLETE WORKOUT F FOR THE FINAL TIME.

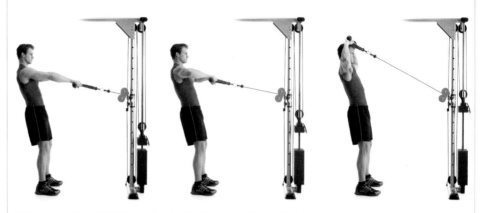

CABLE STANDING MID-PULLEY FACE PULL (PAGE 214)
TOTAL REPS: 50 REST (SECONDS): 75

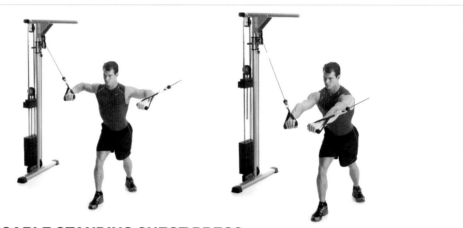

CABLE STANDING CHEST PRESS (PAGE 229)
TOTAL REPS: 50 REST (SECONDS): 75

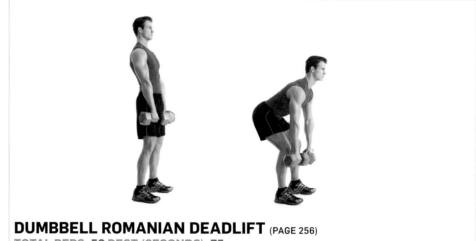

DUMBBELL ROMANIAN DEADLIFT (PAGE 256)
TOTAL REPS: 50 REST (SECONDS): 75

CHAPTER 12

GET STRONG

You could say that my entire career is based on helping people achieve the results they want by making them stronger. One of my first training gigs was at a YMCA in a small town in southern Illinois. I got middle-aged men and women to do deadlifts, squats, presses, and rows with low reps and relatively heavy weights. To everyone's surprise, they built muscle and lost fat by doing what most trainers at the time considered the worst possible system for reaching those goals.

I've come a long way since then, but I've never lost sight of what first made me different from typical trainers in typical health clubs. Whether I'm working with a young bodybuilder who needs to put on pounds of solid muscle, training a mixed-martial-arts fighter to kick more ass without outgrowing his current weight class, or helping a successful businessman lose 6 inches of midlife spread, I always look to increase the trainee's maximal strength. That is, I work with my client to make his nerves, muscles, and joints more adept at handling heavy loads.

And it always works.

NERVES OF STEEL

On the one hand, this is simple stuff: To get bigger, you must get stronger. To get stronger, you must lift progressively heavier weights. To lift progressively heavier weights. . . . well, if you've ever tried it for a sustained period of time—months and years—you know it's not so simple.

Strength training—working out with the goal of increasing your maximal strength—focuses primarily on your nerves. Heavy lifts enhance your ability to recruit your largest motor units. The more motor units you use, the more muscle fibers you stimulate. Since your body always keeps a reserve of motor units for emergency situations, you need to work with near-maximal weights to tap into that reserve. If you don't, you pass up the chance to develop those fibers, along with all the others that you must recruit just to get a chance at the elusive ones.

You can't just jump into lifting max loads and expect good results, which is why you did the 3-week break-in program and 16 weeks of hypertrophy workouts before you got here. By now, you've increased your neural drive by lifting submaximal loads as fast as possible, and you've increased your strength by working with heavy loads, using low-rep sets.

You've also been systematically breaking down and building up muscle tissue, and inducing relatively high levels of muscular fatigue. Now you're going to change your methods. You'll do fewer repetitions per exercise, since you don't want to break down as much muscle tissue as you did during the hypertrophy workouts. And you'll be working with superheavy weights much of the time, which is enormously taxing to your nervous system. Excessive muscle-tissue damage would only slow down your recovery and compromise your success.

"Success" in this 16-week program is defined by increases in neural drive and efficiency, which you'll measure by increases in the amount of weight you can lift. If you're an average gym rat, someone who's never done a serious strength-focused program before, I think it's reasonable to expect to see your strength increase 2 percent a week on the lifts included in my workouts. You'll make faster gains early in the program, with slower gains later, as your body adapts. No two lifters will be able to claim the exact same strength increases after 16 weeks, but everyone should make quantifiable leaps forward in the core lifts.

When you do Get Big and Get Strong back to back, I'd expect you to increase your one-rep max in your core lifts as much as 30 percent. So, if your best-ever squat was 225 before attempting Get Big and Get Strong, you could very well be able to squat more than 300 by the time you finish this program. The gains will come slower for more advanced lifters who are already near the limits of their genetic potential, but even they should make genuine gains in pure strength.

And every lifter, no matter what his level of experience, should also come away from this program with bigger muscles. If you're one of those guys who looks fit when viewed from the front or back but becomes nearly invisible when viewed from the side, this program should fix that: After 16 weeks, you might suggest I change the name of the program from Get Strong to Look Strong.

And, believe it or not, some lifters will also get leaner during this program, with no changes in their diets. I could try to explain why, but it would take a lot of words and would leave us exactly where I started this chapter: It always pays to increase strength, even if the payoff can be dramatically different from one lifter to the next.

THIS IS NOT YOUR FATHER'S STRENGTH-BUILDING WORKOUT

Whenever I talk about strength with people who, for whatever reason, have never focused on it, I get this question: "If strength is so important, how come powerlifters have less muscle and more fat than bodybuilders?" The shorter version of the question: "Why are powerlifters fat?"

I can answer several ways. I can talk about diet (some powerlifters eat what they want when they want, with no restraint), total exercise volume (generally, a competitive powerlifter will do a fraction of the total sets and reps used by a bodybuilder), and/or

workout technique (the powerlifter will take more time between sets and rarely accumulate fatigue for fatigue's sake).

But none of that matters, since this isn't a powerlifting program. If it were, the workouts would focus on improving your performance in the squat, bench press, and deadlift; improvements in functional, total-body strength would be a by-product. I place functional strength first. Boosting your powerlifts is a secondary benefit.

This is what I mean when I talk about functional strength: If you're a fighter, these workouts will help you throw around your opponent. If you're a Strongman competitor, these workouts will help you lift, carry, hold, or flip bigger things than you can handle now. If you're a football player, these workouts will help you overcome and control the guy in front of you.

And if you're primarily a gym rat in search of bigger, stronger muscles, you'll get the former by seeking the latter.

WORKOUT A

LOAD: HEAVY

(4–6 RM)

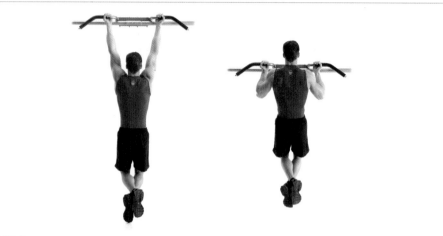

CHINUP (PAGE 207)
TOTAL REPS: 20 REST BETWEEN SETS (SECONDS): 75

WORKOUT B

LOAD: HEAVY

(4–6 RM)

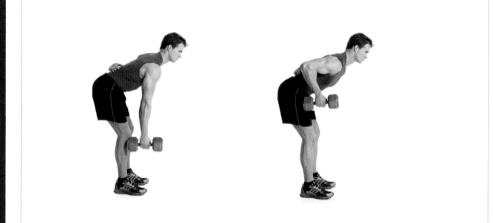

DUMBBELL ONE-ARM BENT-OVER ROW* (PAGE 219)
TOTAL REPS: 20 REST BETWEEN SETS (SECONDS): 75

WORKOUT C

LOAD: MEDIUM

(10–12 RM)

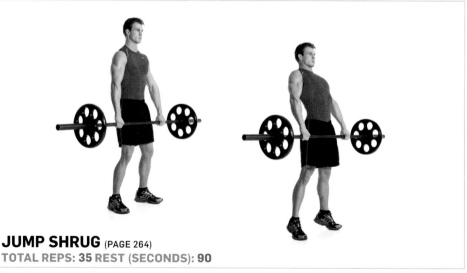

JUMP SHRUG (PAGE 264)
TOTAL REPS: 35 REST (SECONDS): 90

*Start with your weaker side first, then immediately do the same number of reps with your stronger limb. Rest after working both sides.

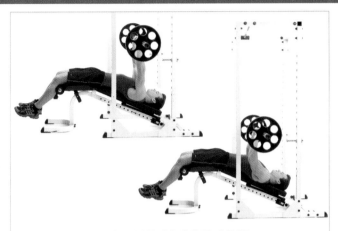

**BARBELL DECLINE CLOSE-GRIP
BENCH PRESS** (PAGE 226)
TOTAL REPS: **20** REST BETWEEN SETS (SECONDS): **75**

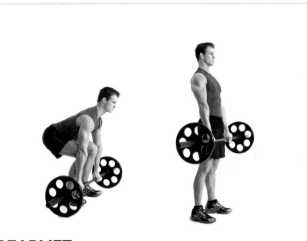

DEADLIFT (PAGE 254)
TOTAL REPS: **20** REST BETWEEN SETS (SECONDS): **75**

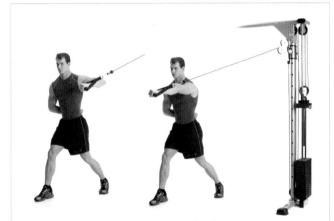

**CABLE STANDING ONE-ARM
CHEST PRESS*** (PAGE 230)
TOTAL REPS: **20** REST BETWEEN SETS (SECONDS): **75**

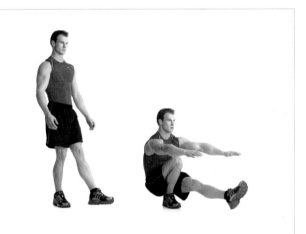

SINGLE-LEG SQUAT* (PAGE 251)
TOTAL REPS: **20** REST BETWEEN SETS (SECONDS): **75**

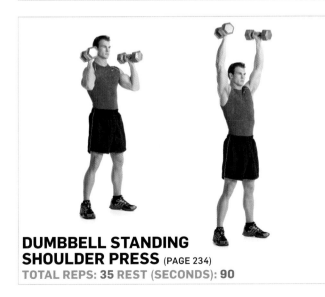

**DUMBBELL STANDING
SHOULDER PRESS** (PAGE 234)
TOTAL REPS: **35** REST (SECONDS): **90**

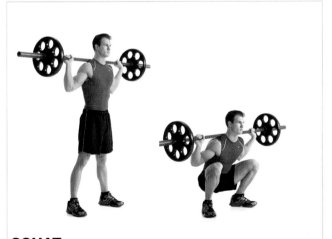

SQUAT (PAGE 241)
TOTAL REPS: **35** REST (SECONDS): **90**

WORKOUT A

LOAD: MEDIUM
(10–12 RM)

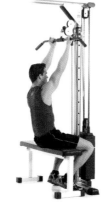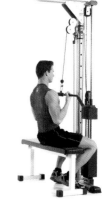

UNDERHAND-GRIP LAT PULLDOWN (PAGE 211)
TOTAL REPS: **30** REST (SECONDS): **45**

WORKOUT B

LOAD: MEDIUM
(10–12 RM)

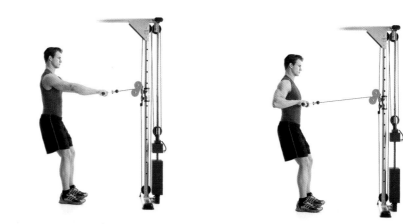

CABLE STANDING MID-PULLEY ROW (PAGE 213)
TOTAL REPS: **30** REST (SECONDS): **45**

WORKOUT C

LOAD: MEDIUM
(10–12 RM)

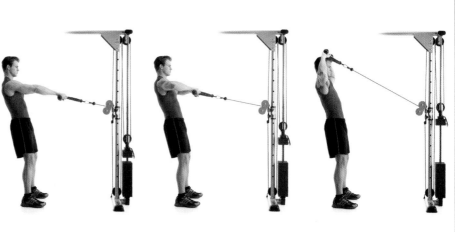

CABLE STANDING MID-PULLEY FACE PULL (PAGE 214)
TOTAL REPS: **30** REST (SECONDS): **45**

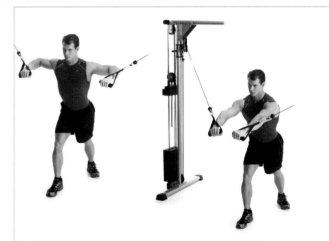

CABLE STANDING CHEST PRESS (PAGE 229)
TOTAL REPS: **30** REST (SECONDS): **45**

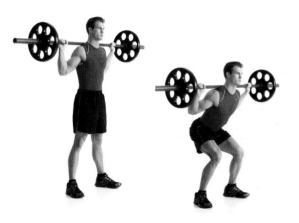

QUARTER SQUAT (PAGE 241)
TOTAL REPS: **30** REST (SECONDS): **45**

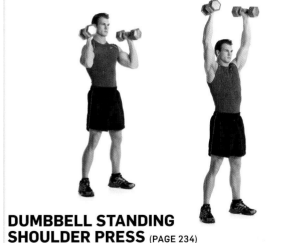

DUMBBELL STANDING SHOULDER PRESS (PAGE 234)
TOTAL REPS: **30** REST (SECONDS): **45**

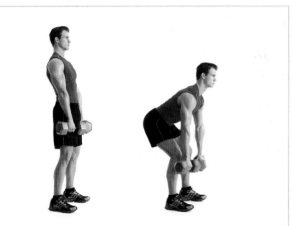

DUMBBELL ROMANIAN DEADLIFT (PAGE 256)
TOTAL REPS: **30** REST (SECONDS): **45**

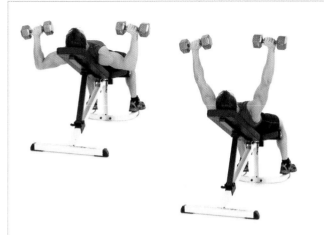

DUMBBELL INCLINE BENCH PRESS (PAGE 227)
TOTAL REPS: **30** REST (SECONDS): **45**

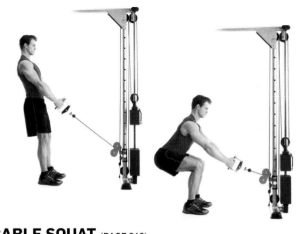

CABLE SQUAT (PAGE 246)
TOTAL REPS: **30** REST (SECONDS): **45**

WORKOUT A

LOAD:
SUPER-HEAVY
(2–3 RM)

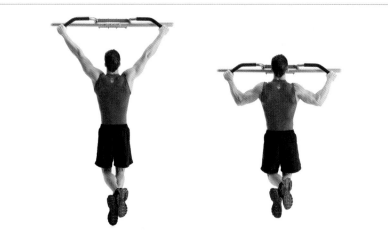

WIDE-GRIP PULLUP (PAGE 209)
TOTAL REPS: 15 REST (SECONDS): 60

WORKOUT B

LOAD:
HEAVY
(4–6 RM)

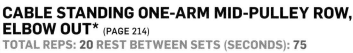

CABLE STANDING ONE-ARM MID-PULLEY ROW, ELBOW OUT* (PAGE 214)
TOTAL REPS: 20 REST BETWEEN SETS (SECONDS): 75

WORKOUT C

LOAD:
MEDIUM
(10–12 RM)

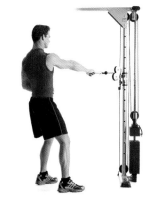

HIGH PULL (PAGE 263)
TOTAL REPS: 35 REST (SECONDS): 90

Start with your weaker side first, then immediately do the same number of reps with your stronger limb. Rest after working both sides.

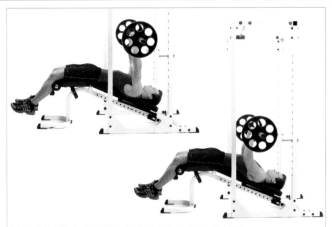

BARBELL DECLINE CLOSE-GRIP
BENCH PRESS (PAGE 226)
TOTAL REPS: 15 REST (SECONDS): 60

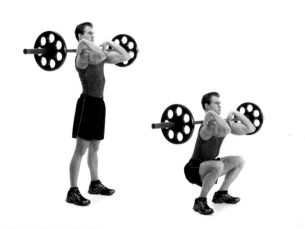

FRONT SQUAT (PAGE 242)
TOTAL REPS: 15 REST (SECONDS): 60

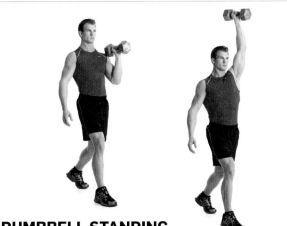

DUMBBELL STANDING
ONE-ARM SHOULDER PRESS* (PAGE 235)
TOTAL REPS: 20 REST BETWEEN SETS (SECONDS): 75

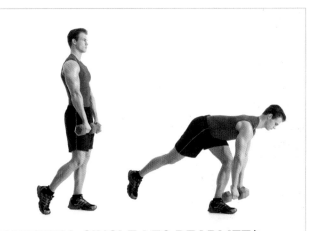

DUMBBELL SINGLE-LEG DEADLIFT*
(PAGE 257)
TOTAL REPS: 20 REST BETWEEN SETS (SECONDS): 75

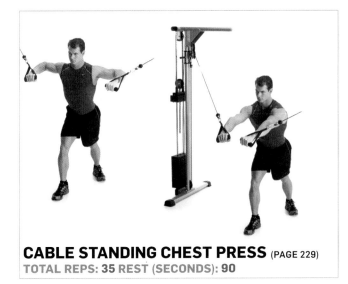

CABLE STANDING CHEST PRESS (PAGE 229)
TOTAL REPS: 35 REST (SECONDS): 90

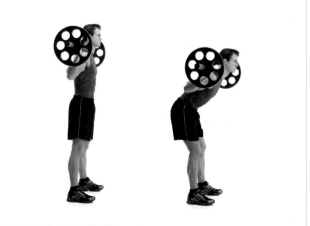

GOOD MORNING (PAGE 258)
TOTAL REPS: 35 REST (SECONDS): 90

157

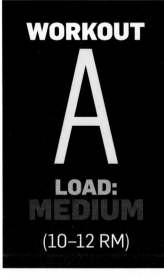

WORKOUT A
LOAD: MEDIUM
(10–12 RM)

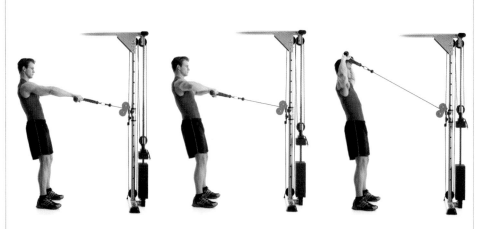

CABLE STANDING MID-PULLEY FACE PULL (PAGE 214)
TOTAL REPS: 30 REST (SECONDS): 40

WORKOUT B
LOAD: MEDIUM
(10–12 RM)

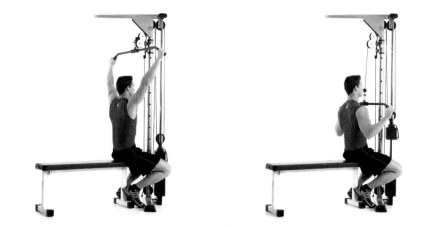

WIDE-GRIP LAT PULLDOWN (PAGE 211)
TOTAL REPS: 30 REST (SECONDS): 40

WORKOUT C
LOAD: MEDIUM
(10–12 RM)

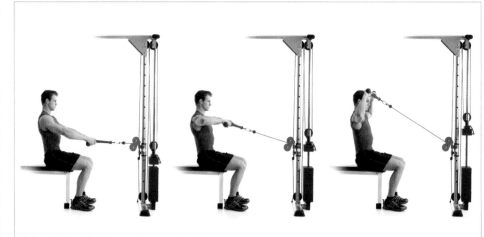

CABLE SEATED FACE PULL (PAGE 217)
TOTAL REPS: 30 REST (SECONDS): 40

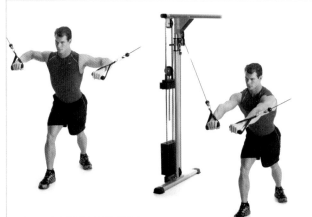

**CABLE STANDING
CHEST PRESS** (PAGE 229)
TOTAL REPS: **30** REST (SECONDS): **40**

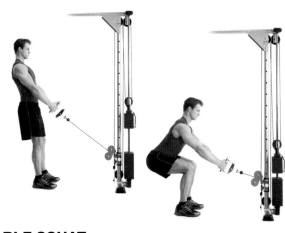

CABLE SQUAT (PAGE 246)
TOTAL REPS: **30** REST (SECONDS): **40**

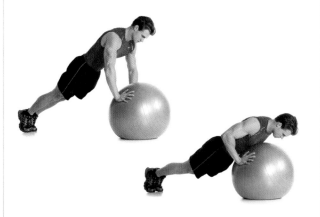

PUSHUP WITH HANDS ON SWISS BALL
(PAGE 232)
TOTAL REPS: **30** REST (SECONDS): **40**

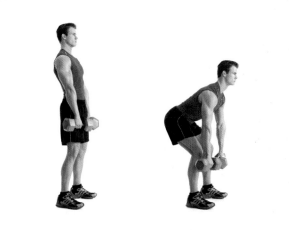

DUMBBELL ROMANIAN DEADLIFT (PAGE 256)
TOTAL REPS: **30** REST (SECONDS): **40**

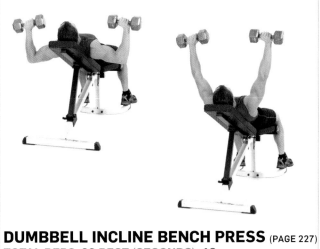

DUMBBELL INCLINE BENCH PRESS (PAGE 227)
TOTAL REPS: **30** REST (SECONDS): **40**

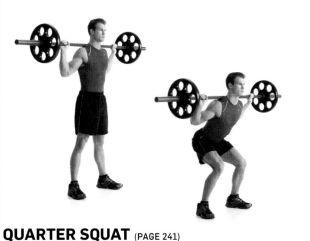

QUARTER SQUAT (PAGE 241)
TOTAL REPS: **30** REST (SECONDS): **40**

WORKOUT A

LOAD: SUPER-HEAVY

(2–3 RM)

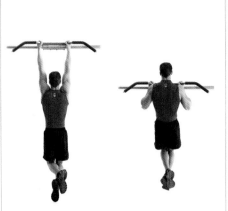

NEUTRAL-GRIP PULLUP (PAGE 209)

TOTAL REPS: 15 REST (SECONDS): 60

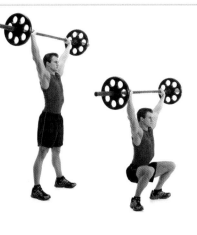

OVERHEAD SQUAT (PAGE 244)

TOTAL REPS: 15 REST (SECONDS): 60

WORKOUT B

LOAD: HEAVY

(4–6 RM)

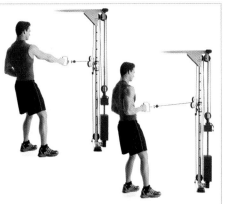

CABLE STANDING ONE-ARM MID-PULLEY ROW, ELBOW IN* (PAGE 213)

TOTAL REPS: 15 REST (SECONDS): 75

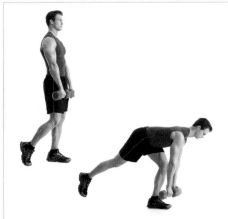

DUMBBELL SINGLE-LEG DEADLIFT* (PAGE 257)

TOTAL REPS: 15 REST (SECONDS): 75

WORKOUT C

LOAD: HEAVY

(4–6 RM)

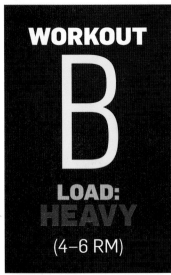

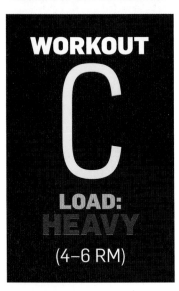

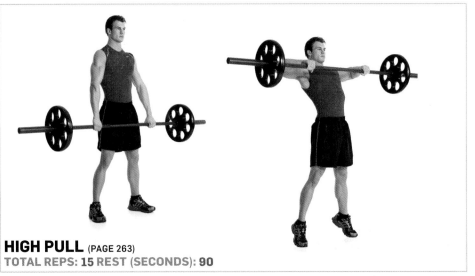

HIGH PULL (PAGE 263)

TOTAL REPS: 15 REST (SECONDS): 90

*Start with your weaker side first, then immediately do the same number of reps with your stronger limb. Rest after working both sides.

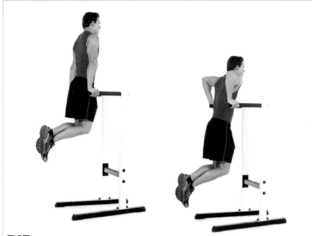

DIP (PAGE 223)
TOTAL REPS: **15** REST (SECONDS): **60**

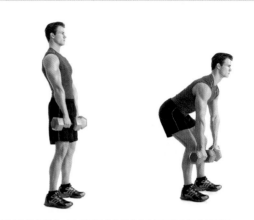

DUMBBELL ROMANIAN DEADLIFT
(PAGE 256)
TOTAL REPS: **15** REST (SECONDS): **60**

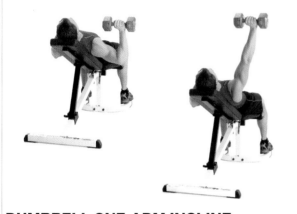

**DUMBBELL ONE-ARM INCLINE
BENCH PRESS*** (PAGE 228)
TOTAL REPS: **15** REST (SECONDS): **75**

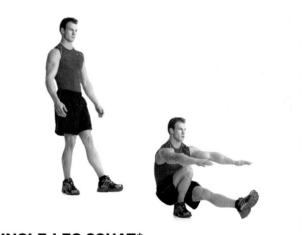

SINGLE-LEG SQUAT* (PAGE 251)
TOTAL REPS: **15** REST (SECONDS): **75**

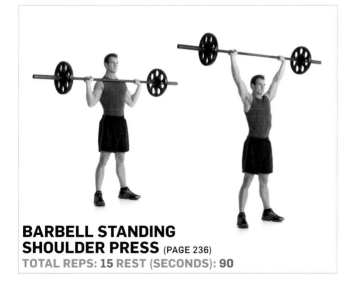

**BARBELL STANDING
SHOULDER PRESS** (PAGE 236)
TOTAL REPS: **15** REST (SECONDS): **90**

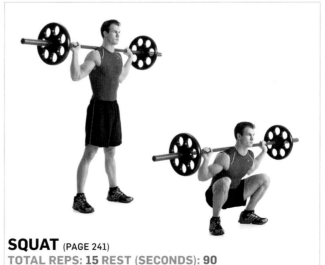

SQUAT (PAGE 241)
TOTAL REPS: **15** REST (SECONDS): **90**

WORKOUT A

LOAD: MEDIUM

(10–12 RM)

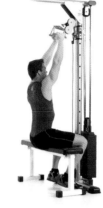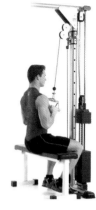

NEUTRAL-GRIP LAT PULLDOWN (PAGE 211)
TOTAL REPS: 30 REST (SECONDS): 35

WORKOUT B

LOAD: MEDIUM

(10–12 RM)

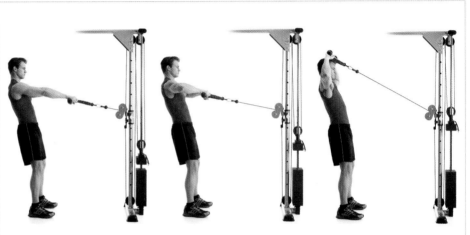

CABLE STANDING MID-PULLEY FACE PULL (PAGE 214)
TOTAL REPS: 30 REST (SECONDS): 35

WORKOUT C

LOAD: MEDIUM

(10–12 RM)

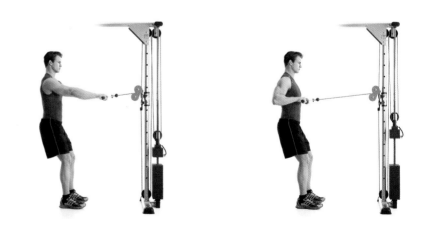

CABLE STANDING MID-PULLEY ROW (PAGE 213)
TOTAL REPS: 30 REST (SECONDS): 35

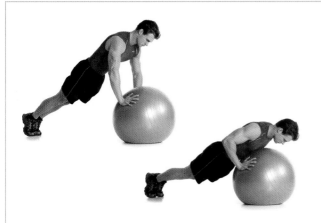

PUSHUP WITH HANDS ON SWISS BALL
(PAGE 232)
TOTAL REPS: 30 REST (SECONDS): 35

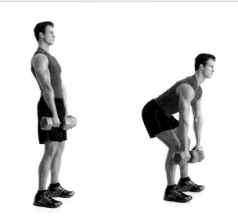

DUMBBELL ROMANIAN DEADLIFT
(PAGE 256)
TOTAL REPS: 30 REST (SECONDS): 35

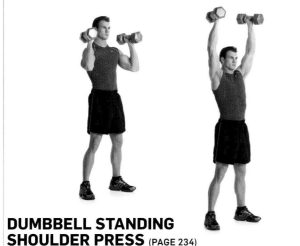

DUMBBELL STANDING
SHOULDER PRESS (PAGE 234)
TOTAL REPS: 30 REST (SECONDS): 35

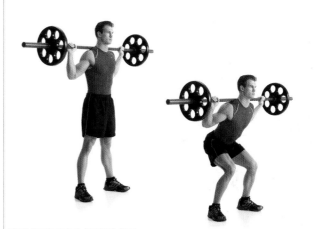

QUARTER SQUAT (PAGE 241)
TOTAL REPS: 30 REST (SECONDS): 35

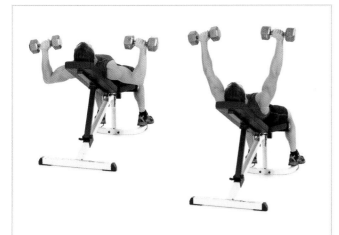

DUMBBELL INCLINE BENCH PRESS (PAGE 227)
TOTAL REPS: 30 REST (SECONDS): 35

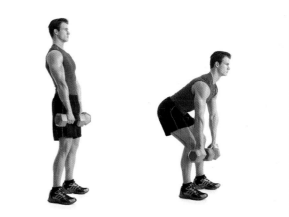

DUMBBELL ROMANIAN DEADLIFT
(PAGE 256)
TOTAL REPS: 30 REST (SECONDS): 35

CHAPTER 13

GET EVEN STRONGER

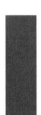f you're considering this program, that means you've finished the 16-week Get Strong program, preceded by 3 weeks of Get Ready. Chances are you've also done Get Big for 16 weeks, and maybe you've even had a go at Get Even Bigger. So that means you're ready for Get Even Stronger, right?

Not necessarily.

These workouts feature three advanced strength-building techniques: supramaximal holds, fast partial reps, and the rest-pause method. They're extremely effective for advanced lifters, but they shouldn't be used by anyone who's *not* advanced. You can consider yourself an advanced lifter if you meet these four criteria:

1. You've been training for at least 4 years without an extended break. (I'll accept 3 years if you've been seriously working toward pure strength.)

2. You've had some instruction on exercise form, preferably from a qualified strength coach. If not, you've worked with advanced-level training partners who corrected your form on the powerlifts. (And if you have to stop and think which exercises are "powerlifts," you *really* aren't ready for this program.)

3. Your total on the three powerlifts—the sum of your one-rep max for bench press, squat, and deadlift—should be at least $4\frac{1}{2}$ times your body weight. To put it another way, you should average at least $1\frac{1}{2}$ times your body weight on the three powerlifts. If you weigh 180 pounds, that means you can bench, squat, and deadlift an average of 270 pounds. That's the minimum.

4. You should be able to use at least twice your body weight on one of those lifts. So if you weigh 180, you should be able to squat or deadlift at least 360.

My first instinct was to make it more stringent, saying you had to bench-press at least $1\frac{1}{2}$ times your body weight and squat and deadlift at least twice your weight. But I know some pretty serious noncompetitive lifters whose body types and genetics keep them from clearing all three hurdles. For example, a 180-pounder with long arms and legs might be really good at deadlifting and capable of pulling upwards of 400 pounds, but because of his biomechanical disadvantages he can't get past 225 on the bench press. I don't want to tell that guy he can't do this program if he's otherwise ready for it.

With the fine print out of the way, let's look at the specific techniques you'll use in this program. In my experience, even the strongest lifters make immediate leaps in strength—5 percent is typical—during the first few weeks of a program using these techniques, due to the fact that they're shocking their muscles with a brand-new stimulus. Gains after that initial shock effect will come much slower, but they should still be real and measurable.

SUPRAMAXIMAL HOLD

What it is: You'll hold a weight near lockout that's heavier than your current one-rep max. (Again, if you don't know what "lockout" means, you really aren't ready for this program.) There's a pretty good psychological reason why a supramaximal hold—which I'll abbreviate as SMH from now on—increases strength: You simply get used to handling heavier weights.

How to do it: Add 20 percent to your one-rep max for the squat, dip, deadlift, or pullup. For the squat, dip, and deadlift, you'll start at the top of the movement and lower a few inches. (This requires that you don't start the deadlift from the floor; you'll need to use a power rack that has adjustable supports for the barbell.) Hold that position for 10 seconds.

For the pullup, place the correct amount of extra weight around your waist with a chin-dip belt, or you can hold a dumbbell between your feet with your legs straight if you have enough room. From the full hang position, pull yourself up just a few inches and hold that position for 10 seconds.

After your SMH, rest for 30 seconds, then do a set with a "heavy" or "superheavy" load for as many reps as possible. Then you'll rest 90 seconds and repeat the sequence.

When to use it: You can perform the supramaximal hold once each week for the squat, dip, deadlift, and pullup. It doesn't matter which day you use it, just make sure it's a day denoted as "heavy" or "superheavy."

REST-PAUSE METHOD

What it is: Rest-pause training is resting the load after each rep for less than 10 seconds. A deadlift uses the rest-pause method by default, since you're resting the barbell on the floor between reps. Remember when I mentioned that your largest muscle fibers can produce maximum force for only 15 seconds? This is due to the limited supply of energy that fuels those fibers. However, that energy system can replenish itself *partially* within 10 seconds. If you simply rest the load for 5 to 10 seconds after each rep, you give the system enough time to replenish some of its energy.

How to do it: Pause for 5 seconds after each repetition by resting the load. You can use this method with any exercise that allows you to rest the load. Unfortunately, there aren't many exercises that are ideal for the rest-pause technique. The best one is the deadlift. A back squat, for example, is difficult. You could set the pins in the power rack so the barbell can rest, but you're not resting in the ideal position, since you're crouched down. The best option with squats is to do one rep, re-rack the load, and do another rep. Of course, this necessitates that you reset your stance with each rep—not bad, but not ideal.

My favorite exercises for the rest-pause method are deadlifts, dips, pullups, and cable exercises. For dips, you need to have a bench or box underneath your legs so you can stand on it between reps (this requires that you keep your legs bent during the exercise). For pullups, you'll drop to the floor between reps.

For cable exercises, simply rest the weight stack between reps.

When to use it: You can use the rest-pause method during any workout that doesn't incorporate the supramaximal hold. Generally, it's best to limit the rest-pause method to loads that are "heavy" or "superheavy," but any load is an option.

FAST PARTIAL REPS

What they are: A fast partial movement is performed by lifting a weight as fast as possible through the strongest half of the movement. Since the range of motion is cut in half, and since you're lifting through the easiest half, you can use a lot more weight and spare your joints. You'll be lifting heavier weights than normal and you'll be lifting them faster—which is, of course, the crux of this book.

How to do them: In the deadlift, your strongest range of motion is the pulling phase from your knees to lockout. For presses and squats, it's the phase from halfway to lockout. For upper-body pulling movements, it's the first half of the repetition, starting with straight arms. So, in a pullup, you'd go from a full hang to the halfway point, when your elbows are flexed about 90 degrees. You'll stick to the target number of reps, but you'll perform the movement with a partial range of motion.

When to use them: You can use fast partials for any workout that doesn't incorporate the supramaximal hold or rest-pause method.

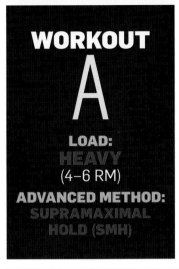

WORKOUT

A

LOAD:
HEAVY
(4–6 RM)
ADVANCED METHOD:
SUPRAMAXIMAL
HOLD (SMH)

USING SUPRAMAXIMAL HOLDS: Use a load that's approximately 20 percent more than your one-rep max. Hold for 5 seconds, rack the weight, and rest for 30 seconds. During that rest period, reduce the weight to one you can lift four to six times on your first work set. Do the set, then rest 90 seconds. During that rest period, add weight for the SMH. Repeat the sequence until you've completed all your reps for that exercise.

Chinup: Start from the hang position, pull yourself up 2 inches, and hold.

Barbell decline close-grip bench press: Lower the barbell 2 inches from the top position, and hold.

Deadlift: Start with the barbell resting on pins at mid-thigh level. Unrack the load, push your hips back slightly to lower the barbell 3 to 4 inches, and hold.

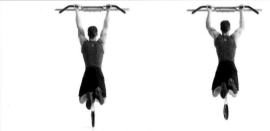

1A SMH FOR CHINUP (PAGE 208)
HOLD: 5 seconds
REST BETWEEN SETS (SECONDS): 30

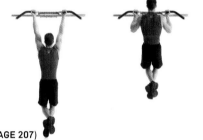

1B CHINUP (PAGE 207)
TOTAL REPS: 15
REST BETWEEN SETS (SECONDS): 90

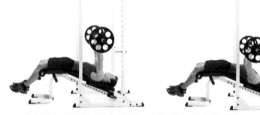

2A SMH FOR BARBELL DECLINE CLOSE-GRIP BENCH PRESS (PAGE 226)
HOLD: 5 seconds
REST BETWEEN SETS (SECONDS): 30

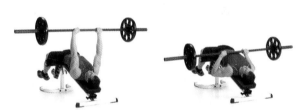

2B BARBELL DECLINE CLOSE-GRIP BENCH PRESS (PAGE 226)
TOTAL REPS: 15
REST BETWEEN SETS (SECONDS): 90

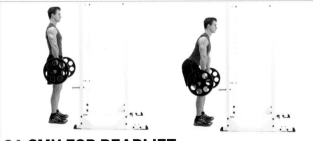

3A SMH FOR DEADLIFT (PAGE 255)
HOLD: 5 seconds
REST BETWEEN SETS (SECONDS): 30

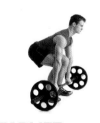
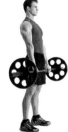

3B DEADLIFT (PAGE 254)
TOTAL REPS: 15
REST BETWEEN SETS (SECONDS): 90

(CONTINUED)

WORKOUT
B
LOAD:
HEAVY
(4–6 RM)

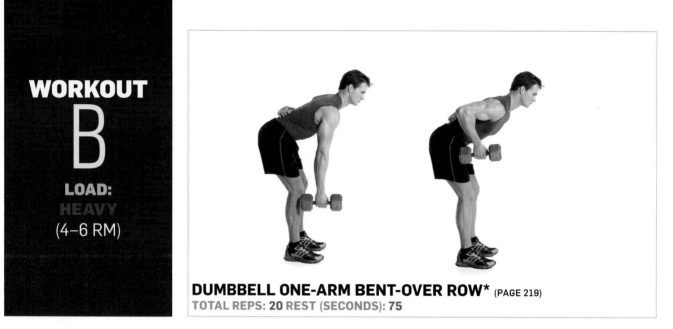

DUMBBELL ONE-ARM BENT-OVER ROW* (PAGE 219)
TOTAL REPS: 20 REST (SECONDS): 75

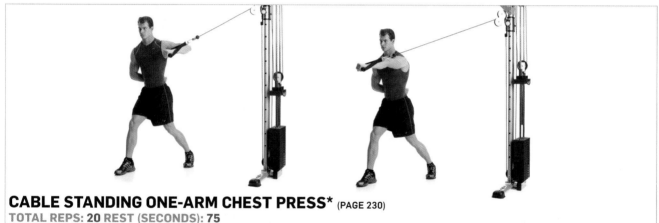

CABLE STANDING ONE-ARM CHEST PRESS* (PAGE 230)
TOTAL REPS: 20 REST (SECONDS): 75

SINGLE-LEG SQUAT* (PAGE 251)
TOTAL REPS: 20 REST (SECONDS): 75

LATERAL RAISE* (PAGE 292)
TOTAL REPS: 20 REST (SECONDS): 75

* Start with your weaker side first, then immediately do the same number of reps with your stronger limb. Rest after working both sides.

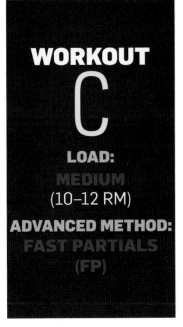

WORKOUT C

LOAD:
MEDIUM
(10–12 RM)

ADVANCED METHOD:
FAST PARTIALS
(FP)

USING FAST PARTIALS: The purpose of fast partials is to allow you to use a heavier weight than you normally could, since you're lifting only through the strongest part of the range of motion. Here, the load is "medium," which means a weight you could lift 10 to 12 times on your first work set. You should be able to use 15 percent more weight than you could with the full range of motion. If you'd normally use 135 on the front squat for 10 to 12 reps, you should be able do fast partials with 155.

Good morning: Use the first half of the range of motion—from the top position to where your torso is about 45 degrees relative to the floor.

Dumbbell seated shoulder press: Go from lockout to the top of your head.

Front squat: From lockout, go halfway toward the point at which your upper thighs would be parallel to the floor.

Cable standing mid-pulley face pull: Starting with straight arms, pull halfway; your elbows won't reach the point at which they're bent 90 degrees.

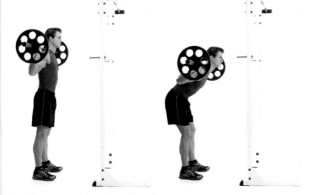

1 FP GOOD MORNING (PAGE 259)
TOTAL REPS: 30 REST (SECONDS): 90

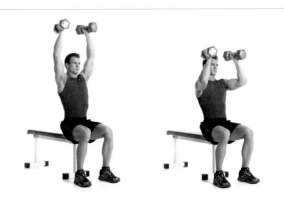

2 FP DUMBBELL SEATED SHOULDER PRESS (PAGE 235)
TOTAL REPS: 30 REST (SECONDS): 90

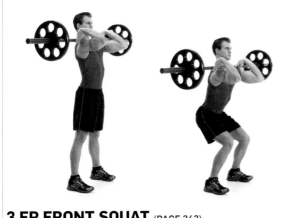

3 FP FRONT SQUAT (PAGE 243)
TOTAL REPS: 30 REST (SECONDS): 90

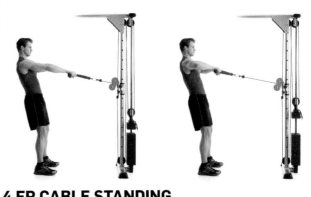

4 FP CABLE STANDING MID-PULLEY FACE PULL (PAGE 215)
TOTAL REPS: 30 REST (SECONDS): 90

WORKOUT A

LOAD: MEDIUM

(10–12 RM)

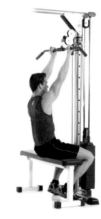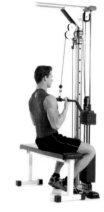

UNDERHAND-GRIP LAT PULLDOWN (PAGE 211)
TOTAL REPS: 30 REST (SECONDS): 45

WORKOUT B

LOAD: MEDIUM

(10–12 RM)

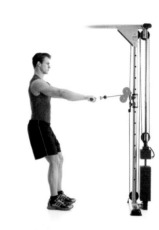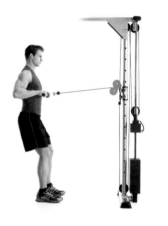

CABLE STANDING MID-PULLEY ROW (PAGE 213)
TOTAL REPS: 30 REST (SECONDS): 45

WORKOUT C

LOAD: MEDIUM

(10–12 RM)

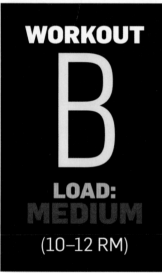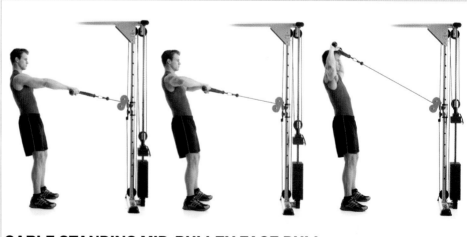

CABLE STANDING MID-PULLEY FACE PULL (PAGE 214)
TOTAL REPS: 30 REST (SECONDS): 45

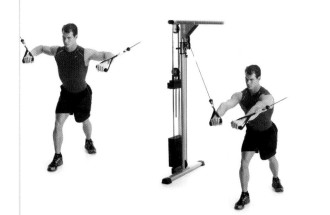

CABLE STANDING CHEST PRESS (PAGE 229)
TOTAL REPS: **30** REST (SECONDS): **45**

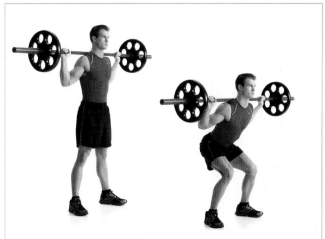

QUARTER SQUAT (PAGE 241)
TOTAL REPS: **30** REST (SECONDS): **45**

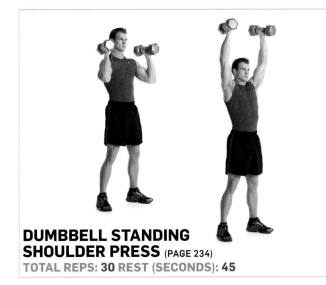

DUMBBELL STANDING SHOULDER PRESS (PAGE 234)
TOTAL REPS: **30** REST (SECONDS): **45**

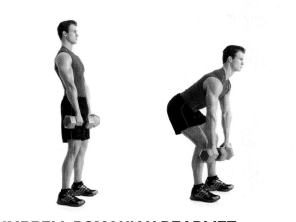

DUMBBELL ROMANIAN DEADLIFT (PAGE 256)
TOTAL REPS: **30** REST (SECONDS): **45**

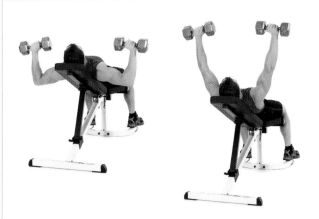

DUMBBELL INCLINE BENCH PRESS (PAGE 227)
TOTAL REPS: **30** REST (SECONDS): **45**

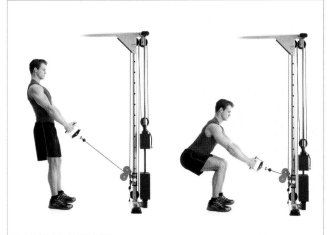

CABLE SQUAT (PAGE 246)
TOTAL REPS: **30** REST (SECONDS): **45**

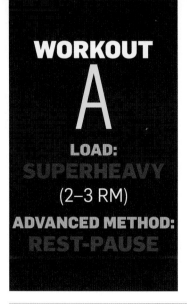

WORKOUT

A

LOAD:
SUPERHEAVY
(2–3 RM)
ADVANCED METHOD:
REST-PAUSE

USING THE REST-PAUSE METHOD: Rest for 5 seconds between repetitions in Workout A. That is, do your first rep, rest 5 seconds. Do your second, rest. Then do your third (if you make it to three). Use this technique until you've done all 15 reps for each exercise.

Pullup: Drop to the floor between reps.

Dip: You can drop to the floor or rest your feet on a bench or box between reps.

Deadlift: Easiest of all—just rest the barbell on the floor between reps.

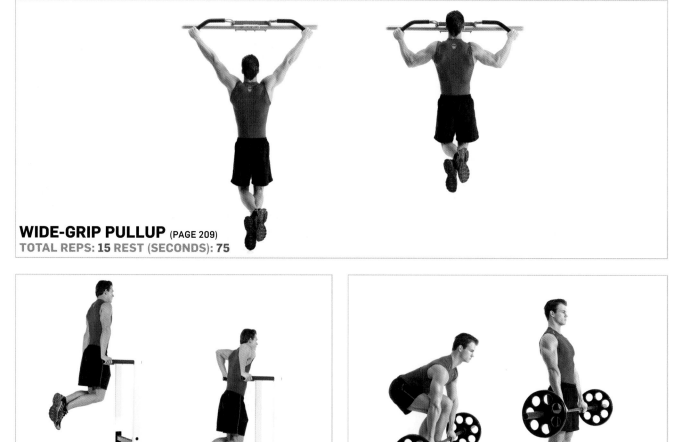

WIDE-GRIP PULLUP (PAGE 209)
TOTAL REPS: 15 REST (SECONDS): 75

DIP (PAGE 223)
TOTAL REPS: 15 REST (SECONDS): 75

DEADLIFT (PAGE 254)
TOTAL REPS: 15 REST (SECONDS): 75

Start with your weaker side first, then immediately do the same number of reps with your stronger limb. Rest after working both sides.

WORKOUT
B
LOAD:
HEAVY
(4–6 RM)

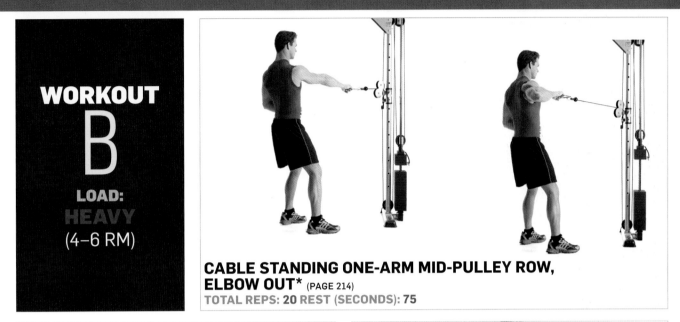

CABLE STANDING ONE-ARM MID-PULLEY ROW, ELBOW OUT* (PAGE 214)
TOTAL REPS: 20 REST (SECONDS): 75

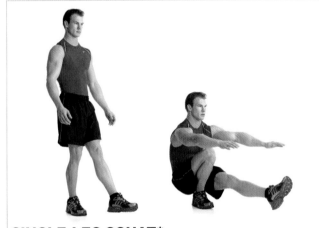

SINGLE-LEG SQUAT* (PAGE 251)
TOTAL REPS: 20 REST (SECONDS): 75

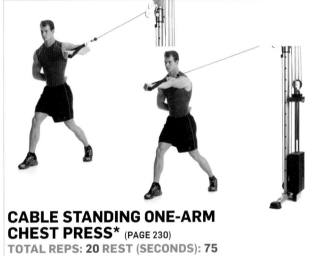

CABLE STANDING ONE-ARM CHEST PRESS* (PAGE 230)
TOTAL REPS: 20 REST (SECONDS): 75

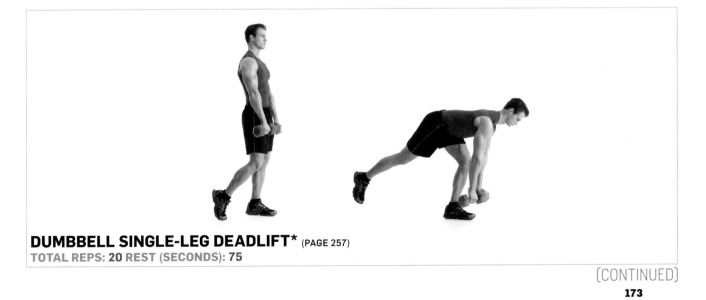

DUMBBELL SINGLE-LEG DEADLIFT* (PAGE 257)
TOTAL REPS: 20 REST (SECONDS): 75

(CONTINUED)

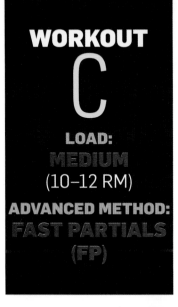

WORKOUT

C

LOAD:
MEDIUM
(10–12 RM)
ADVANCED METHOD:
FAST PARTIALS
(FP)

USING FAST PARTIALS:

Cable standing high-pulley row with V bar: Starting with straight arms, pull halfway; your elbows won't reach the point at which they're bent 90 degrees.

Dumbbell Romanian deadlift: Start at the top position, push your hips back, and lower the dumbbells until they're a few inches above your knees.

Dumbbell standing shoulder press: As with the seated version, you'll lower the weights from lockout to the top of your head, and do your reps from there.

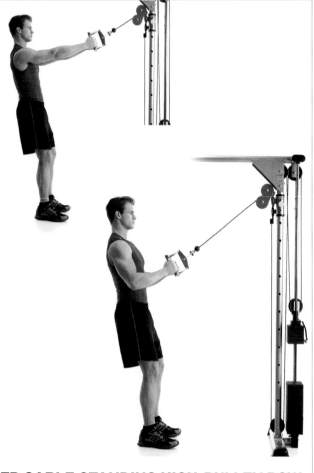

FP CABLE STANDING HIGH-PULLEY ROW WITH V BAR (PAGE 216)
TOTAL REPS: 30 REST (SECONDS): 90

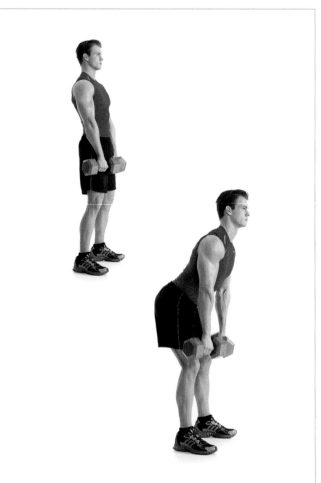

FP DUMBBELL ROMANIAN DEADLIFT
(PAGE 257)
TOTAL REPS: 30 REST (SECONDS): 90

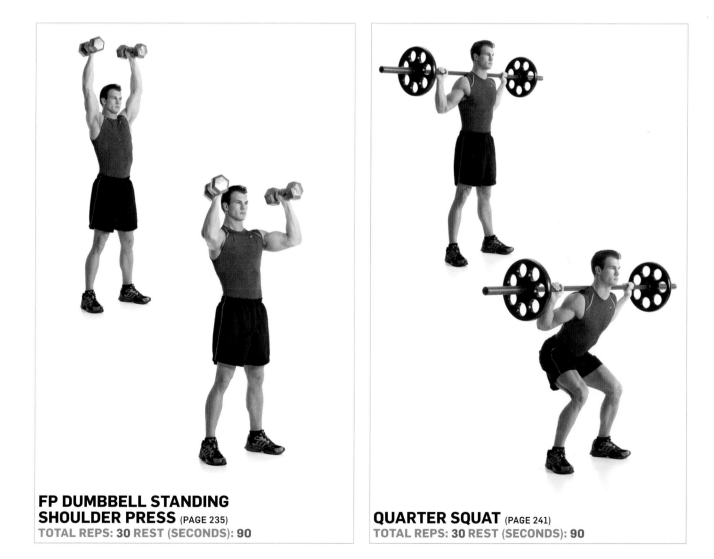

**FP DUMBBELL STANDING
SHOULDER PRESS** (PAGE 235)
TOTAL REPS: 30 REST (SECONDS): 90

QUARTER SQUAT (PAGE 241)
TOTAL REPS: 30 REST (SECONDS): 90

WORKOUT A
LOAD: MEDIUM
(10–12 RM)

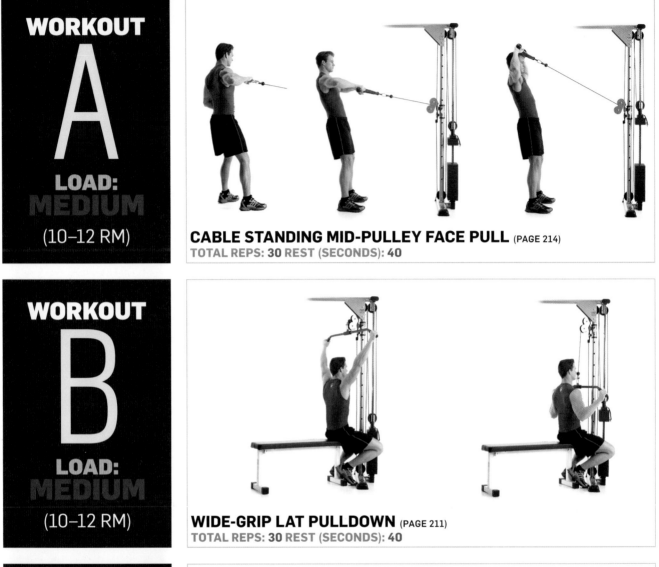

CABLE STANDING MID-PULLEY FACE PULL (PAGE 214)
TOTAL REPS: **30** REST (SECONDS): **40**

WORKOUT B
LOAD: MEDIUM
(10–12 RM)

WIDE-GRIP LAT PULLDOWN (PAGE 211)
TOTAL REPS: **30** REST (SECONDS): **40**

WORKOUT C
LOAD: MEDIUM
(10–12 RM)

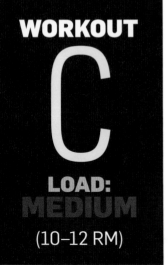
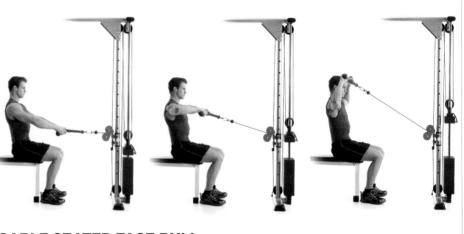

CABLE SEATED FACE PULL (PAGE 217)
TOTAL REPS: **30** REST (SECONDS): **40**

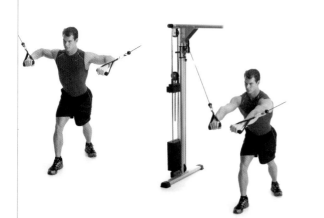

CABLE STANDING CHEST PRESS (PAGE 229)
TOTAL REPS: 30 REST (SECONDS): 40

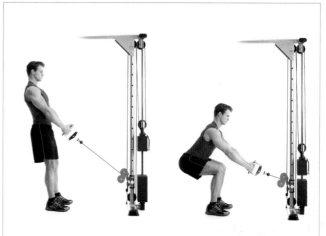

CABLE SQUAT (PAGE 246)
TOTAL REPS: 30 REST (SECONDS): 40

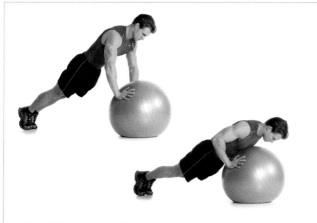

PUSHUP WITH HANDS ON SWISS BALL
(PAGE 232)
TOTAL REPS: 30 REST (SECONDS): 40

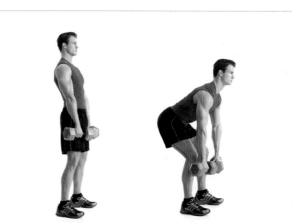

DUMBBELL ROMANIAN DEADLIFT
(PAGE 256)
TOTAL REPS: 30 REST (SECONDS): 40

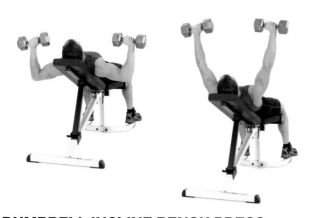

DUMBBELL INCLINE BENCH PRESS
(PAGE 227)
TOTAL REPS: 30 REST (SECONDS): 40

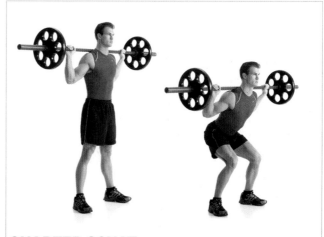

QUARTER SQUAT (PAGE 241)
TOTAL REPS: 30 REST (SECONDS): 40

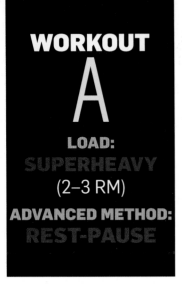

WORKOUT

A

LOAD:
SUPERHEAVY
(2–3 RM)

ADVANCED METHOD:
REST-PAUSE

USING THE REST-PAUSE METHOD: This workout makes it simple—two cable exercises (just return the weight to the stack), one deadlift (rest the bar on the floor), and the floor press, in which you can rest your upper arms on the floor for 5 seconds between reps.

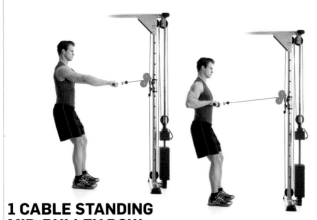

**1 CABLE STANDING
MID-PULLEY ROW** (PAGE 213)
TOTAL REPS: 15 REST (SECONDS): 60

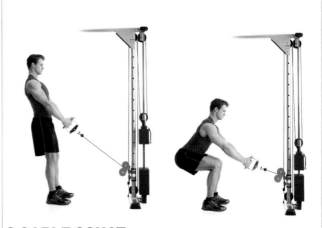

2 CABLE SQUAT (PAGE 246)
TOTAL REPS: 15 REST (SECONDS): 60

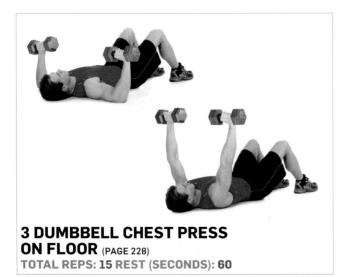

**3 DUMBBELL CHEST PRESS
ON FLOOR** (PAGE 228)
TOTAL REPS: 15 REST (SECONDS): 60

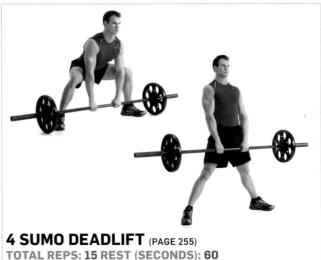

4 SUMO DEADLIFT (PAGE 255)
TOTAL REPS: 15 REST (SECONDS): 60

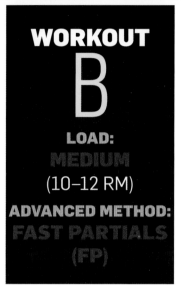

WORKOUT B

LOAD:
MEDIUM
(10–12 RM)

ADVANCED METHOD:
FAST PARTIALS
(FP)

USING FAST PARTIALS:

Chinup: Starting with straight arms, pull yourself halfway up.

Dip: From lockout, lower yourself halfway.

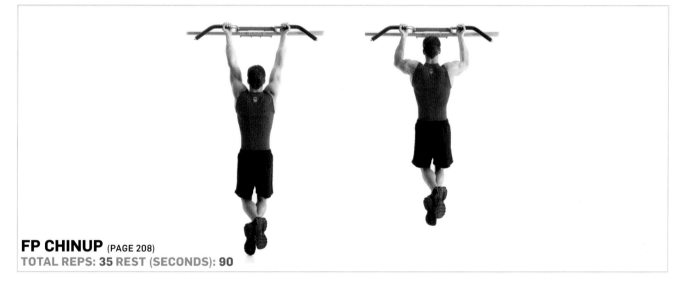

FP CHINUP (PAGE 208)
TOTAL REPS: 35 REST (SECONDS): 90

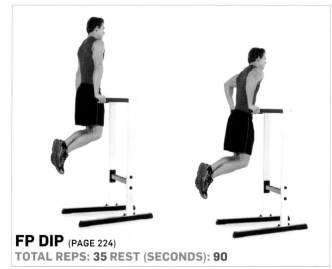

FP DIP (PAGE 224)
TOTAL REPS: 35 REST (SECONDS): 90

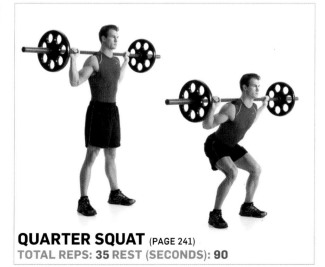

QUARTER SQUAT (PAGE 241)
TOTAL REPS: 35 REST (SECONDS): 90

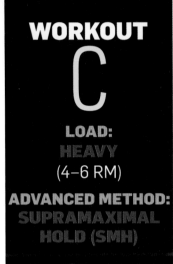

WORKOUT C

LOAD: HEAVY
(4–6 RM)

ADVANCED METHOD: SUPRAMAXIMAL HOLD (SMH)

USING SUPRAMAXIMAL HOLDS:

Pullup: Start from the hang position, pull yourself up 2 inches, and hold.

Barbell decline close-grip bench press: Lower the barbell 2 inches from the top position, and hold.

Front squat: Start with the barbell resting on pins at chest level. Set the bar on the top of your chest, unrack it, push your hips back slightly to lower the barbell 3 to 4 inches, and hold.

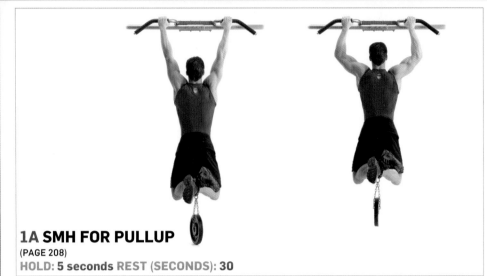

1A SMH FOR PULLUP
(PAGE 208)
HOLD: **5 seconds** REST (SECONDS): **30**

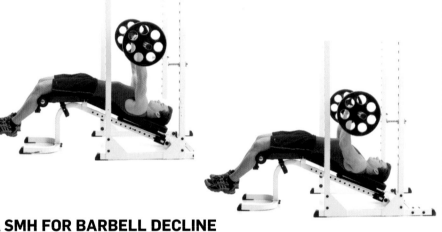

2A SMH FOR BARBELL DECLINE CLOSE-GRIP BENCH PRESS (PAGE 226)
HOLD: **5 seconds** REST (SECONDS): **30**

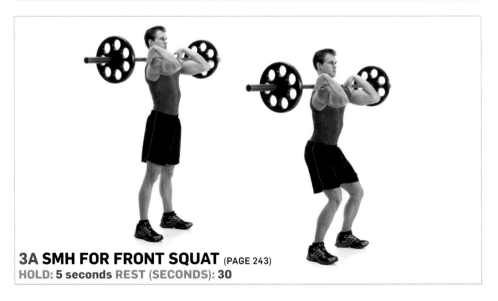

3A SMH FOR FRONT SQUAT (PAGE 243)
HOLD: **5 seconds** REST (SECONDS): **30**

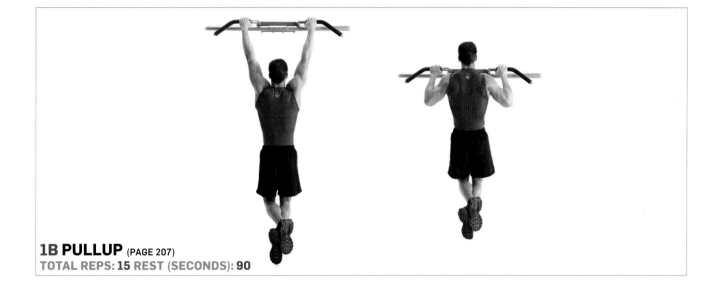

1B PULLUP (PAGE 207)
TOTAL REPS: **15** REST (SECONDS): **90**

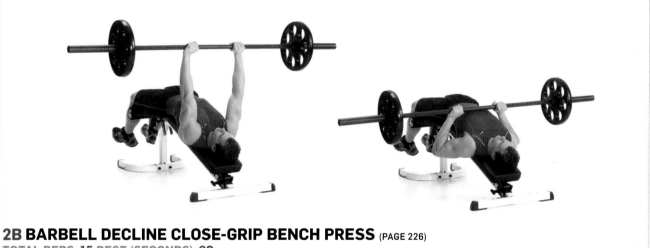

2B BARBELL DECLINE CLOSE-GRIP BENCH PRESS (PAGE 226)
TOTAL REPS: **15** REST (SECONDS): **90**

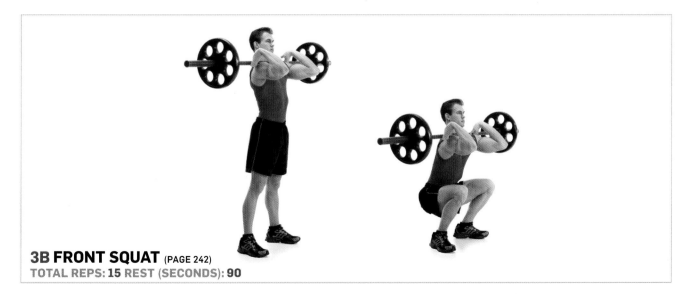

3B FRONT SQUAT (PAGE 242)
TOTAL REPS: **15** REST (SECONDS): **90**

WORKOUT A

LOAD: MEDIUM

(10–12 RM)

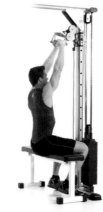

NEUTRAL-GRIP LAT PULLDOWN (PAGE 211)
TOTAL REPS: 30 REST (SECONDS): 35

WORKOUT B

LOAD: MEDIUM

(10–12 RM)

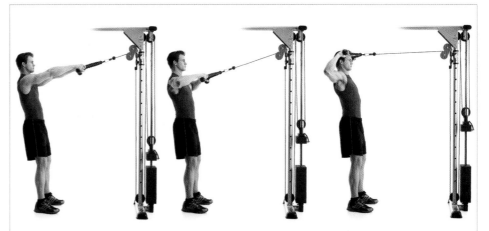

CABLE STANDING HIGH-PULLEY FACE PULL (PAGE 216)
TOTAL REPS: 30 REST (SECONDS): 35

WORKOUT C

LOAD: MEDIUM

(10–12 RM)

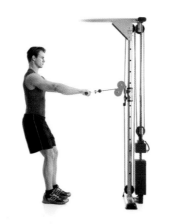

CABLE STANDING MID-PULLEY ROW (PAGE 213)
TOTAL REPS: 30 REST (SECONDS): 35

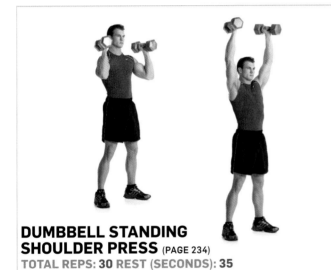

PUSHUP WITH HANDS ON SWISS BALL
(PAGE 232)
TOTAL REPS: 30 REST (SECONDS): 35

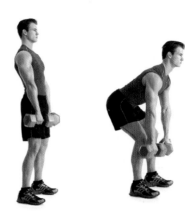

DUMBBELL ROMANIAN DEADLIFT
(PAGE 256)
TOTAL REPS: 30 REST (SECONDS): 35

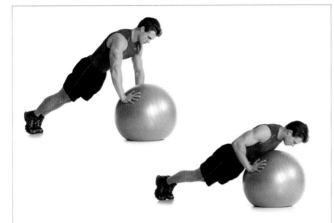

DUMBBELL STANDING SHOULDER PRESS (PAGE 234)
TOTAL REPS: 30 REST (SECONDS): 35

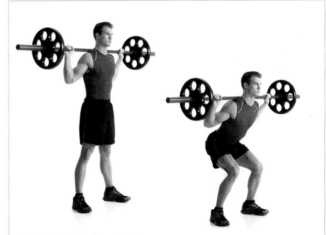

QUARTER SQUAT (PAGE 241)
TOTAL REPS: 30 REST (SECONDS): 35

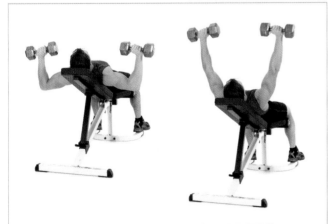

DUMBBELL INCLINE BENCH PRESS
(PAGE 227)
TOTAL REPS: 30 REST (SECONDS): 35

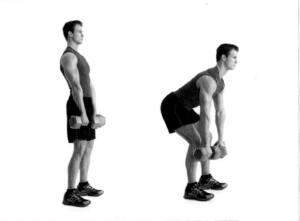

DUMBBELL ROMANIAN DEADLIFT
(PAGE 256)
TOTAL REPS: 30 REST (SECONDS): 35

CHAPTER 14

GET LEAN

Nobody's impressed by muscles they can't see. Being big, strong, and fat is better than being small, weak, and fat, but you don't have to settle for that kind of compromise. I've never known a lifter who set out to build muscles with no intention of ever seeing them—or of showing them off from time to time.

The question is, how do you lose the fat covering your muscles without sacrificing the muscles themselves?

For starters, I'll concede this point up front: Any good workout routine can help you lose fat. You could take any of the workouts in Chapters 9 through 13, use them in conjunction with the nutrition guidelines in Chapters 22 and 23, and strip some tallow off your torso.

Consider the hypertrophy-focused workouts in Chapters 10 and 11. More muscle means a faster metabolism, which is a crucial component of successful fat loss. Looking at it from the opposite direction, the best way to ensure you *won't* lose fat is to allow your metabolism to slow down—exactly what happens when you follow conventional weight-loss advice by eating less and doing low-intensity exercise. You inevitably lose muscle mass along with whatever fat comes off, and that slows down your metabolism.

But a muscle-building workout presents some serious problems when your goal is fat loss. It requires a high volume of exercise to break down as much muscle protein as possible, and it only works if you're eating so much food that you not only replace that protein but end up with more of it. You also accumulate a lot of fatigue in the process. Without the extra food, you won't be able to recover sufficiently between workouts, meaning you could lose strength and size over time.

Now consider the strength-focused programs in Chapters 12 and 13. On the plus side, you're doing fewer sets and reps, so there's less chance of overtraining due to the pure volume of exercise. But you're also cranking up the intensity of the workouts by using heavier loads. That puts extra stress on your nervous system, not to mention the strain on your joints. You're also breaking down a lot of muscle protein. Once again, less food means longer and less complete recovery from one workout to the next.

So hypertrophy programs are too high in volume, and strength programs demand too much from your joints and nervous system. That means, by default, you're left with lower-volume workouts using lighter weights. In what universe is less exercise, at lower intensity, a formula for successful training for any goal—especially fat loss?

Now you know why I devoted an entire chapter to this subject, including a unique, specialized workout system.

THE MEETING OF MINDS (AND BEERS)

One of the privileges of my position as a fitness professional is that I have interesting friends, including Alwyn Cosgrove, a fat-loss specialist who's coauthor of *The New Rules of Lifting* books, among many other accomplishments and distinctions. When we got together for lunch a while back, the conversation turned to fat loss. The 1-hour lunch stretched into 2 hours, then 3. Beers mysteriously showed up on our table. (Like I said, we were *talking* about fat loss, not actively pursuing it.)

We decided to make a list of the essential components of fat-loss training. It went something like this.

1. CREATE A CALORIC DEFICIT

Everyone agrees that fat loss requires burning more calories than you take in. The disagreements begin when you try to figure out *how*. Your body won't release stored fat without a good reason.

But if you give it too good a reason—a big caloric deficit—your body will make critical adjustments to hang on to that fat and get back to its comfort level. Your metabolism will almost certainly slow down, and you might sacrifice some of your metabolically expensive muscle tissue as well.

So your first goal is to keep your metabolism running at least as fast as it was before you created the caloric deficit. You do that in two ways:

>> Eating frequently, with plenty of protein, healthy fats, and vegetables at each meal

>> Doing kick-ass workouts that force your body to continue burning calories at a faster speed long after you leave the gym

The latter phenomenon is called *excess postexercise oxygen consumption*, or EPOC. Lots of people, including Alwyn, refer to it as the "afterburn." Your body uses more oxygen than usual when you exercise, which makes sense when you consider that exercise speeds up your heart and your rate of breathing. A really hard workout requires a lot more oxygen, consistent with the greater increase in heart rate and respiration. Your body temperature also goes higher with a more challenging workout.

The bigger the changes, the more time it takes to return to your preexercise baseline, and the more calories your body burns in order to get there.

That's why EPOC is crucial to fat loss,

which brings us to Steps Two, Three, and Four.

2. INCREASE THE METABOLIC COST OF EACH EXERCISE

In terms of metabolic demand, there's a massive difference between a squat and an arm curl. The former challenges hundreds of muscle groups and sends your heart rate sky-high. The latter doesn't. The more muscle you use on an exercise, and the more difficult it is to perform, the higher its metabolic cost.

3. INCREASE THE METABOLIC COST OF EACH WORKOUT

No matter how difficult the exercises are, you can negate their metabolic cost by resting longer between sets. On the other hand, if you make your rest periods shorter than usual, you increase the difficulty and boost EPOC.

4. PERFORM HIGH-INTENSITY INTERVAL TRAINING (HIIT)

There's a pretty good reason why traditional weight-loss advice includes lots of steady-pace endurance exercise. That type of workout burns a lot of calories. The more you do, the more you burn. Problem is, you can't generate a lot of EPOC if your workouts are long and slow. It's better to make them short and fast, and even better to make them short, fast, and intermittent—go hard for a designated period (typically 30 to 60 seconds, although I prefer all-out sprints for 15 seconds), then recover by going easy for a period that's two or three times as long as your hard effort. Then you do it again, and again.

The shift from slow to fast and back again is much more demanding than steady-pace exercise, which is why HIIT creates a bigger oxygen deficit and leads to more fat loss. You can't do a lot of it—15 to 30 minutes two or three times a week is the max for all but elite athletes—but you also don't need a lot to see the benefits.

5. SURROUND YOURSELF WITH PEOPLE WHO SUPPORT YOUR EFFORTS

Now we're back to something everyone agrees on. Exercise psychologists have shown that your social network can mean the difference between success and failure. Supportive friends, co-workers, relatives, spouses, and spousal equivalents understand what you're trying to do, offer encouragement when you need it most, and help when they can.

Believe me, you need all the support you can get when you're serious about changing your physique.

You might have co-workers who slip doughnuts onto your desk when you aren't looking. Your friends might pressure you to hit happy hour buffets and then drink until closing time. Your wife or girlfriend might insist on keeping the cabinets stocked with chips and the freezer filled with Ben and Jerry's. Your mother might make snide remarks about how you're getting too big or too skinny, with Dad noting how unusual it is for a father of three to spend so much time in the gym.

At the end of the day, it's difficult for anyone to stick to a healthy routine, and it's especially difficult when you're trying to lose fat.

SWEATING: THE DETAILS

All of my fat-loss workouts employ a simple premise: The sooner you start perspiring, the better. If you aren't sweating within the first 10 minutes of a workout, you aren't working hard enough. Put another way, you're not creating an oxygen debt fast enough. There's only so much time you can devote to fat-burning exercise when you're also following a strict eating plan, and you can't afford to waste any of it. Time is EPOC.

I like to start this type of workout with 5 minutes of rope jumping, followed by 5 minutes of squat thrusts. (In case the words "squat thrust" don't give you PE flashbacks, it's a simple four-part exercise. From a standing position: 1. Drop down until your hands touch the floor. 2. Thrust your legs back so you're in a pushup position. 3. Return to the #1 position. 4. Stand.) Both challenge your entire body, and you can't cheat on either one.

You probably won't be able to do either exercise for 5 minutes without a break, but you don't have to. Just do as much as you can of each exercise in the allotted time, stopping when you need to. Count the repetitions, and try to increase the number of jumps and squat thrusts you can do in subsequent workouts. Over time, you should be able to complete 5 minutes of rope jumping and squat thrusts with minimal rest.

If you don't have the desire or coordination to jump rope, do jumping jacks instead.

THE PROGRAM

Even the best fat-loss programs have one big shortcoming: You lose strength. Since the biggest benefits of strength training come when you tap into your biggest motor units, any loss of strength presents a serious handicap. Ideally, you want to increase your strength, but workouts designed for that purpose rarely work for fat loss, as I explained earlier.

Which brings me to the most unique feature of my fat-loss program: the loading week.

If you've done either or both of the strength programs, you know that I included an unloading week after each phase, in order to give your joints a break and allow your body to catch up on its recovery. Here I use the same strategy, but flip it 180 degrees: Instead of using lighter weights for a week to unload, you'll use superheavy weights between phases to reload. That ensures you don't lose strength—and the all-important ability to tap into your biggest motor units—as you take inches off your waist. In fact, you should actually gain some strength.

The volume during the loading week is kept low to avoid overtraining. That's why there are just two workouts per loading week, which is a switch from the three-a-week unloading programs I used in the Get Big and Get Strong programs. Any strength you gain in your loading weeks will come into play when you return to fat-loss workouts. You'll be able to work with heavier weights, which makes the programs more effective.

A quick note about HIIT: You'll see in the charts that I prescribe 15-second sprints, with 45 seconds of easy-pace exercise before and after. Most of you will choose to run or use a bike outdoors, or run or ride indoors on a treadmill or exercise bike. But I want to emphasize that you can use any piece of equipment or type of exercise for HIIT. You could even do calisthenics, although I don't think it's a particularly good idea right after lifting weights, since your muscles are already fatigued and depleted of nutrients. Inducing more fatigue makes recovery from one workout to the next a lot more problematic, setting you up for poor workouts, at a minimum, and injuries and burnout in the worst-case scenario. Since you'll be doing HIIT after every workout for 15 consecutive weeks, I recommend mixing it up to keep it fresh and interesting. And make sure you get outdoors as often as possible, weather permitting.

You can expect to see rapid fat loss in the early weeks of Get Lean. Most of my clients start off losing at least 2 pounds a week. I don't expect many of you to keep up that rate of fat loss for the entire 16 weeks—that would be 32 pounds of fat, a hell of a trick for anyone who isn't excessively overweight to begin with. (And what are the odds that someone that big picks up a book called *Huge in a Hurry* to begin with?) But 10 pounds of fat loss could be realistic for you, with most of that happening in the first few weeks.

WORKOUT A

LOAD:
HEAVY
(4–6 RM)

HIIT
DURATION: 15 SECONDS
RECOVERY: 45 SECONDS
TOTAL TIME: 10 MINUTES

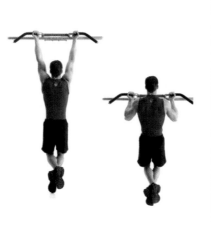

CHINUP (PAGE 207)
TOTAL REPS: 20 REST BETWEEN SETS (SECONDS): 45

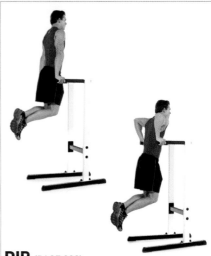

DIP (PAGE 233)
TOTAL REPS: 20 REST BETWEEN SETS (SECONDS): 45

WORKOUT B

LOAD:
MEDIUM
(10–12 RM)

HIIT
DURATION: 15 SECONDS
RECOVERY: 45 SECONDS
TOTAL TIME: 10 MINUTES

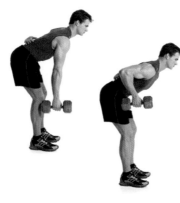

DUMBBELL ONE-ARM BENT-OVER ROW* (PAGE 219)
TOTAL REPS: 35 REST (SECONDS): 60

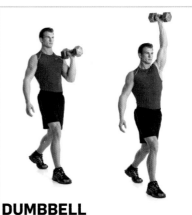

DUMBBELL STANDING ONE-ARM SHOULDER PRESS* (PAGE 235)
TOTAL REPS: 35 REST (SECONDS): 60

WORKOUT C

LOAD:
LIGHT
(20–22 RM)

HIIT
DURATION: 15 SECONDS
RECOVERY: 45 SECONDS
TOTAL TIME: 10 MINUTES

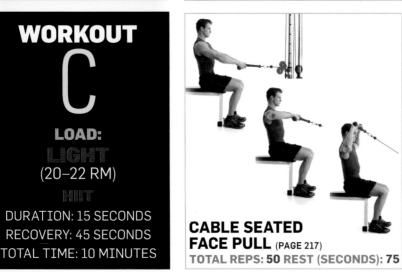

CABLE SEATED FACE PULL (PAGE 217)
TOTAL REPS: 50 REST (SECONDS): 75

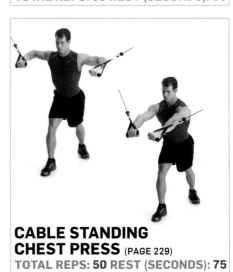

CABLE STANDING CHEST PRESS (PAGE 229)
TOTAL REPS: 50 REST (SECONDS): 75

*Start with your weaker side first, then immediately do the same number of reps with your stronger limb. Rest after working both sides.

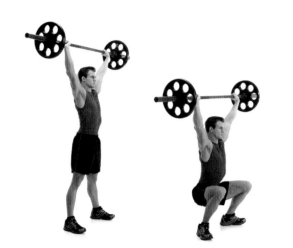

OVERHEAD SQUAT (PAGE 244)
TOTAL REPS: **20** REST BETWEEN SETS (SECONDS): **45**

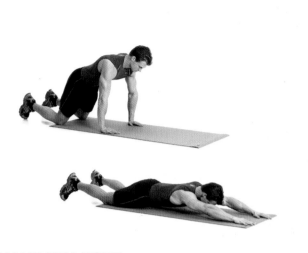

HAND WALKOUT (PAGE 271)
TOTAL REPS: **20** REST BETWEEN SETS (SECONDS): **45**

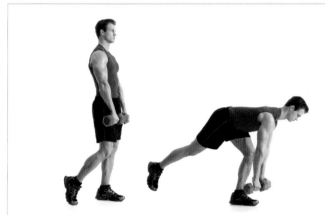

DUMBBELL SINGLE-LEG DEADLIFT*
(PAGE 257)
TOTAL REPS: **35** REST (SECONDS): **60**

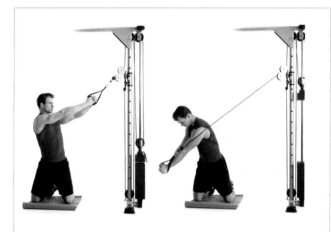

CABLE WOODCHOP ON KNEES* (PAGE 273)
TOTAL REPS: **35** REST (SECONDS): **60**

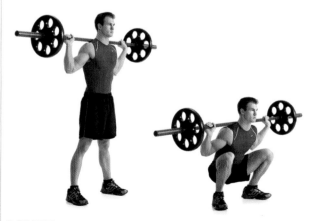

SQUAT (PAGE 241)
TOTAL REPS: **50** REST (SECONDS): **75**

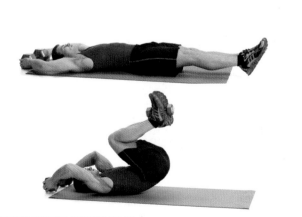

REVERSE CRUNCH (PAGE 275)
TOTAL REPS: **50** REST (SECONDS): **75**

WORKOUT A

LOAD:
SUPERHEAVY
(2–3 RM)

HIIT

DURATION: 15 SECONDS
RECOVERY: 45 SECONDS
TOTAL TIME: 16 MINUTES

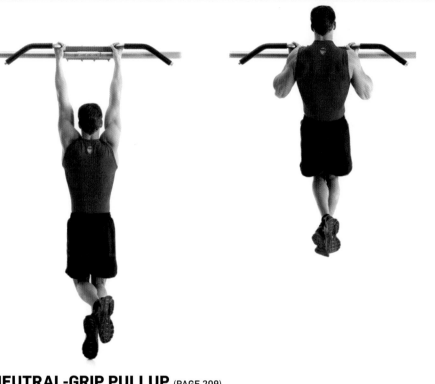

NEUTRAL-GRIP PULLUP (PAGE 209)
TOTAL REPS: 10 REST (SECONDS): 75

WORKOUT B

LOAD:
SUPERHEAVY
(2–3 RM)

HIIT

DURATION: 15 SECONDS
RECOVERY: 45 SECONDS
TOTAL TIME: 16 MINUTES

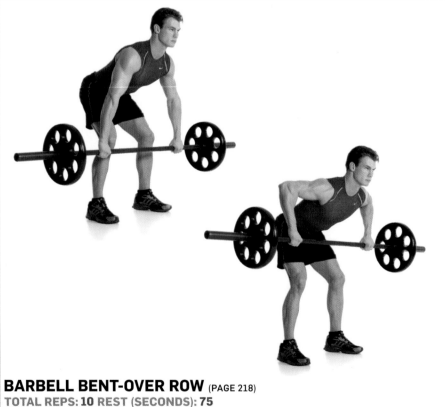

BARBELL BENT-OVER ROW (PAGE 218)
TOTAL REPS: 10 REST (SECONDS): 75

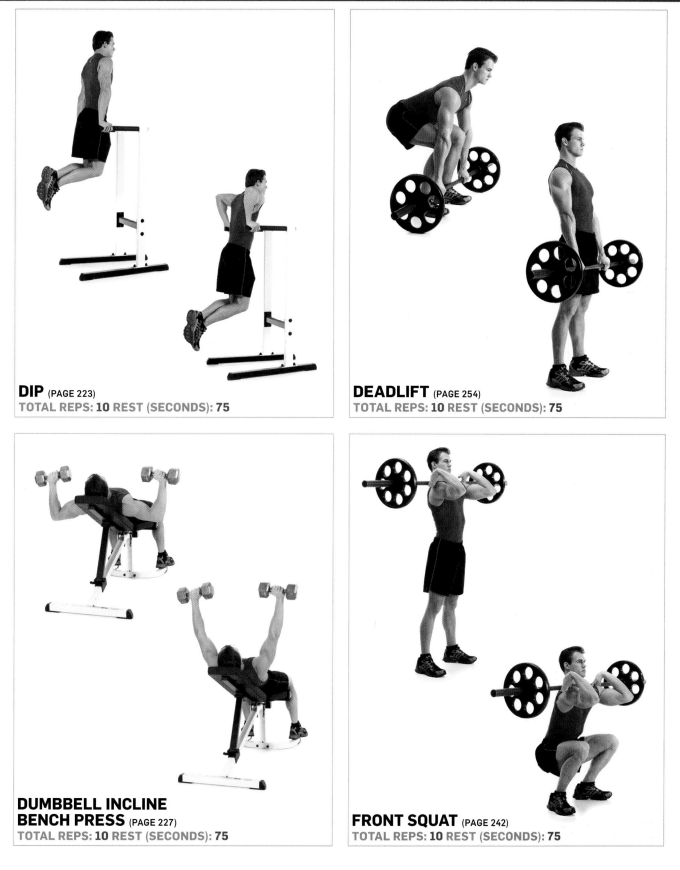

DIP (PAGE 223)
TOTAL REPS: **10** REST (SECONDS): **75**

DEADLIFT (PAGE 254)
TOTAL REPS: **10** REST (SECONDS): **75**

**DUMBBELL INCLINE
BENCH PRESS** (PAGE 227)
TOTAL REPS: **10** REST (SECONDS): **75**

FRONT SQUAT (PAGE 242)
TOTAL REPS: **10** REST (SECONDS): **75**

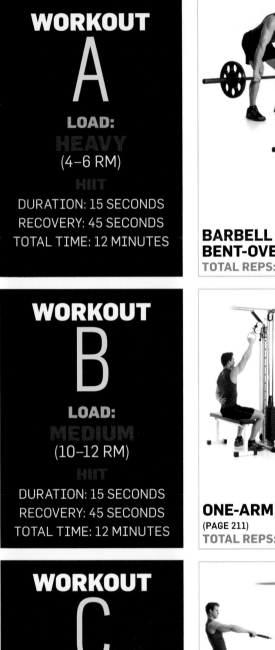

WORKOUT A

LOAD:
HEAVY
(4–6 RM)

HIIT

DURATION: 15 SECONDS
RECOVERY: 45 SECONDS
TOTAL TIME: 12 MINUTES

WORKOUT B

LOAD:
MEDIUM
(10–12 RM)

HIIT

DURATION: 15 SECONDS
RECOVERY: 45 SECONDS
TOTAL TIME: 12 MINUTES

WORKOUT C

LOAD:
LIGHT
(20–22 RM)

HIIT

DURATION: 15 SECONDS
RECOVERY: 45 SECONDS
TOTAL TIME: 12 MINUTES

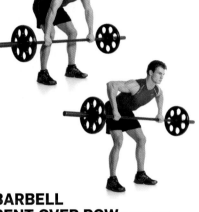

BARBELL BENT-OVER ROW (PAGE 218)
TOTAL REPS: 20 REST (SECONDS): 40

PUSH PRESS (PAGE 237)
TOTAL REPS: 20 REST (SECONDS): 40

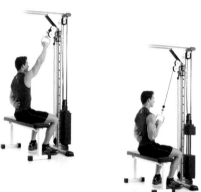

ONE-ARM LAT PULLDOWN*
(PAGE 211)
TOTAL REPS: 35 REST (SECONDS): 55

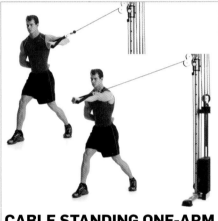

CABLE STANDING ONE-ARM CHEST PRESS* (PAGE 230)
TOTAL REPS: 35 REST (SECONDS): 55

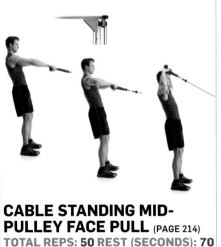

CABLE STANDING MID-PULLEY FACE PULL (PAGE 214)
TOTAL REPS: 50 REST (SECONDS): 70

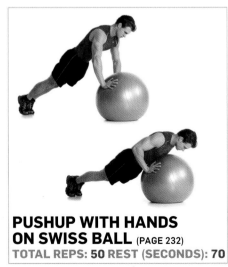

PUSHUP WITH HANDS ON SWISS BALL (PAGE 232)
TOTAL REPS: 50 REST (SECONDS): 70

Start with your weaker side first, then immediately do the same number of reps with your stronger limb. Rest after working both sides.

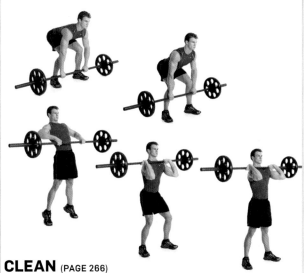

CLEAN (PAGE 266)
TOTAL REPS: **20** REST (SECONDS): **40**

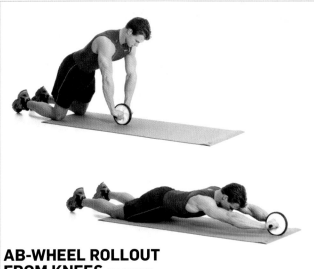

AB-WHEEL ROLLOUT FROM KNEES (PAGE 272)
TOTAL REPS: **20** REST (SECONDS): **40**

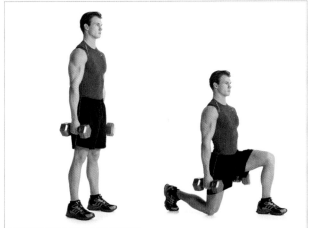

REVERSE LUNGE* (PAGE 250)
TOTAL REPS: **35** REST (SECONDS): **55**

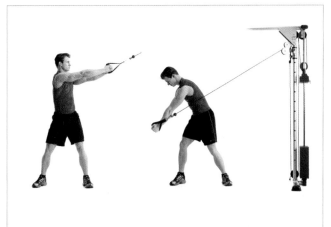

CABLE STANDING WOODCHOP* (PAGE 274)
TOTAL REPS: **35** REST (SECONDS): **55**

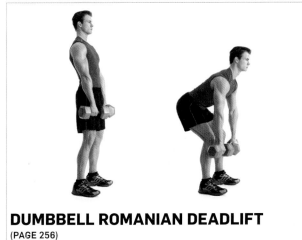

DUMBBELL ROMANIAN DEADLIFT
(PAGE 256)
TOTAL REPS: **50** REST (SECONDS): **70**

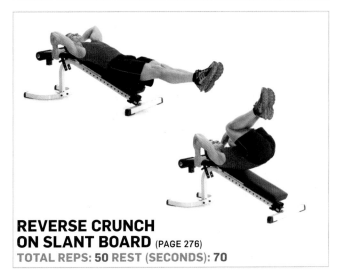

REVERSE CRUNCH ON SLANT BOARD (PAGE 276)
TOTAL REPS: **50** REST (SECONDS): **70**

WORKOUT
A

LOAD:
SUPERHEAVY
(2–3 RM)

HIIT

DURATION: 15 SECONDS
RECOVERY: 45 SECONDS
TOTAL TIME: 18 MINUTES

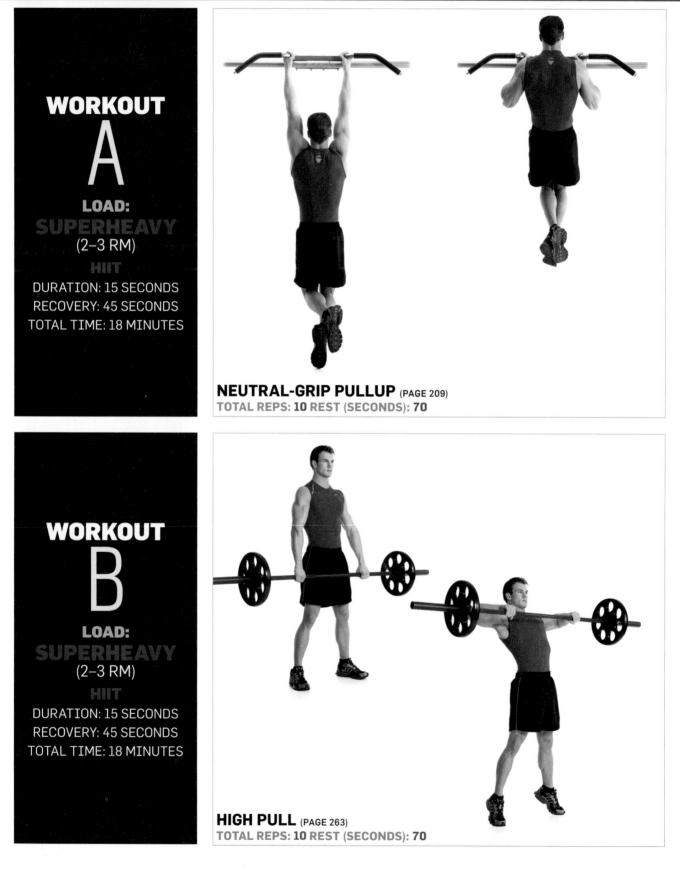

NEUTRAL-GRIP PULLUP (PAGE 209)
TOTAL REPS: 10 REST (SECONDS): 70

WORKOUT
B

LOAD:
SUPERHEAVY
(2–3 RM)

HIIT

DURATION: 15 SECONDS
RECOVERY: 45 SECONDS
TOTAL TIME: 18 MINUTES

HIGH PULL (PAGE 263)
TOTAL REPS: 10 REST (SECONDS): 70

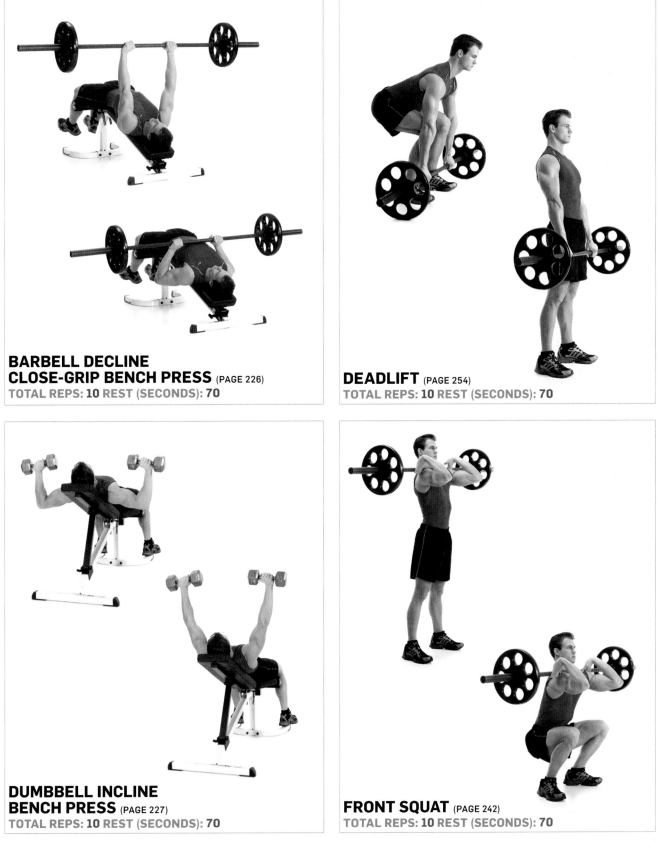

**BARBELL DECLINE
CLOSE-GRIP BENCH PRESS** (PAGE 226)
TOTAL REPS: 10 REST (SECONDS): 70

DEADLIFT (PAGE 254)
TOTAL REPS: 10 REST (SECONDS): 70

**DUMBBELL INCLINE
BENCH PRESS** (PAGE 227)
TOTAL REPS: 10 REST (SECONDS): 70

FRONT SQUAT (PAGE 242)
TOTAL REPS: 10 REST (SECONDS): 70

WORKOUT A

LOAD:
HEAVY
(4–6 RM)
HIIT
DURATION: 15 SECONDS
RECOVERY: 45 SECONDS
TOTAL TIME: 14 MINUTES

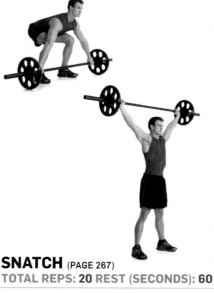
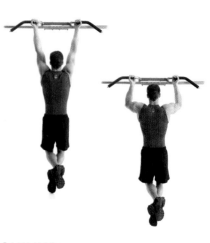

SNATCH (PAGE 267)
TOTAL REPS: 20 REST (SECONDS): 60

CHINUP (PAGE 207)
TOTAL REPS: 20 REST (SECONDS): 35

WORKOUT B

LOAD:
MEDIUM
(10–12 RM)
HIIT
DURATION: 15 SECONDS
RECOVERY: 45 SECONDS
TOTAL TIME: 14 MINUTES

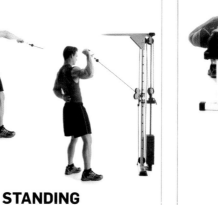
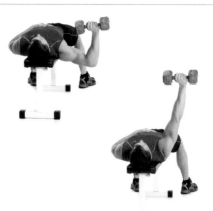

CABLE STANDING ONE-ARM MID-PULLEY FACE PULL* (PAGE 215)
TOTAL REPS: 35 REST (SECONDS): 50

DUMBBELL ONE-ARM BENCH PRESS* (PAGE 228)
TOTAL REPS: 35 REST (SECONDS): 50

WORKOUT C

LOAD:
LIGHT
(20–22 RM)
HIIT
DURATION: 15 SECONDS
RECOVERY: 45 SECONDS
TOTAL TIME: 14 MINUTES

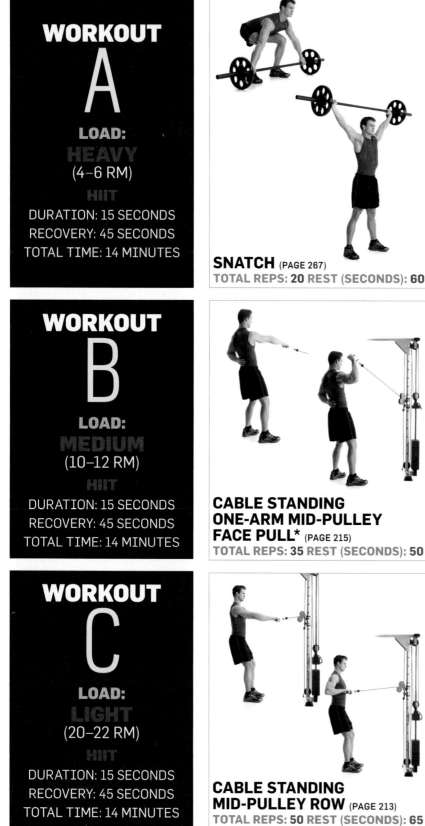
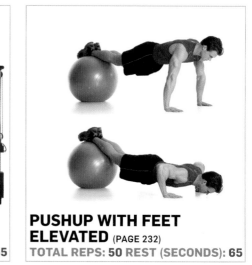

CABLE STANDING MID-PULLEY ROW (PAGE 213)
TOTAL REPS: 50 REST (SECONDS): 65

PUSHUP WITH FEET ELEVATED (PAGE 232)
TOTAL REPS: 50 REST (SECONDS): 65

*Start with your weaker side first, then immediately do the same number of reps with your stronger limb. Rest after working both sides.

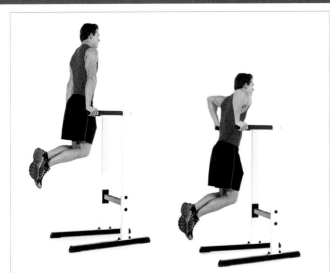

DIP (PAGE 223)
TOTAL REPS: **20** REST (SECONDS): **35**

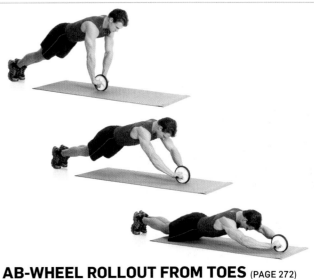

AB-WHEEL ROLLOUT FROM TOES (PAGE 272)
TOTAL REPS: **20** REST (SECONDS): **35**

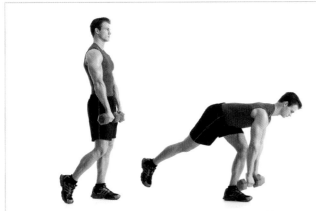

DUMBBELL SINGLE-LEG DEADLIFT*
(PAGE 257)
TOTAL REPS: **35** REST (SECONDS): **50**

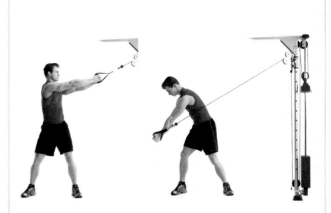

CABLE STANDING WOODCHOP* (PAGE 274)
TOTAL REPS: **35** REST (SECONDS): **50**

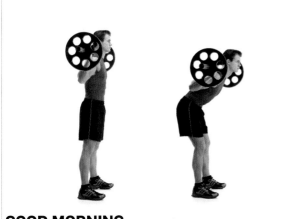

GOOD MORNING (PAGE 258)
TOTAL REPS: **50** REST (SECONDS): **65**

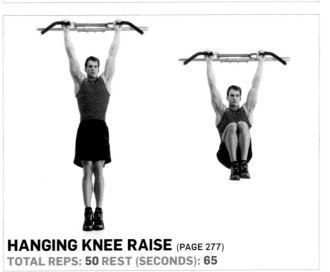

HANGING KNEE RAISE (PAGE 277)
TOTAL REPS: **50** REST (SECONDS): **65**

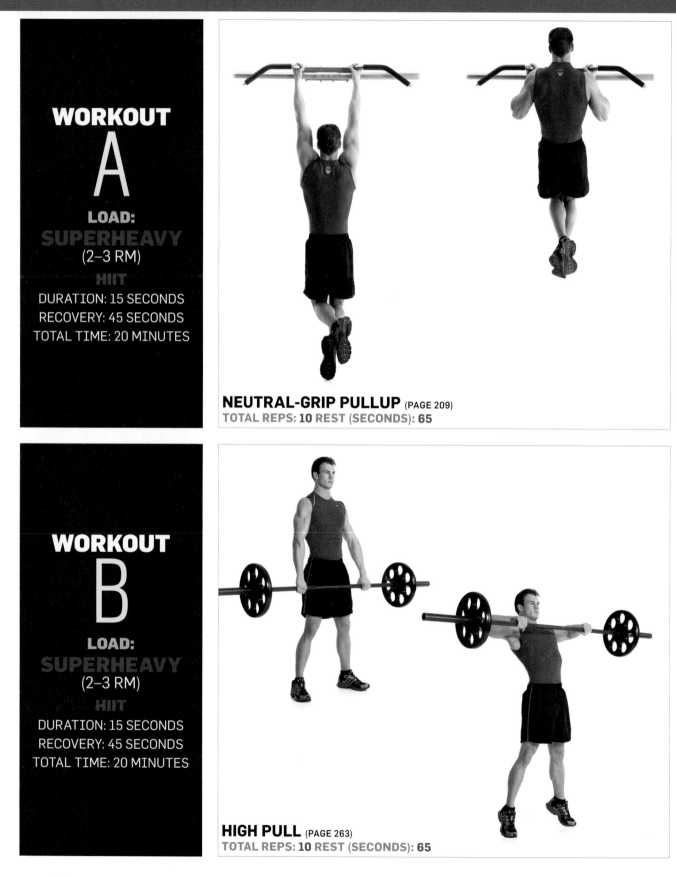

WORKOUT

A

LOAD:
SUPERHEAVY
(2–3 RM)

HIIT
DURATION: 15 SECONDS
RECOVERY: 45 SECONDS
TOTAL TIME: 20 MINUTES

NEUTRAL-GRIP PULLUP (PAGE 209)
TOTAL REPS: **10** REST (SECONDS): **65**

WORKOUT

B

LOAD:
SUPERHEAVY
(2–3 RM)

HIIT
DURATION: 15 SECONDS
RECOVERY: 45 SECONDS
TOTAL TIME: 20 MINUTES

HIGH PULL (PAGE 263)
TOTAL REPS: **10** REST (SECONDS): **65**

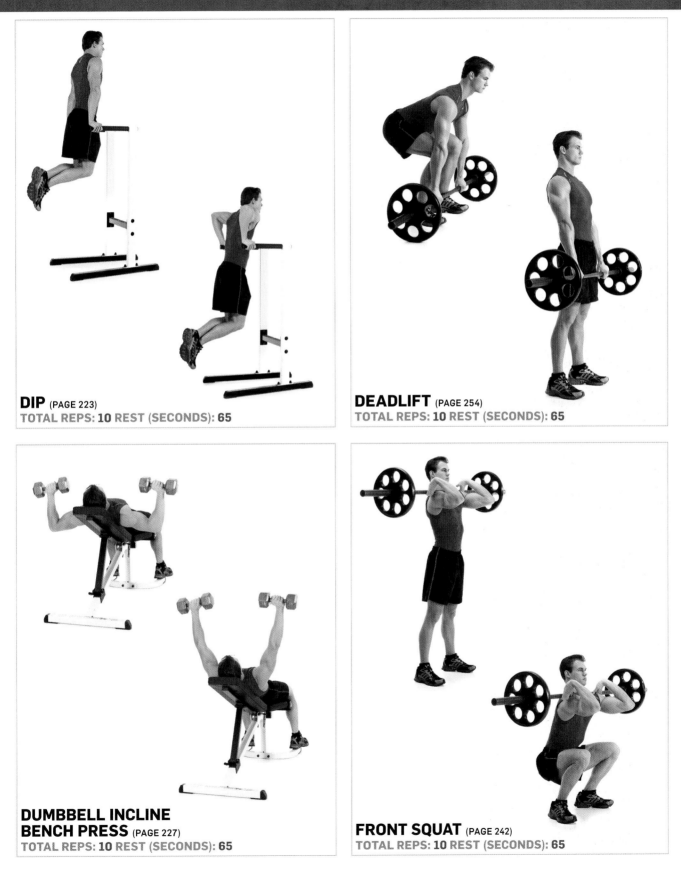

DIP (PAGE 223)
TOTAL REPS: 10 REST (SECONDS): 65

DEADLIFT (PAGE 254)
TOTAL REPS: 10 REST (SECONDS): 65

DUMBBELL INCLINE BENCH PRESS (PAGE 227)
TOTAL REPS: 10 REST (SECONDS): 65

FRONT SQUAT (PAGE 242)
TOTAL REPS: 10 REST (SECONDS): 65

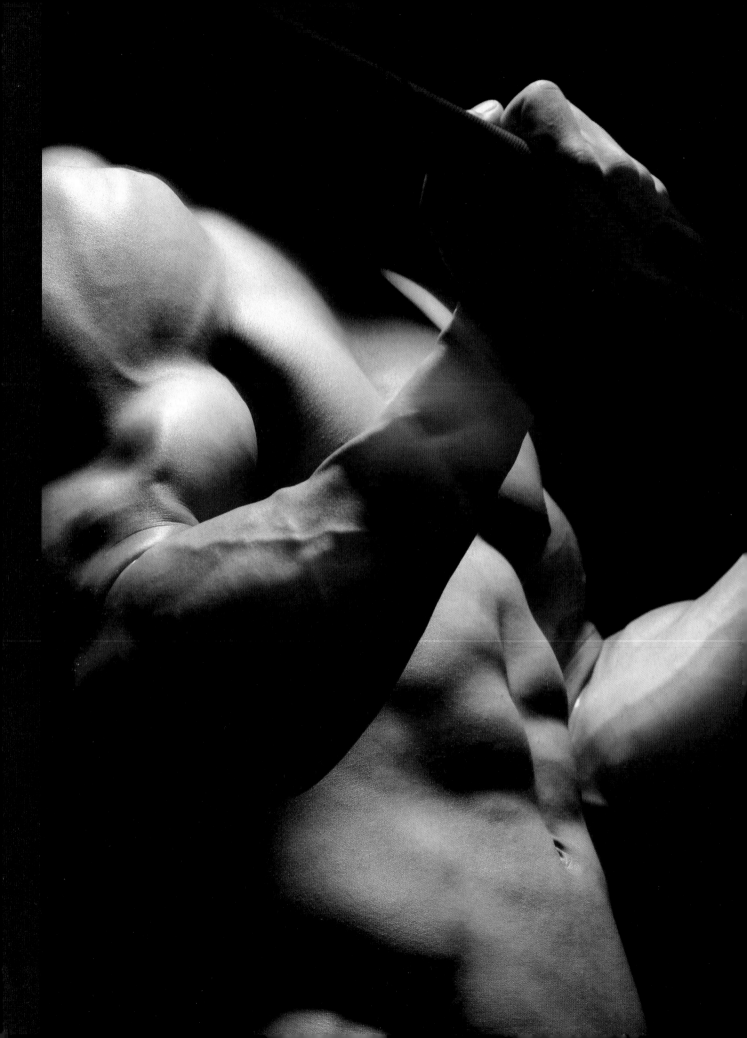

PART 4: THE EXERCISES

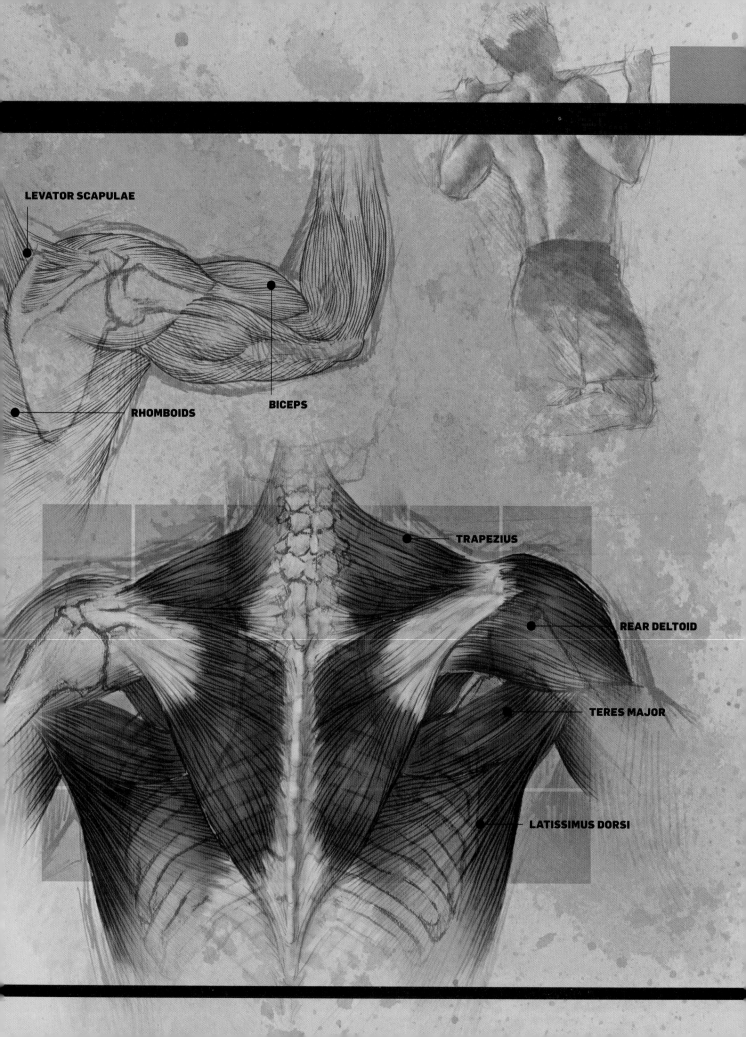

LEVATOR SCAPULAE

RHOMBOIDS

BICEPS

TRAPEZIUS

REAR DELTOID

TERES MAJOR

LATISSIMUS DORSI

CHAPTER 15

UPPER-BODY PULLS

The exercises in this chapter work the muscles that act on three major joints:

SHOULDERS

Your **LATISSIMUS DORSI** are the prime movers for your ball-and-socket shoulder joints when you pull your upper arms down or in toward your body, aided by your **REAR DELTOIDS.** Classic exercises for these muscles include lat pulldowns, pullups, and rows.

SHOULDER BLADES

The diamond-shaped **TRAPEZIUS** muscle starts at the base of your skull, spreads out to the back of your shoulders, then runs down to the middle of your back. The upper part of the muscle pulls your shoulder blades upward, as in shrugs and upright rows. The middle part brings them in toward each other, an important part of rowing exercises. The lower part pulls your shoulder blades down and toward each other, which happens when you do pullups and lat pulldowns. Beneath the traps are your **LEVATOR SCAPULAE** and **RHOMBOIDS**, which assist in most of these actions.

ELBOWS

I don't need to remind anyone reading this book that your **BICEPS** flex your arms at the elbow joints. You probably figured this out in kindergarten. Beneath the biceps is a thick, strong muscle called the **BRACHIALIS**. It works hardest when you pull with a grip that's neutral (your palms facing each other) or overhand. Your biggest forearm muscle, the **BRACHIORADIALIS**, assists your brachialis.

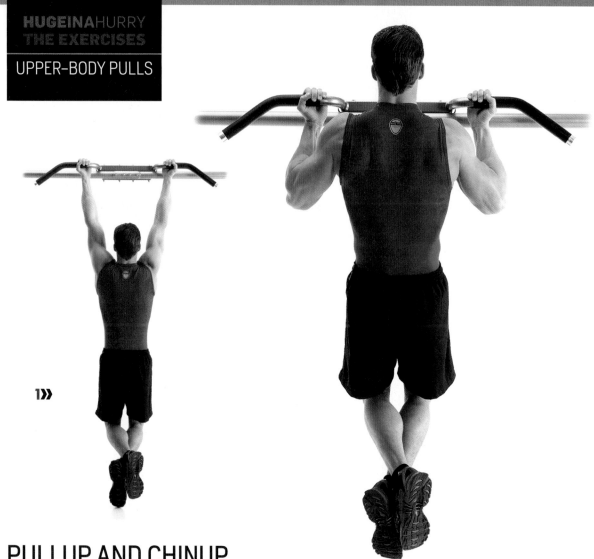

1»

PULLUP AND CHINUP

PREP: You'll need a bar strong enough to hold your weight and high enough to allow a full range of motion; the kind of bar that you twist into a door frame won't work unless you're really short or the door is really tall. You'll start each repetition hanging from the bar with your arms fully extended overhead. You can keep your legs straight, or bend your knees and cross your feet behind you.

If you need to use more weight for low-rep sets, use a chin-dip belt (which looks like a regular weight belt but has a chain in front to which you attach weight plates or a dumbbell), or hold a dumbbell between your feet.

UP: Pull yourself up until your chin is over the bar.

DOWN: Lower yourself to the starting position.

VARIATIONS:

1» CHINUP

WHERE IT IS: Get Big, Phase 1; Get Even Bigger; Get Strong, Phase 1; Get Even Stronger, Phases 1 and 3; Get Lean, Phase 1

HOW TO DO IT: Use a shoulder-width, underhand grip.

WHAT IF I CAN'T DO ENOUGH PULLUPS OR CHINUPS?

With the advent of Universal machines in the 1960s and '70s, the chinup became a forgotten exercise. Even lifters who were strong enough for them opted for lat pulldowns. And, of course, many novice lifters aren't yet strong enough.

If you can't do enough pullups or chinups with your body weight to complete the workouts as written, you have two options: One is to use an assisted-chinup machine, a staple of newer gyms, which allows you to replicate the body-weight exercise. If you have access to one and need to use it, push yourself to reduce the amount of assistance you get from the machine, with the goal of working with your own body weight as soon as possible.

Without access to that machine, you can use an advanced technique called rest-pause, which I describe in Chapter 13. You'll get on the bar and do two or three reps, drop off, catch your breath, then jump back up and do the next. When you've done enough to complete a set (four to six, if the workout calls for "heavy" weights), take the full rest period. After the first set, do as many as you can per set—even if it's just one or two—and then take the designated rest period.

That's only practical if you can do a couple of reps at a time. If you can only do one at a time, you could spend a half-hour trying to reach your target on a single exercise, which isn't a good way to invest your time.

Try this instead: Set up a chair or bench beneath the bar. Grab the bar, and lift your feet off the chair. From a dead hang, do as many reps as you can, even if it's just one. Then lower your feet to the chair, and do the rest of the reps in that set, pushing off with your feet to assist your back and arm muscles. The only way this works is if you use the push-off as little as possible—each rep should feel difficult, as if you're lifting almost all your body weight.

The last and worst option is to use lat pulldowns as substitutes for pullups and chinups, using appropriate weights and grips that match the ones I prescribe. It's still a decent exercise, but not nearly as beneficial to your entire body as the exercises you're replacing.

PULLUP AND CHINUP
(CONTINUED)

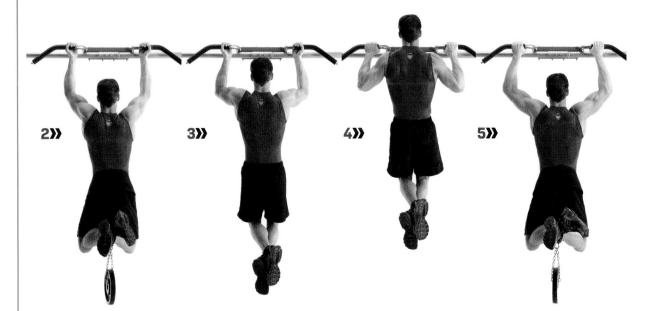

2»

3»

4»

5»

2»
SUPRAMAXIMAL CHINUP

WHERE IT IS: Get Even Stronger, Phase 1

HOW TO DO IT: Use a load that's approximately 20 percent more than your one-rep max. You can add weight with a chin-dip belt, or hold a dumbbell with your feet. Start from the hang position, pull yourself up 2 inches, and hold.

3» FAST PARTIAL CHINUP

WHERE IT IS: Get Even Stronger, Phase 3

HOW TO DO IT: Starting with straight arms, pull yourself halfway up.

4» PULLUP

WHERE IT IS: Get Big, Phase 2; Get Even Bigger, Total-Body HFT; Get Even Stronger, Phase 3

HOW TO DO IT: Use an overhand grip that's narrow—your hands should be slightly less than shoulder-width apart.

5»
SUPRAMAXIMAL PULLUP

WHERE IT IS: Get Even Stronger, Phase 3

HOW TO DO IT: Use a load that's approximately 20 percent more than your one-rep max. Start from the hang position, pull yourself up 2 inches, and hold.

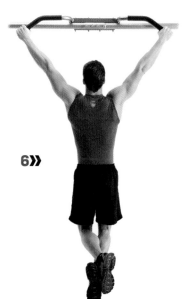

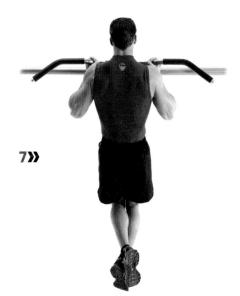

6»

7»

6» WIDE-GRIP PULLUP

WHERE IT IS: Get Strong, Phase 2; Get Even Stronger, Phase 2

HOW TO DO IT: Use an overhand grip that's as wide as comfortably possible.

7» NEUTRAL-GRIP PULLUP

WHERE IT IS: Get Big, Phase 3; Get Even Bigger, HFT for Arms; Get Strong, Phase 3; Get Lean, Phases 1A, 2A, and 3A

HOW TO DO IT: Most gyms will have a pullup station with handles that allow your palms to face each other. If you have multiple neutral-grip choices, select the one that comes closest to shoulder width. If you don't have access to fixed neutral-grip handles, borrow a V bar from the lat-pulldown station (it's shaped like a triangle that's open on one side). Rest the hinge of the V bar lengthwise on a regular chinup bar, with the gripping handles below it on either side. Grab it and alternate your reps so that your head goes above the bar to the left on one rep and to the right on the next.

Caution: If you have to resort to using a V bar, make sure you keep one hand on it at the end of your set. If you let go with both hands, it'll fall off the chinup bar, with a high likelihood of hitting you on the head.

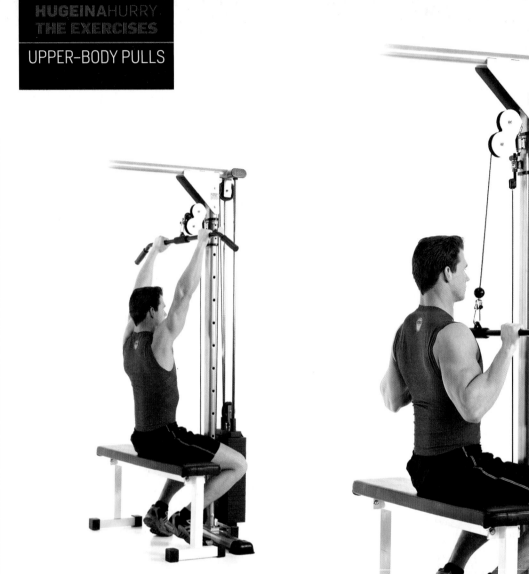

LAT PULLDOWN

WHERE IT IS: Get Big, Phase 1A

PREP: Attach the long, straight bar to the high cable of the lat-pulldown station. Sit on the seat and adjust the knee supports for comfort. (You can also lift the knee supports so they're above your actual knee height, to avoid using them altogether. This adds some challenge to your core muscles.) Now stand, grab the bar overhand with a grip that's just less than shoulder width, and return to the seat.

DOWN: Pull the bar down until it touches your chest. A good self-coaching cue is to imagine you're pushing your chest out to meet the bar. You want to keep your torso vertical and your lower back in its natural arch, but you also want your upper back—the thoracic spine—to arch as you contract your upper-back muscles.

UP: Return the bar to the starting position.

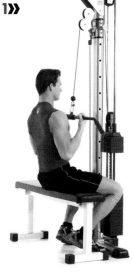

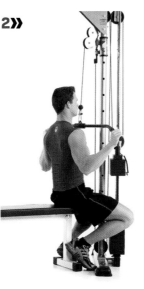

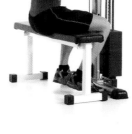

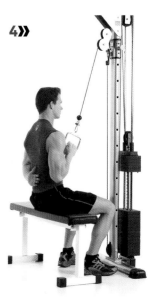

VARIATIONS:

1》 UNDERHAND-GRIP LAT PULLDOWN

WHERE IT IS: Get Ready; Get Big, Phase 3A; Get Even Bigger, HFT for Arms; Get Strong, Phase 1A; Get Even Stronger, Phase 1A

HOW TO DO IT: Grab the bar with an underhand, shoulder-width grip.

2》 WIDE-GRIP LAT PULLDOWN

WHERE IT IS: Get Big, Phase 2A; Get Strong, Phase 2A; Get Even Stronger, Phase 2A

HOW TO DO IT: Grab the bar overhand, with your hands as wide as the bar allows.

3》 NEUTRAL-GRIP LAT PULLDOWN

WHERE IT IS: Get Strong, Phase 3A; Get Even Stronger, Phase 3A

HOW TO DO IT: Use the V-bar attachment (it's shaped like a triangle that's open on one side).

4》 ONE-ARM LAT PULLDOWN

WHERE IT IS: Get Even Bigger, Total-Body HFT; Get Lean, Phase 2

HOW TO DO IT: Attach the D-shaped handle to the cable. Start with your weaker side (usually the left, if you're right-handed), and grab the handle with a neutral grip. Hold your nonworking arm behind your back. Pull the handle down to the outside of your chest, keeping your torso vertical and your elbow in as close as possible to your torso.

CABLE STANDING ROW

PREP: Essentially, there are four categories of standing rows:

>> **Mid-pulley rows, in which you set the cable pulley at chest height**

>> **Low-pulley rows, in which you use the lowest setting on the cable station**

>> **High-pulley rows, in which you use the highest setting**

>> **Face pulls, in which you use a rope attachment (for the standard version) or a D-shaped handle (for the one-arm version) and pull the cable toward your chin before finishing with a movement called external rotation**

It gets a little complicated when gyms have limited equipment options. Some gyms don't have cable machines that allow adjustments to chest height. In those situations, you're limited to low or high settings, and I'd rather you use the low setting, unless the exercise specifies "high-pulley."

In some gyms, the only low cables will be the seated-row station, in which you have to straddle the bench, or the cable-crossover station, where you may not have enough room to stand back far enough to do the exercise without bumping buttocks with a guy who's using the other side of the machine for curls or extensions. If the gym's crowded, it's going to be awkward either way, so choose whichever one is easiest and pisses off fewer people.

You have more options for high-cable standing rows: the lat-pulldown station, the two cables on the crossover station, and the triceps-pushdown station. You'll still be the only one using them for standing rows, but at least you're less likely to make unintentional contact.

Use whatever attachment is specified, with the assigned grip. Stand with your feet about shoulder-width apart, toes pointed forward, with your glutes and abs tight and your head and neck aligned with your back. You want to be back far enough from the weight stack that there's tension in the cable throughout the range of motion, and you want to feel as if you're in a strong, balanced position, with your knees flexed and your lower back in its natural arch.

At the start of each rep, your arms are extended toward the pulley, and your torso is either vertical or leaning back slightly.

UP: Pull the bar to your chest on rows, and the attachment toward your chin on face pulls. (See individual exercise descriptions for specific instructions.)

DOWN: Return to the starting position.

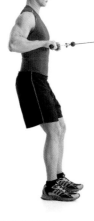

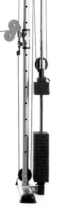

VARIATIONS:

1» CABLE STANDING MID-PULLEY ROW

WHERE IT IS: Get Ready; Get Strong, Phases 1A and 3A; Get Even Stronger, Phases 1A, 3, and 3A; Get Lean, Phase 3

HOW TO DO IT: Attach a straight bar to the cable, and grab the bar with a shoulder-width, palms-down grip. Pull the bar to your chest.

2» CABLE STANDING MID-PULLEY ROW WITH NEUTRAL GRIP

WHERE IT IS: Get Big, Phase 2

HOW TO DO IT: Use a V-bar attachment.

3» CABLE STANDING ONE-ARM MID-PULLEY ROW, ELBOW IN

WHERE IT IS: Get Even Bigger, HFT for Arms and Total-Body HFT; Get Strong, Phase 3

HOW TO DO IT: Attach the D-shaped handle, and grab it with a neutral grip. Keeping your elbow in, pull until your hand reaches the side of your torso.

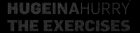
CABLE STANDING ROW
(CONTINUED)

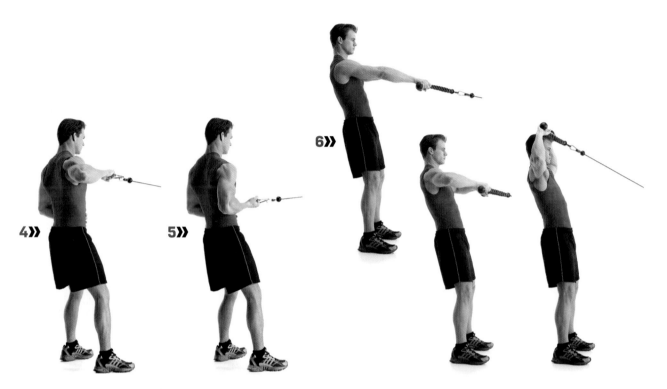

4» CABLE STANDING ONE-ARM MID-PULLEY ROW, ELBOW OUT

WHERE IT IS: Get Strong, Phase 2; Get Even Stronger, Phase 2A

HOW TO DO IT: Start with your palm facing down, and pull until your hand is in line with your torso, allowing your elbow to flare out to the side.

5» CABLE STANDING ONE-ARM MID-PULLEY ROW, PALM UP

WHERE IT IS: Get Big, Phases 2 and 3; Get Even Bigger, HFT for Arms

HOW TO DO IT: Same as "elbow in," except your palm is facing up.

6» CABLE STANDING MID-PULLEY FACE PULL

WHERE IT IS: Get Big, Phases 1A, 2A, and 3A; Get Even Bigger, HFT for Arms and Total-Body HFT; Get Strong, Phases 1A, 2A, and 3; Get Even Stronger, Phases 1A, 2A, and 3; Get Lean, Phase 2

HOW TO DO IT: Use a rope attachment, and grab the ends with overhand grips. Pull the rope toward your chin, keeping your palms down and elbows up. When your upper arms reach the plane of your torso, externally rotate your upper arms: that is, without lifting your arms any higher or moving them backward, rotate your upper-arm bones until your forearms are perpendicular to the floor. Reverse that motion as you return to the starting position.

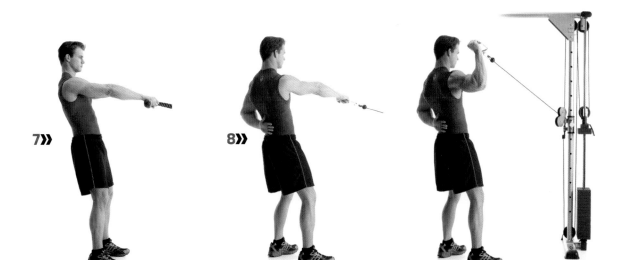

7›› FAST PARTIAL CABLE STANDING MID-PULLEY FACE PULL

WHERE IT IS: Get Even Stronger, Phase 1

HOW TO DO IT: Use a rope attachment, and grab the ends with overhand grips. Starting with straight arms, pull halfway; your elbows won't reach the point at which they're bent 90 degrees.

8›› CABLE STANDING ONE-ARM MID-PULLEY FACE PULL

WHERE IT IS: Get Lean, Phase 3

HOW TO DO IT: Attach the D-shaped handle, and grab it with your palm down. Your nonworking arm should be behind your back. Pull the handle toward your chin, with your palm down and elbow up. When your upper arm reaches the plane of your torso, externally rotate until your forearm is perpendicular to the floor.

CABLE STANDING ROW
(CONTINUED)

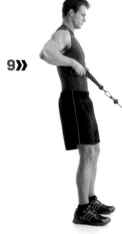

9》

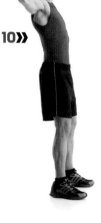

10》

11》

9》 CABLE STANDING LOW-PULLEY ROW WITH ROPE ATTACHMENT

WHERE IT IS: Get Ready

HOW TO DO IT: Attach the rope to the pulley and adjust it to the lowest setting. (If you're using the seated-row station, you don't have to worry about the setting.) Grab the ends of the rope attachment with your palms facing each other, and pull until your hands touch the sides of your midsection.

10》 CABLE STANDING HIGH-PULLEY FACE PULL

WHERE IT IS: Get Even Stronger, Phase 3A

HOW TO DO IT: Use a rope attachment, and grab the ends with overhand grips. Pull the rope toward your chin, keeping your palms down and elbows up. When your upper arms reach the plane of your torso, externally rotate your upper arms.

11》 FAST PARTIAL CABLE STANDING HIGH-PULLEY ROW WITH V BAR

WHERE IT IS: Get Even Stronger, Phase 2

HOW TO DO IT: Set the pulley to its highest position and attach the V bar. Grab the handles and step back so you're in the shoulder-width stance described earlier, with your arms extended and tension on the cable. Pull until your hands are halfway to your lower chest; your elbows won't reach the point at which

they're bent 90 degrees. (In a full-range-of-motion version of this exercise, which is not featured in any of the *Huge in a Hurry* workout programs, you would pull the V bar all the way to your lower chest.)

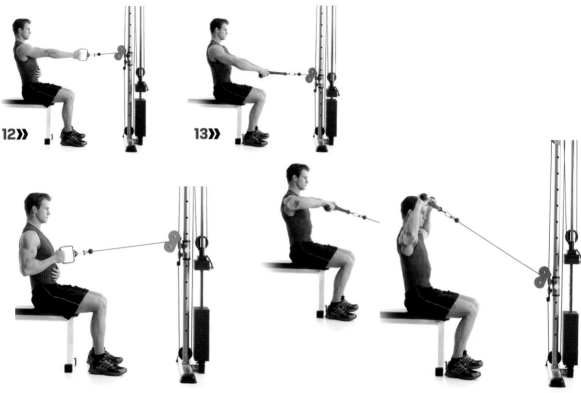

12» CABLE SEATED ONE-ARM ROW WITH NEUTRAL GRIP

WHERE IT IS: Get Big, Phase 1

HOW TO DO IT: Set the pulley at the lowest position (if you have a choice at the seated-row station). Attach the D-shaped handle to the cable. Grab the handle with a neutral grip and sit on the bench with your feet against the supports, knees bent, and torso upright. You want your abs tight, your neck and head aligned with your torso, your working arm straight, and tension in the cable. Place your nonworking arm on your abdomen. Pull until your hand touches the side of your torso, keeping your elbow in.

13» CABLE SEATED FACE PULL

WHERE IT IS: Get Big, Phases 1A, 2A, and 3A; Get Even Bigger, HFT for Arms; Get Strong, Phase 2; Get Even Stronger, Phase 2A; Get Lean, Phase 1

HOW TO DO IT: Set the pulley at the lowest position (if you have a choice at the seated-row station). Attach the rope handles, and grab the ends with your palms down. Sit on the bench with your feet against the supports, knees bent, and torso upright. You want your abs tight and your neck and head aligned with your torso. Your arms should be fully extended in front with tension on the cable. Pull the rope toward your chin, keeping your palms down and elbows up. When your upper arms reach the plane of your torso, externally rotate your upper arms. That is, without lifting your arms any higher, or moving them backwards, rotate your upper-arm bones until your forearms are perpendicular to the floor. Reverse that motion as you return to the starting position.

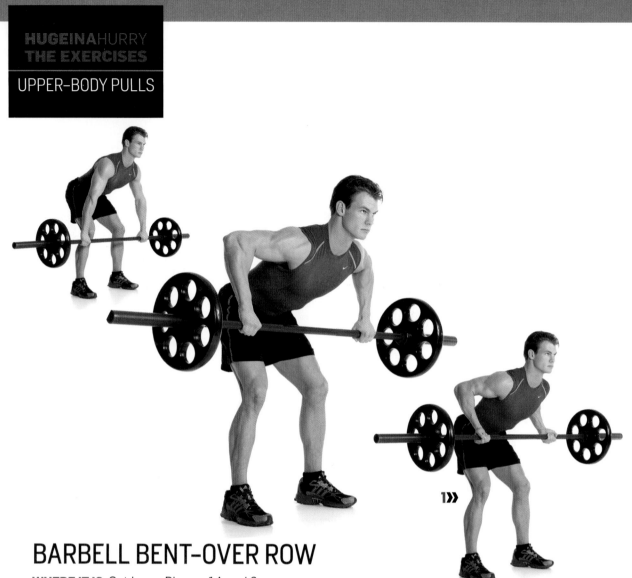

BARBELL BENT-OVER ROW

WHERE IT IS: Get Lean, Phases 1A and 2

PREP: Load a barbell with the appropriate weight. Grab the bar with an overhand grip that's just less than shoulder width. Stand holding the barbell at arm's length in front of your thighs, with your feet about shoulder-width apart. Tighten up your abs and lower back. Now push your hips back, folding your torso forward as if your thighs and torso were two parts of a jackknife and your hips were the hinge. Your knees will bend slightly as your hips shift backward. You want your torso just above parallel to the floor, with the barbell directly below your abdomen, and your neck and head aligned with your back.

UP: Pull the bar up until it touches your abdominals, without moving your legs or torso out of the position described above.

DOWN: Lower the bar to arm's length.

VARIATION:

1》 BARBELL BENT-OVER ROW, PALMS UP

WHERE IT IS: Get Even Bigger, HFT for Arms

HOW TO DO IT: Use a shoulder-width, underhand grip. Everything else is the same.

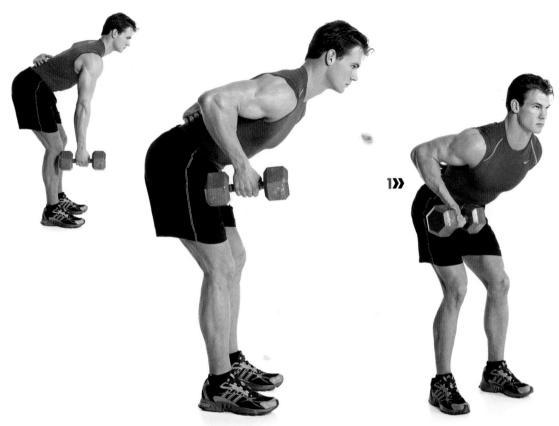

DUMBBELL ONE-ARM BENT-OVER ROW

WHERE IT IS: Get Even Bigger, HFT for Other Muscle Groups; Get Strong, Phase 1; Get Even Stronger, Phase 1; Get Lean, Phase 1

PREP: Grab a dumbbell with your weaker hand (usually your left if you're right-handed), and hold it at arm's length in front of your legs, palm facing in. Place your nonworking arm behind your back. Tighten your core and push your hips back until your torso is at a 45-degree angle to the floor. Your knees will bend slightly. Make sure your neck and head align with your back.

UP: Pull the dumbbell up to the side of your abdomen.

DOWN: Lower the dumbbell to arm's length.

VARIATION:

1» DUMBBELL ONE-ARM BENT-OVER ROW, PALM UP

WHERE IT IS: Get Even Bigger, HFT for Other Muscle Groups, and Total-Body HFT

HOW TO DO IT: Same as above, except with an underhand grip. Pull until the edge of the dumbbell touches the side of your abdomen.

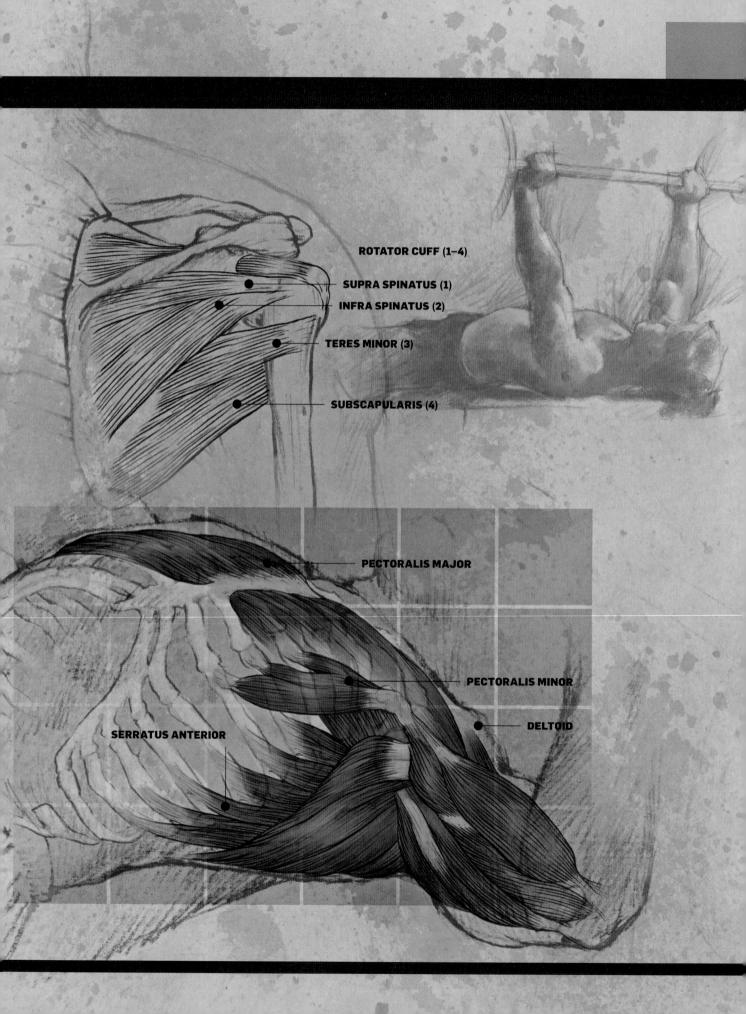

ROTATOR CUFF (1–4)

SUPRA SPINATUS (1)

INFRA SPINATUS (2)

TERES MINOR (3)

SUBSCAPULARIS (4)

PECTORALIS MAJOR

PECTORALIS MINOR

DELTOID

SERRATUS ANTERIOR

CHAPTER 16

UPPER-BODY PUSHES

The exercises in this chapter work muscles that act on three major joints:

SHOULDERS

Your **PECTORALIS MAJOR** pulls your upper arms closer to your torso. So even though the movement is generally described as a "push"—as in pushups, bench presses, or shoving someone in a bar fight—the key action involves your pectoral muscles *pulling* your upper arms horizontally or diagonally toward or across your torso. Your pecs also pull your upper arms down when they're raised behind your torso, as in a dip.

Bodybuilders have bought into the fundamentally ridiculous notion that exercises such as flies and cable crossovers somehow isolate the pecs and thus are necessary to build them. But if you compare the upper-arm movement of crossovers with bench presses, you see they're exactly the same. The only difference is that your elbow joints are in a fixed position in the former and straighten in the latter. To get that "benefit," you do exercises that involve less weight and, in the case of flies using devices like the pec-deck machine, more risk to your shoulders.

Your **DELTOIDS** are responsible for lifting your arms overhead, as in a shoulder press, or up from your sides, as in a lateral raise. The front part of the muscle assists your pecs in their duties on pushups, dips, and bench presses.

SHOULDER BLADES

We don't usually think of our shoulder blades as playing a key role in pushing exercises. But something has to pull and rotate them when you do chest and shoulder presses. Those jobs fall to your **PECTORALIS MINOR,** which is below your pec major, and your **SERRATUS ANTERIOR,** the fingerlike muscles on the sides of your rib cage. I include standing chest presses—with one or both arms—to make sure those muscles get the work they need to keep your shoulders healthy and strong. Pushups and dips also allow unfettered use of those muscles. Just as important is the fact that I deliberately avoid some exercises that don't allow enough movement of the shoulder blades, as I'll explain later in this chapter.

ELBOWS

Your **TRICEPS** straighten your arms at the elbow joints, which is, of course, a key part of exercises such as the pushup, bench press, dip, and shoulder press. Just about everybody who's ever entered a gym is convinced they need to do special elbow-straightening exercises to build their triceps. The main impetus for this belief seems to be the sheer investment gym owners make in triceps-isolating equipment. Every cable apparatus has a dedicated triceps-pushdown station, and benches are typically crowded by people doing triceps kickbacks and extensions with dumbbells or EZ-curl bars. But the notion is as flawed as the idea that pecs need to be isolated with special exercises that don't involve the elbow joint. Do your chest presses, shoulder presses, and dips with serious weights and you won't have to think twice about isolation exercises for your pecs or your triceps.

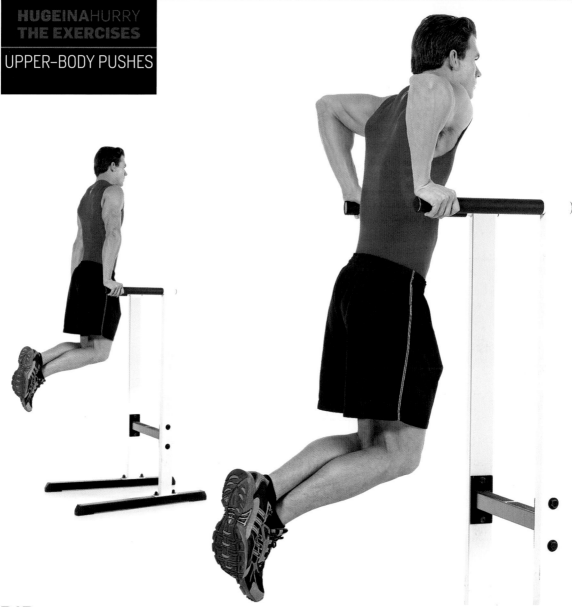

DIP

WHERE IT IS: Get Ready; Get Big, Phases 2 and 3; Get Even Bigger, HFT for Arms, Total-Body HFT; Get Strong, Phase 3; Get Even Stronger, Phases 2 and 3; Get Lean, Phases 1, 1A, 3, and 3

PREP: First you have to locate the dip station in your gym. Many gyms, if not most, keep it well-hidden. Sometimes you'll find a stand-alone dip station. Other times it's part of a device called the "captain's chair" that is used for an ab exercise resembling the hanging leg raise. Newer gyms have a machine for assisted dips and pullups that allows you to work with less than your body weight.

It's unlikely, though, that you'll need assistance on dips—most of you reading this should be able to use your body weight for the number of reps specified. More likely, you'll need to add resistance. For that you'll need a chin-dip belt, described in the previous chapter.

If you have a choice of several dip bars, you'll probably want to use the set that's narrower. Doing dips with a wider grip could put more stress on your shoulder joints. But this is completely up to you. The best choice is the one that feels best. No exercise should hurt while you're performing it.

DIP
(CONTINUED)

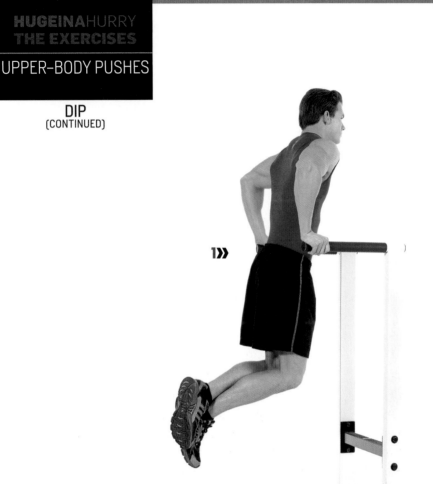

1»

DIP (CONTINUED)

Hop up on the bars and set yourself with your arms straight and torso leaning forward slightly. You can work with straight legs or with your ankles crossed behind you with knees bent. (The latter is probably a better choice if you're adding resistance with a chin-dip belt.)

DOWN: Bend at the elbows and lower yourself as far as your mobility and comfort allow. A good target for most lifters is to descend until your upper arms are parallel to the floor. There's no real benefit to going lower than that, even if you can without discomfort. If you can't go that low, no problem. There's no rule here that everyone has to use the exact same range of motion.

UP: Push back up until your elbows are fully locked.

Caution: Dips are generally safe for your shoulder joints, since they allow free movement of your shoulder blades. But if you've ever had an injury to your acromioclavicular (AC) joint—the place where your collarbone meets the tippy-top of your shoulder blade—you could find the exercise uncomfortable as well as hard to do with any serious resistance. Lots of current and former contact-sport athletes, particularly football players and grapplers, have lingering AC-joint injuries.

The solution is easy enough: Just substitute dumbbell decline bench presses with a neutral grip when the workout calls for dips with a load that would create shoulder-joint discomfort.

VARIATION:

1» FAST PARTIAL DIP

WHERE IT IS: Get Even Stronger, Phase 3

HOW TO DO IT: From lockout, lower yourself halfway.

BENCH PRESS

PREP: One feature of the *Huge in a Hurry* programs that's unique is the lack of traditional barbell bench presses on a flat bench. It's not an oversight. I certainly understand the exercise's appeal and its blunt efficacy, but I think you'll get more out of the variations I use in its place. My biggest concern with the flat barbell press is the restriction of shoulder-blade movement; heavy bench pressing, over time, can change the natural movement patterns of your shoulder blades. Once their movement is dysfunctional, any number of back, neck, and shoulder problems can result.

In my experience, the classic barbell press on a flat bench is an invitation to break all the rules of the program. A lifter's ego is tied up in the amount of weight he can use on the barbell bench press, which leads to overreaching and compromised form, both of which are distractions from his goals. Conversely, nobody's self-esteem hinges on the amount of weight he uses on the decline close-grip bench press. So if I make that the pushing exercise in any particular workout, you're more likely to use the right amount of weight and adhere to the recommended form.

The actual setup is easy enough: Find the appropriate bench (one with uprights for a barbell, or without them for dumbbells) and adjust it to the prescribed position (flat, incline, decline). Load the barbell or grab the dumbbell or dumbbells you need. When working with a barbell and superheavy weights, find a spotter.

If you're using a flat or incline bench, set your body in an athletic position, with your feet shoulder-width apart and flat on the floor. (You'll have to hook your feet behind supports on a decline bench.) You want three points of contact on a flat or incline bench: the back of your head, your shoulder blades, and your glutes. On a decline bench, you'll have those same three points of contact, plus parts of your legs.

Your hand position is determined by the grip required; the specifics are described with those particular exercise variations. On all free-weight chest presses, you'll start with your arms extended and the weights straight up over your chest.

One more complication: Unless you work out in a fully equipped bodybuilding gym, you may not be able to find a decline bench with uprights for bench presses. The solution is easy: Just slip two 25- or 45-pound weight plates under each leg at one end of a flat bench, and you have a decline bench.

DOWN: Lower the weights to your upper abdomen on decline presses, to your lower chest on flat presses, and to your upper chest on incline presses. A barbell has an obvious stopping point (i.e., *you*), while dumbbells should go to the sides of your torso.

UP: Push the weights straight up to the starting position.

BENCH PRESS
(CONTINUED)

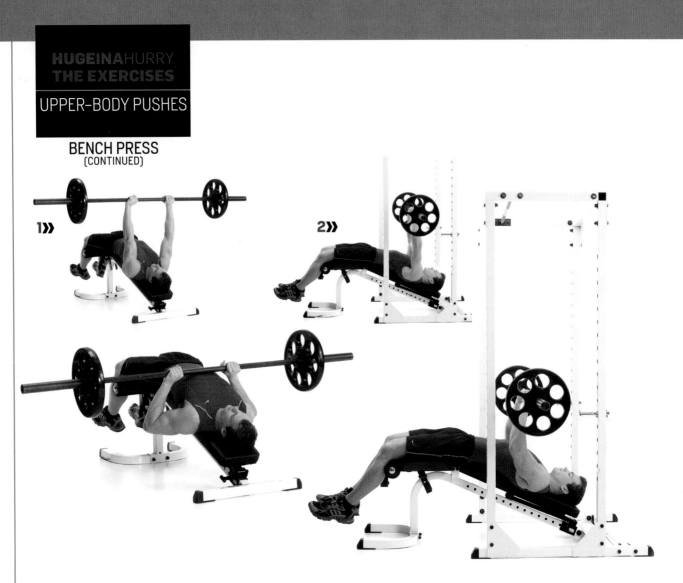

VARIATIONS:

1» BARBELL DECLINE CLOSE-GRIP BENCH PRESS

WHERE IT IS: Get Big, Phase 1; Get Strong, Phases 1 and 2; Get Even Stronger, Phases 1 and 3; Get Lean, Phase 2A

HOW TO DO IT: Find a decline bench or create one as described. Grab the bar with your hands about shoulder-width apart—that means about 10 to 15 inches from thumb to thumb. It's okay to adjust for comfort, but don't go any narrower than that, and don't go all the way out to normal bench-press width, which is about one and a half times the width of your shoulders. Also, make sure you wrap your thumbs around the bar—don't do the "false grip" with your fingers and thumbs on the same side of the bar.

Unrack the load by yourself or with the help of a spotter. Hold the barbell directly over your chest with your arms locked. Lower it to your upper abs, then press back up to the starting position.

2» SUPRAMAXIMAL BARBELL DECLINE CLOSE-GRIP BENCH PRESS

WHERE IT IS: Get Even Stronger, Phases 1 and 3

HOW TO DO IT: Use a load that's approximately 20 percent more than your one-rep max. Lower the barbell 2 inches from the top position, and hold.

3»

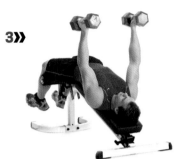

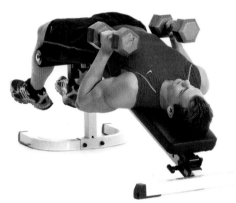

4»

3» DUMBBELL DECLINE BENCH PRESS WITH NEUTRAL GRIP

WHERE IT IS: Get Ready

HOW TO DO IT: Hold the dumbbells over your chest with your arms locked and your palms facing each other. Keep your elbows in toward your torso as you lower the dumbbells until they touch the sides of your midsection.

4» DUMBBELL INCLINE BENCH PRESS

WHERE IT IS: Get Big, Phases 1 and 3; Get Even Bigger, HFT for Arms and Total-Body HFT; Get Strong, Phases 1A, 2A, and 3A; Get Even Stronger, Phases 1A, 2A, and 3A; Get Lean, Phases 1A, 2A, and 3A

HOW TO DO IT: Set the bench to a 45-degree incline. Grab two dumbbells and lie faceup on the bench with your arms extended over your chest and your palms facing forward. Your hands should be about shoulder-width apart at the top. As you lower the weights, your elbows will flare out to your sides. Your hands should stay over your elbows throughout the movement. Lower the weights as far as your shoulder mobility allows.

BENCH PRESS
(CONTINUED)

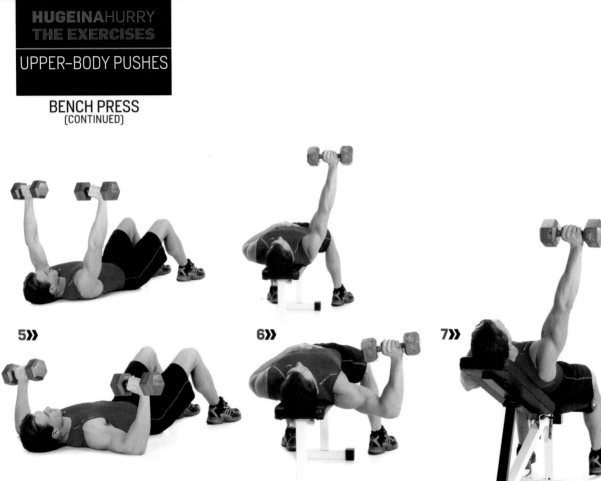

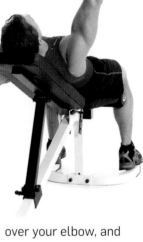

5»

6»

7»

5» DUMBBELL CHEST PRESS ON FLOOR

WHERE IT IS: Get Even Stronger, Phase 3

HOW TO DO IT: Grab two dumbbells and lie faceup on the floor, with your hips and knees bent and feet flat on the floor. (This exercise is often called a "floor press," for obvious reasons.) Start and finish with your hands shoulder-width apart and your palms forward. In the middle, your upper arms will rest on the floor, for reasons that become apparent when you do the workouts in which this variation appears.

6» DUMBBELL ONE-ARM BENCH PRESS

WHERE IT IS: Get Big, Phase 2; Get Even Bigger; Get Lean, Phase 3

HOW TO DO IT: Grab one dumbbell and lie on your back on a flat bench, holding the weight in your weaker or nondominant hand (usually your left if you're right-handed). Hold the weight straight up over your chest with your working arm, palm facing forward. Rest your nonworking hand on your abdomen. For balance, you'll need to spread your feet wider than normal. Lower the weight as far as your mobility allows, keeping your hand over your elbow, and return to the starting position, making sure to straighten your arm fully on each repetition.

7» DUMBBELL ONE-ARM INCLINE BENCH PRESS

WHERE IT IS: Get Strong, Phase 3

HOW TO DO IT: Use a bench inclined to 45 degrees. Otherwise, it's the same as the flat-bench version.

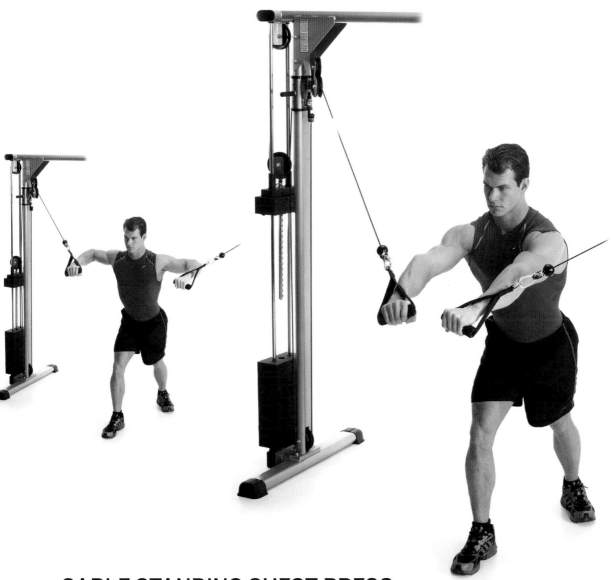

CABLE STANDING CHEST PRESS

WHERE IT IS: Get Big, Phases 1A, 2A, and 3A; Get Even Bigger, HFT for Arms and Total-Body HFT; Get Strong, Phases 1A, 2, and 2A; Get Even Stronger, Phases 1A and 2A; Get Lean, Phase 1

PREP: You'll need the cable-crossover station and two D-shaped handles. If the pulleys are fully adjustable (rather than limiting you to a choice of either high or low), set them at shoulder height. Grab one handle with each hand and pull them to the sides of your chest. Stand between the stacks, and split your stance (one leg ahead of the other). Lean forward slightly, with a tight core and your neck and head in line with your back. Now adjust your starting position so that your elbows are bent 90 degrees and your upper arms are parallel to the floor. You want tension in the cables at the starting point, so you may need to adjust your stance forward a bit to achieve that.

UP: Press the handles straight out in front of you so they come together as your elbows lock out.

DOWN: Return to the starting position, using the longest range of motion your shoulder mobility allows.

CABLE STANDING
CHEST PRESS
(CONTINUED)

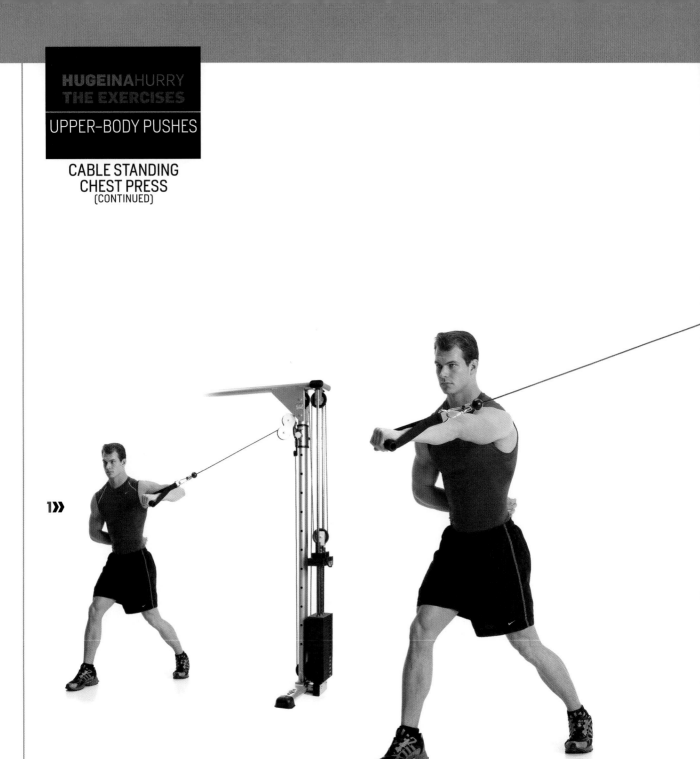

1»

VARIATION:

1» CABLE
STANDING ONE-ARM
CHEST PRESS

WHERE IT IS: Get Big, Phase 3; Get Even Bigger, HFT for Arms and Total-Body HFT; Get Strong, Phase 1; Get Even Stronger, Phases 1 and 2; Get Lean, Phase 2

HOW TO DO IT: Same as for standard cable standing chest press, starting with your weaker or non-dominant arm. Hold your nonworking arm behind your back.

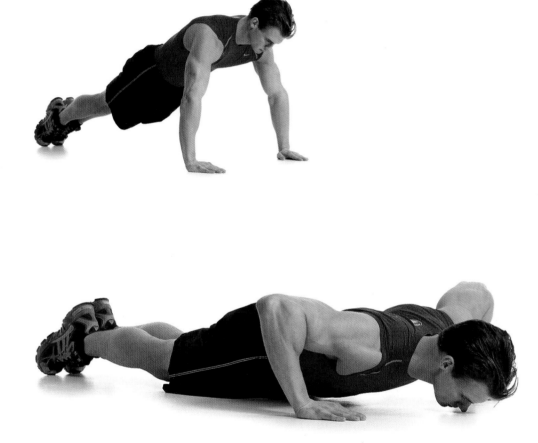

PUSHUP

WHERE IT IS: Get Ready

PREP: Get into classic pushup position: your hands flat on the floor and directly below your shoulders, your weight resting on your hands and toes. Your body should form a straight line from your neck through your ankles. Your abs should be tight.

DOWN: Bend at the elbows and lower yourself until your chest touches the floor, while keeping your body in the exact same alignment.

UP: Push up *past* the starting position, adding an extra inch or two as you pull your shoulder blades apart. That ensures a full range of motion for your pec minor and serratus muscles.

PUSHUP
(CONTINUED)

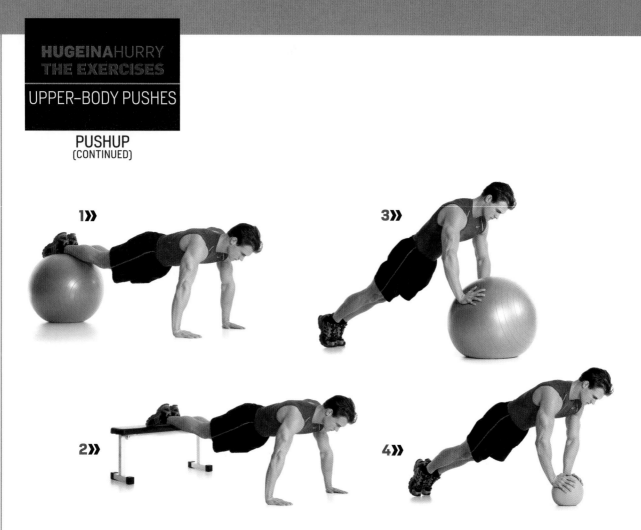

1»

2»

3»

4»

VARIATIONS:

1» PUSHUP WITH FEET ELEVATED

WHERE IT IS: Get Lean, Phase 3

HOW TO DO IT: Same as for standard pushup, except you start with your toes resting on a bench, chair, or ball.

2» PUSHUP WITH WIDE HAND POSITION, FEET ELEVATED

WHERE IT IS: Get Even Bigger, HFT for Other Muscle Groups

HOW TO DO IT: Same as for standard pushup, except your hands are spread beyond shoulder width.

3» PUSHUP WITH HANDS ON SWISS BALL

WHERE IT IS: Get Big, Phases 1A, 2A, and 3A; Get Even Bigger, HFT for Arms and HFT for Other Muscle Groups; Get Strong, Phases 2A and 3A; Get Even Stronger, Phases 2A and 3A; Get Lean, Phase 2

HOW TO DO IT: Same as for standard pushup, except your hands are on a Swiss ball, which adds an element of balance. More muscles in your shoulder girdle and core will work to keep you in place. You can use any Swiss ball you have available, as long as it's fully inflated. If you have several choices, you might want to start with a smaller one and work your way up.

4» PUSHUP WITH HANDS ON MEDICINE BALL

WHERE IT IS: Get Even Bigger, HFT for Arms

HOW TO DO IT: The challenge here varies with the size of the medicine ball. (You can also use a basketball if you're working out at home and don't have a medicine ball handy.) The smaller the ball you use, the closer your hands will be to each other; your thumbs and index

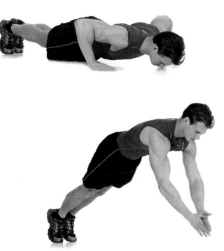

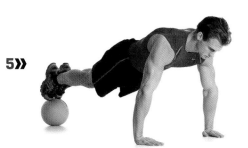

fingers might actually touch with a 3-kilogram ball, while they'll be a couple inches apart on a 5-kilogram ball (depending, of course, on the size of your hands). You want to stay in the standard pushup position, with your body in a straight line from neck to ankles and your core tight. But instead of letting your elbows flare out, you'll keep them tucked in to your sides. So you'll feel more of the work in your triceps and shoulders.

5» PUSHUP WITH FEET ON MEDICINE BALL

WHERE IT IS: Get Even Bigger, HFT for Arms

HOW TO DO IT: It's exactly what you think it is: keeping your feet balanced on a ball, instead of a bench, adds a challenge to your core, as well as to the stabilizing muscles of your shoulder girdle.

6» PUSHUP WITH CLAP

WHERE IT IS: Get Even Bigger, HFT for Other Muscle Groups

HOW TO DO IT: Start with a slight variation on the standard pushup position: Instead of placing your hands directly below your shoulders, set them slightly beyond shoulder width. After you lower your chest to the floor, push up explosively, with enough power to get your hands all the way off the floor. Clap your hands, then land in the starting position and immediately drop down for the next repetition.

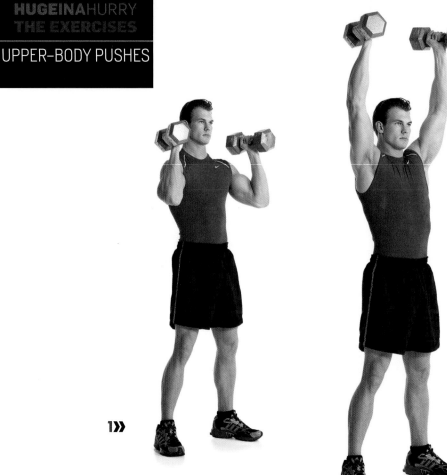

1»

SHOULDER PRESS

PREP: On all shoulder presses—barbell or dumbbell, standing or seated—you start with the bar or dumbbells at shoulder level, with your feet shoulder-width apart, legs straight but not locked at the knees, and your core muscles tight. Most of us think of this as a "shoulder" exercise (understandable, considering the name), but in reality it involves almost all your muscles.

UP: Push the weight straight up from your shoulders, locking your elbows at the top. Do not cheat yourself by shortening your range at the top of the movement; shoulder presses are great triceps-building exercises, as long as you straighten your arms on each rep.

DOWN: Lower the bar until it touches the top of your chest, or the dumbbells until they touch the edges of your shoulders.

VARIATIONS:

1» DUMBBELL STANDING SHOULDER PRESS

WHERE IT IS: Get Ready; Get Big, Phases 1A, 2, 2A, and 3A; Get Even Bigger, HFT for Arms; Get Strong, Phases 1, 1A and 3A; Get Even Stronger, Phases 1A and3A

HOW TO DO IT: Stand holding dumbbells at the edges of your shoulders with your palms facing each other. This neutral grip opens up your shoulder joints and allows you to work more productively with heavier weights. Press the weights straight up from your shoulders—there's no need to bring them together overhead—until your elbows lock out, then lower them to the edges of your shoulders.

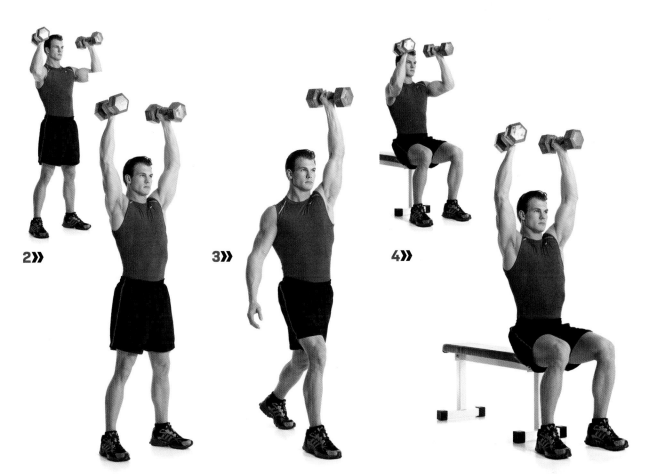

2» FAST PARTIAL DUMBBELL STANDING SHOULDER PRESS

WHERE IT IS: Get Even Stronger, Phase 2

HOW TO DO IT: Lower the weights from lockout to the top of your head, and do your reps from there.

3» DUMBBELL STANDING ONE-ARM SHOULDER PRESS

WHERE IT IS: Get Big, Phase 1; Get Even Bigger, HFT for Arms and Total-Body HFT; Get Strong, Phase 2; Get Lean, Phase 1

HOW TO DO IT: Hold the dumbbell with your weaker or non-dominant hand (usually your left if you're right-handed) at the edge of your corresponding shoulder, palm facing in. Your nonworking arm should be at your side. With heavier loads, it's a good idea to split your stance, with your right leg in front if you're pressing with your left arm, and vice versa.

4» FAST PARTIAL DUMBBELL SEATED SHOULDER PRESS

WHERE IT IS: Get Even Stronger, Phase 1

HOW TO DO IT: Sit upright on a flat bench with your feet flat on the floor. Lower the weights from lockout to the top of your head, and do your reps from there. The exercise is the same as the standing version; your challenge is to keep your torso and shoulder girdle tight and stable without any help from your lower body.

SHOULDER PRESS
(CONTINUED)

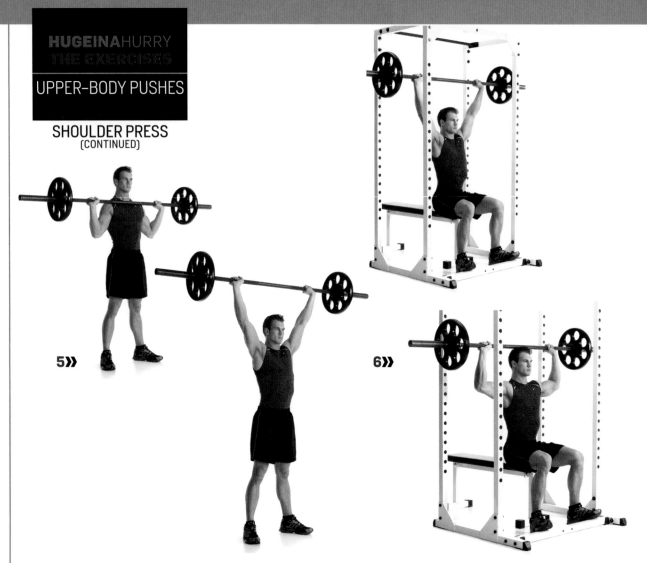

5»

6»

5» BARBELL STANDING SHOULDER PRESS

WHERE IT IS: Get Strong, Phase 3

HOW TO DO IT: Hold the barbell with your hands beyond shoulder-width apart. Press straight up, moving your chin back to avoid contact. Finish with the bar directly over the middle of your head. Reverse the motion on the way down, moving your head just enough to allow the bar to get past.

6» BARBELL SEATED PARTIAL SHOULDER PRESS

WHERE IT IS: Get Even Bigger, HFT for Arms

HOW TO DO IT: You can start with the barbell off the floor by using a squat rack. Maneuver a flat bench (or a flat bench with a vertical back support) in front of the pins, which you set at what will be eye level while you sit on the bench. Place the barbell on the pins and grab it overhand with a shoulder-width grip. Sit on the bench, unrack the bar, and hold it overhead with straight arms. Make sure your core is tight. Lower the bar until it grazes the top of your head (for obvious reasons, you need to lower the bar slowly on this exercise), then push it back up until your arms are straight again.

If you don't want to use the squat rack, you can start with the bar on the floor in front of the bench. Stand and clean the bar to your shoulders, then sit on the bench. (The clean and power clean are described and shown in Chapter 19.) Push the bar overhead, and start the exercise from there.

7>> PUSH PRESS

WHERE IT IS: Get Even Bigger, Total-Body HFT; Get Lean, Phase 2

PREP: Set up as you would for a barbell standing shoulder press.

UP: Instead of pushing the bar straight up, push your hips back so your body descends a few inches. Now use your lower body to generate momentum as you drive the bar upward until your arms are locked out.

DOWN: Reverse the motion as you lower the bar. Instead of stopping at the original position, drop right into the next repetition.

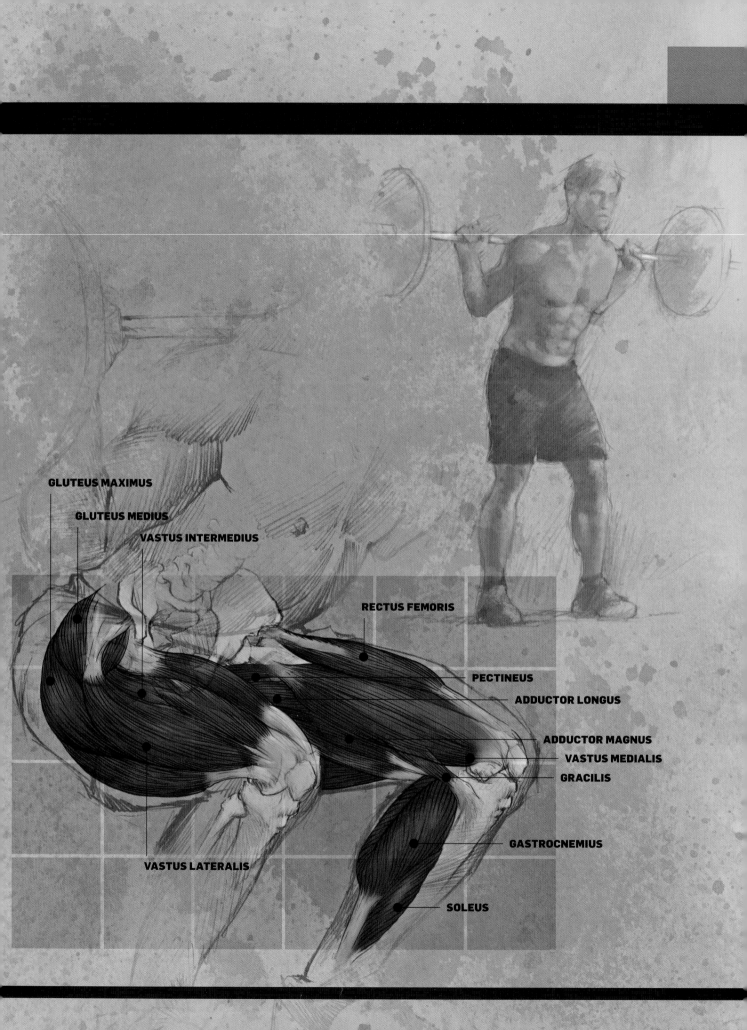

GLUTEUS MAXIMUS

GLUTEUS MEDIUS

VASTUS INTERMEDIUS

RECTUS FEMORIS

PECTINEUS

ADDUCTOR LONGUS

ADDUCTOR MAGNUS

VASTUS MEDIALIS

GRACILIS

GASTROCNEMIUS

VASTUS LATERALIS

SOLEUS

CHAPTER 17

SQUATS AND SQUAT VARIATIONS

Lifting heavy objects from a squat involves just about every muscle in your lower body.

KNEES

Squats are often called a "knee-dominant" or "quad-dominant" exercise. So you'd think that the **QUADRICEPS**, the muscles responsible for straightening your knees when they're bent, would be the main players. You're welcome to test that theory by doing heavy squats and heavy deadlifts in back-to-back workouts (although I certainly wouldn't recommend it). You'd quickly realize, if it weren't already apparent, that the mighty muscles of your hip joints are equal partners in squats, and the muscles in your lower back are fatigued by both exercises.

Which isn't to diminish the importance of your quadriceps, a group made up of the **VASTUS LATERALIS, VASTUS INTERMEDIUS, VASTUS MEDIALIS,** and **RECTUS FEMORIS.** You don't have to worry about the individual contributions of these four muscles in the exercises I describe in this chapter; although they have individual functions (the medialis, for example, helps stabilize your kneecap), they'll grow bigger and stronger as a unit without any special intervention on your part.

HIPS

The force employed by the hip joint comes from the **GLUTEUS MAXIMUS** and **HAMSTRINGS**. On the outside of your hip, the **GLUTEUS MEDIUS** works to maintain stability (along with the **GLUTEUS MINIMUS,** which is directly beneath it and therefore not shown in the illustration on page

238). Similarly, your inner-thigh muscles—**PECTINEUS, ADDUCTOR LONGUS, GRACILIS,** and **ADDUCTOR MAGNUS**—provide strength and stability. The wider your stance on squats and deadlifts (especially sumo deadlifts, described in the next chapter), the more those inner-thigh muscles come into play.

ANKLES

When a lifter switches from machine-based exercises for his lower body—leg presses, extensions, and curls—and starts doing squats instead, he quickly notices that all the muscles of his lower body get bigger, including his calves. No, calves aren't the prime movers in the squat or any of its variations, but they still benefit from being in the line of fire. All lower-body movements—whether you're walking, running, jumping, or rising out of a squat with 225 pounds on your shoulders—start with your big toe. Your calves will get bigger by virtue of the fact they're the conduit between your feet and your knees. In a squat or lunge, there's not a lot of movement in your ankle joints, but your calf muscles still have to support your body weight along with the barbell and whatever plates you've loaded onto it.

You have two main calf muscles: The **GASTROCNEMIUS** is the one on the outside that's shaped like a salmon fillet. Beneath it is the **SOLEUS,** which is flatter and more flounder-shaped.

Bodybuilders like to obsess over their ability to isolate their individual calf muscles, which is a pretty good sign of having too much time on their hands. Functionally, the soleus is more of a postural muscle, working to help keep you upright when you're standing around. (If you've ever wondered why some obese people have calves the size of boiled hams, it's largely because their soleus muscles are forced to do heavy-resistance training every time they stand up.) The gastroc is more responsible for generating lower-leg strength and power.

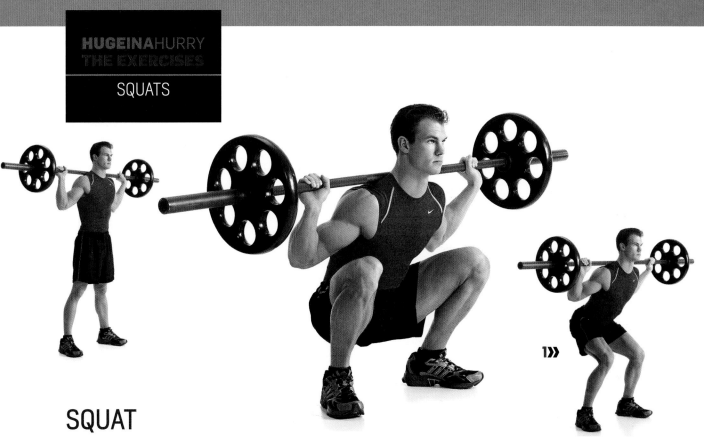

SQUAT

WHERE IT IS: Get Ready; Get Big, Phase 2; Get Strong, Phases 1 and 3; Get Lean, Phase 1

PREP: You'll need to set up in a squat rack (also called a power rack or power cage). Set the barbell on pins just below shoulder height. Duck your head under the bar, and set it on your upper back/lower traps, in the groove at the base of your rear deltoid muscles. Grab the bar overhand at whatever width is comfortable for you (narrower is generally better), and rotate your arms backward, lifting your elbows as high as they'll go and locking the bar into place on your back.

Lift the bar off the pins and take one step back. Set your feet so they're just wider than your shoulders and angled out slightly.

DOWN: Take a deep breath and hold it in your stomach as you push your hips back to start the squat. As you descend, focus on your hips, sitting back as if you're aiming for a chair behind you, and let your knees bend on their own. When they start to bend, try to pull them outward; this activates the outer-hip muscles, which act as stabilizers for your lower back. (It also prevents your knees from buckling inward, which is a weak position for your knees as well as your back.)

Squat down as far as possible while keeping your core tight and your back in its natural arch. A good target is to get your upper thighs parallel to the floor, or slightly below that point.

UP: Press down through your heels and push your upper back up into the bar as you return to the starting position. Exhale when your hips and knees are straight.

VARIATION:

1» QUARTER SQUAT

WHERE IT IS: Get Big, Phase 2A; Get Strong, Phases 1A, 2A, and 3A; Get Even Stronger, Phases 1A, 2A, and 3A

HOW TO DO IT: Do everything the same, except with one-half your normal range of motion.

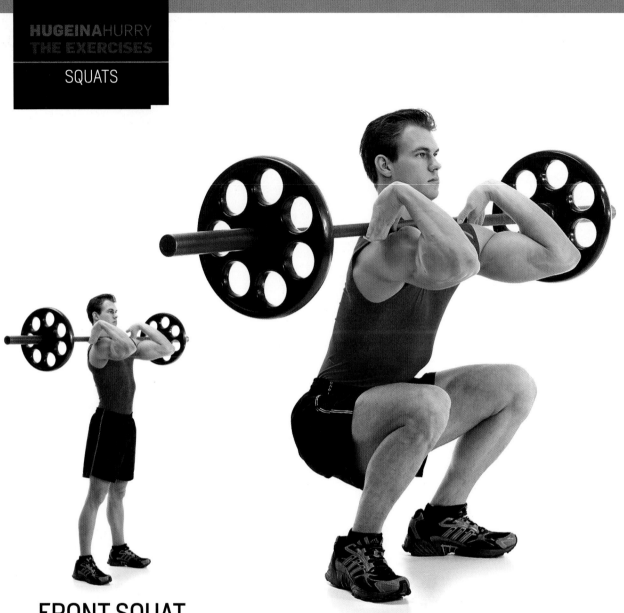

FRONT SQUAT

WHERE IT IS: Get Big, Phases 1 and 3; Get Even Bigger, HFT for Arms and Total-Body HFT; Get Strong, Phase 2; Get Even Stronger, Phase 3; Get Lean, Phases 1A, 2A, and 3A

PREP: Set up the barbell in the squat rack with the pins at chest level. Grab the barbell with a shoulder-width, underhand grip. Walk under the bar, rotating your arms under it so that the bar is on your upper chest and your palms. Your upper arms will be parallel to the floor. Lift the bar off the pins and step back into a shoulder-width stance with your feet pointing straight ahead. Pull your elbows up as high as possible, allowing the barbell to shift back onto your fingers. (If you've never done this before, it will feel awkward the first few times. Don't panic; your wrist and shoulder flexibility will improve over time, making the position feel more natural.)

DOWN: Take a deep breath and hold it as you push your hips back and squat down as far as possible while keeping your core tight and your lower back in its natural arch. You'll be able to keep your torso more vertical than you can with a traditional squat, and thus increase your range of motion.

UP: Return to the starting position and exhale.

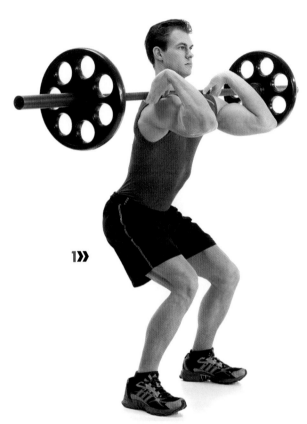

1»

VARIATIONS:

1» FAST PARTIAL FRONT SQUAT

WHERE IT IS: Get Even Stronger, Phase 1

HOW TO DO IT: From lockout, go halfway toward the point at which your upper thighs would be parallel to the floor.

2» SUPRAMAXIMAL FRONT SQUAT

WHERE IT IS: Get Even Stronger, Phase 3

HOW TO DO IT: Use a load that's approximately 20 percent more than your one-rep max. Push your hips back slightly to lower the barbell 3 to 4 inches, and hold.

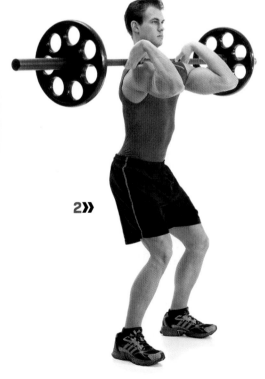

2»

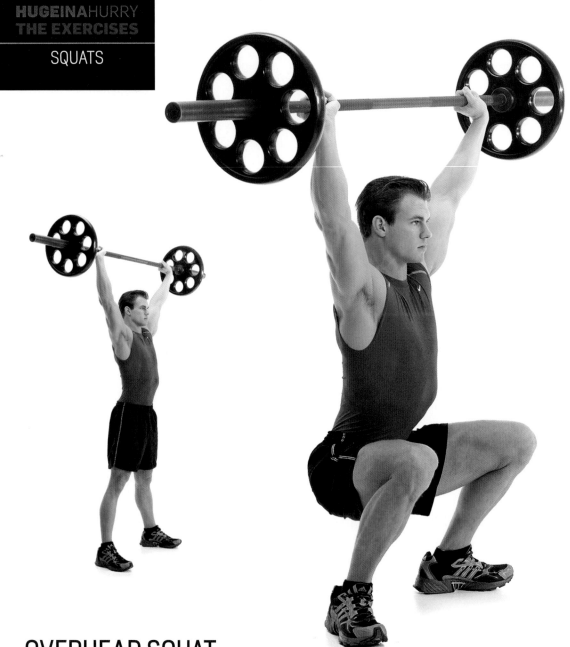

OVERHEAD SQUAT

WHERE IT IS: Get Big, Phase 3, Get Strong, Phase 3; Get Lean, Phase 1

PREP: You've already practiced the unloaded version of this lift in your warmups (if you skipped that part, you'll find it in Chapter 7). Now it's time to advance to the serious version. Set up a barbell in the squat rack with the pins at shoulder height. Grab the barbell with a very wide grip, and press it overhead until your arms are straight. Step back into a stance that's beyond shoulder width, with your feet angled out.

DOWN: Take a deep breath and hold it as you push your hips back, keeping your chest up and your core as tight as possible. Squat down as far as your mobility allows while holding the bar overhead, or just behind your head, with your arms locked.

UP: Stand up to the starting position and exhale.

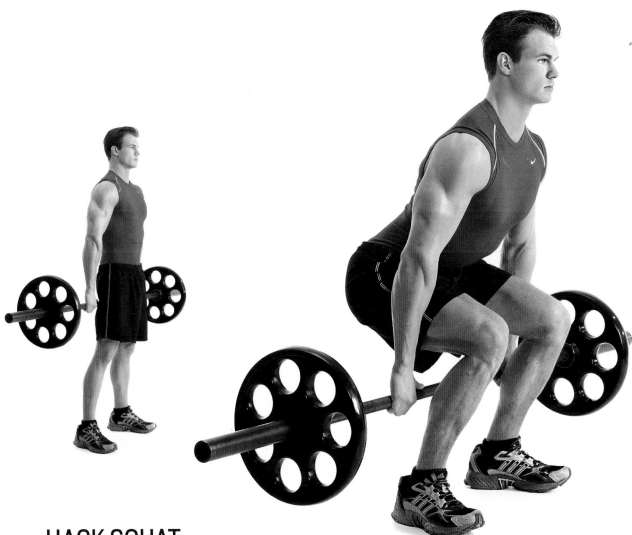

HACK SQUAT

WHERE IT IS: Get Big, Phase 2; Get Even Bigger, Total-Body HFT

PREP: Set the barbell in the squat rack on pins at mid-thigh level. Stand with your back to the barbell, squat down slightly, and grab the barbell underhand with a shoulder-width grip. Stand up with the barbell held behind you.

DOWN: Suck air into your stomach, hold your breath, then push your hips back and squat down until the barbell touches your calves. Keep your core tight and your torso as vertical as possible.

UP: Return to the starting position and exhale.

Quick tip: If you have short legs, the weights may hit the floor before the bar hits your calves. You can increase your range of motion by loading the barbell with smaller plates—25-pounders instead of 45s.

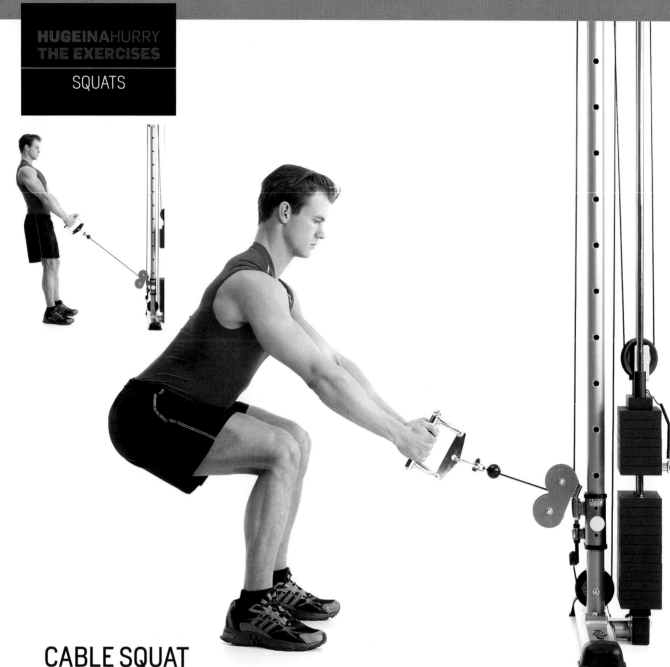

CABLE SQUAT

WHERE IT IS: Get Big, Phases 1A and 3A; Get Even Bigger, HFT for Arms; Get Strong, Phases 1A and 2A; Get Even Stronger, Phases 1A, 2A, and 3

PREP: Set a cable pulley on its lowest position and attach a straight bar, V handle, or rope. Grab the bar, handle, or rope and step back so that your arms are straight and there's tension on the cable. (The cable should be at a 45- to 60-degree angle to the floor.) Stand with your feet just beyond shoulder width, your toes pointing straight ahead. You should be leaning back slightly, both for balance and to keep tension on the cable.

DOWN: Suck air into your stomach, hold your breath, then push your hips back and squat down as far as possible while keeping your arms straight and angled down slightly. Your torso should shift slightly forward as you squat down.

UP: Return to the starting position—that is, upright and leaning back slightly—and exhale.

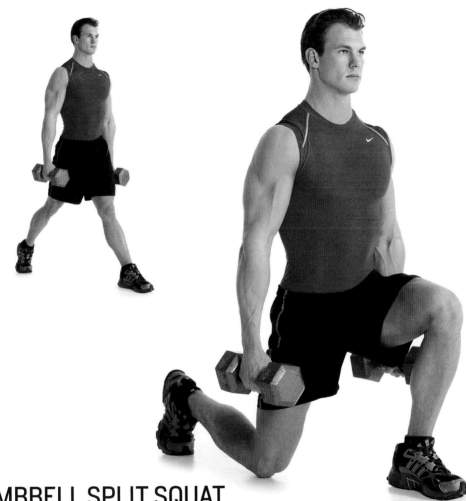

DUMBBELL SPLIT SQUAT

WHERE IT IS: Get Ready

PREP: Stand holding dumbbells at your sides. Take a long step forward with your weaker or non-dominant leg (probably your left, if you're right-handed). Your back leg should be slightly bent at the knee, with your back heel elevated. This is your starting position.

DOWN: Lower yourself until your rear knee grazes the floor, while keeping your torso as upright as possible.

UP: Lift back up to the starting position, and finish all your reps with your nondominant leg before doing the same number of reps with your dominant leg forward.

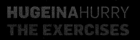
BULGARIAN SPLIT SQUAT

WHERE IT IS: Get Big, Phases 1 and 3; Get Even Bigger, HFT for Arms and Total-Body HFT

PREP: You'll need a pair of dumbbells and a flat bench or chair. Hold the dumbbells at arm's length at your sides, and stand facing away from the bench. Rest the top of your stronger or dominant foot on the bench, and place your other foot as far forward as possible. Your back knee should be slightly bent and your torso as upright as possible. This is the starting position.

DOWN: Squat down as far as you can while keeping your torso upright.

UP: Return to the starting position. Finish all your reps with your nondominant leg before doing the same number of reps with your dominant leg forward.

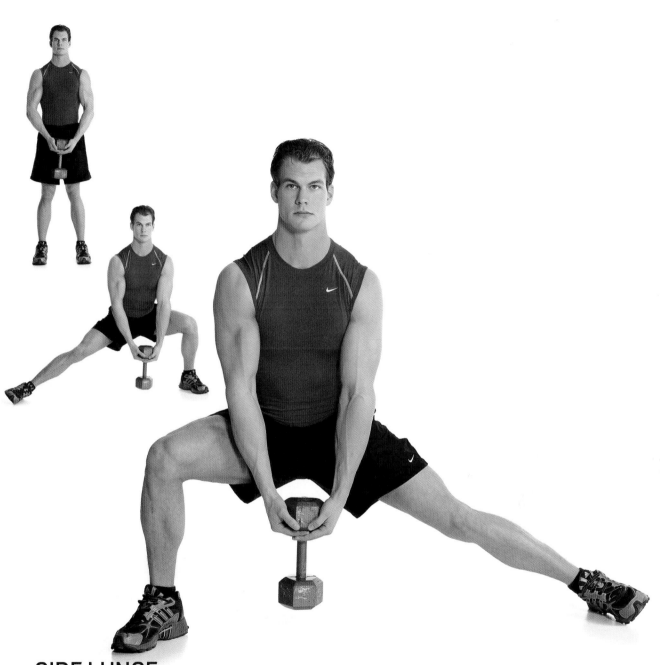

SIDE LUNGE

WHERE IT IS: Get Big, Phases 1A, 2A, and 3A; Get Even Bigger, HFT for Arms

PREP: Grab a single dumbbell or weight plate and hold it with both hands in front of your chest as you stand with your feet shoulder-width apart.

DOWN: Step as far as you can to your weaker or nondominant side, keeping that foot pointing straight ahead. Push your hips back and squat down as far as possible, keeping your bent knee directly over your corresponding foot.

UP: Push through your left heel to return to the starting position, then immediately lunge to your other side. That's one repetition.

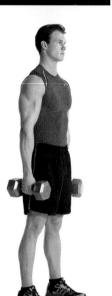

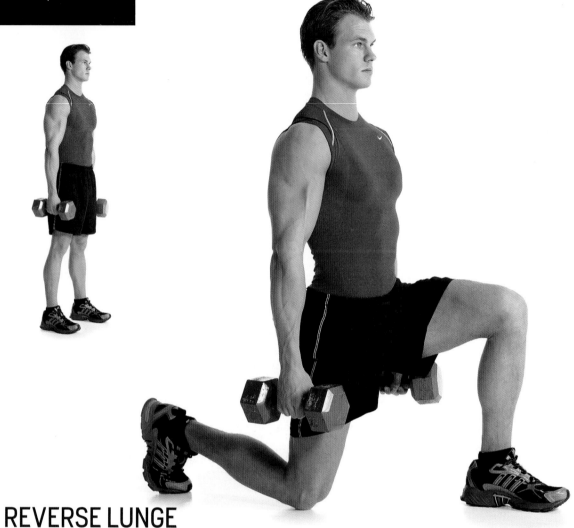

REVERSE LUNGE

WHERE IT IS: Get Even Bigger, HFT for Other Muscle Groups and Total-Body HFT; Get Lean, Phase 2

PREP: Hold a pair of dumbbells at arm's length at your sides as you stand with your feet shoulder-width apart, toes pointing forward.

DOWN: Step back as far as possible with your dominant leg and drop down until that knee grazes the floor, keeping your torso as upright as possible.

UP: Push through your forward heel to return to the starting position, then immediately lunge back with that leg. That's one repetition.

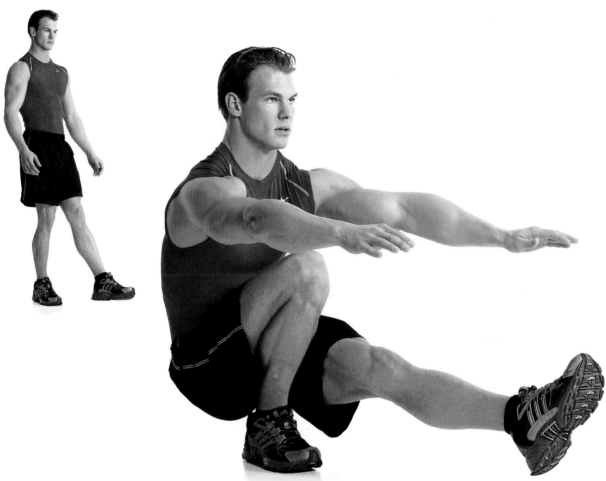

SINGLE-LEG SQUAT

WHERE IT IS: Get Even Bigger, HFT for Other Muscle Groups; Get Strong, Phases 1 and 3; Get Even Stronger, Phases 1 and 2

PREP: Stand with your feet shoulder-width apart. Lift your stronger or dominant leg straight out in front of you, as high as possible. If you need added resistance (and believe me, not many of us do), you have two options:

»Hold a weight plate at chest level with both hands

»Hold a dumbbell in one hand at arm's length (in your left hand while squatting down with your left leg, and vice versa)

DOWN: Suck air into your stomach, then push your hips back and squat down as far as possible while keeping your torso as upright as possible. The heel of your front leg can touch the floor at the bottom of the squat, if you can get down that far.

UP: Return to the starting position and exhale. Do all your reps with your nondominant leg, then repeat with your dominant leg.

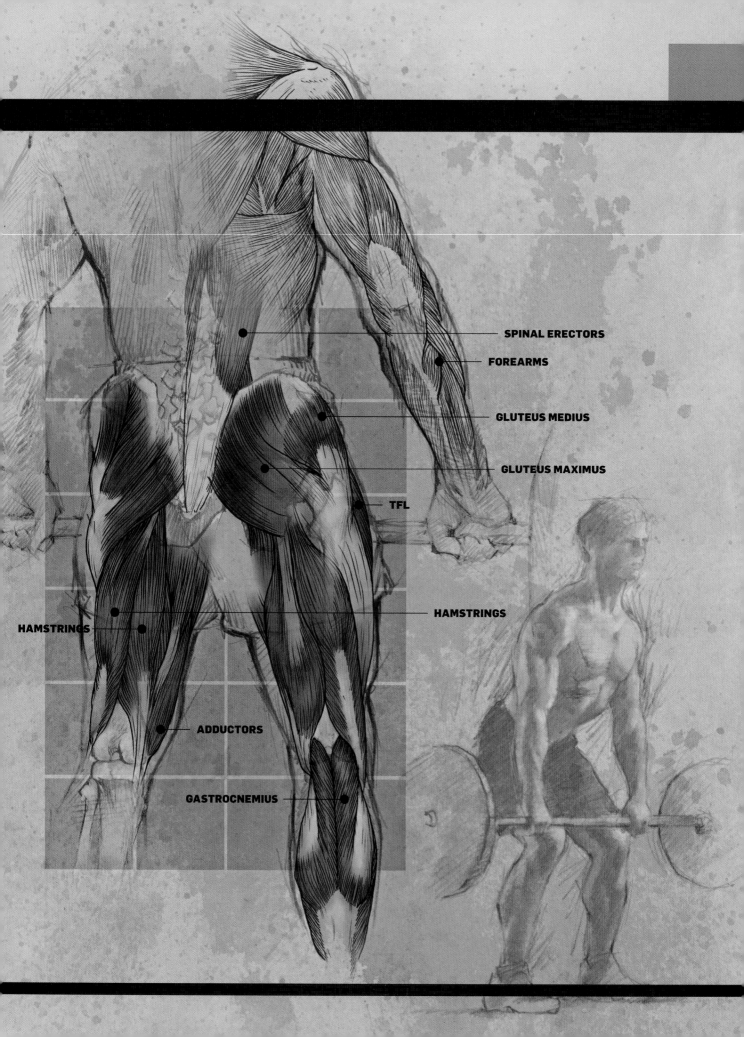

SPINAL ERECTORS

FOREARMS

GLUTEUS MEDIUS

GLUTEUS MAXIMUS

TFL

HAMSTRINGS

HAMSTRINGS

ADDUCTORS

GASTROCNEMIUS

CHAPTER 18

DEADLIFTS AND DEADLIFT VARIATIONS

Most of the force behind exercises in the deadlift category comes from muscles that act on the hip joints. But those muscles aren't the only ones that come into play.

HIPS

Your body's thickest, strongest muscles—the **GLUTEUS MAXIMUS** and **HAMSTRINGS**—are responsible for straightening your body when it's bent at the hips. If you're picking something heavy up off the floor—as in a deadlift—your torso is bent forward. If you're jumping, sprinting, or climbing, your legs are out in front of your torso, and the powerful muscles surrounding your hip joints pull them back to drive your body upward or forward.

SPINE

A network of muscles called the **SPINAL ERECTORS** runs vertically up your back, on either side of your spine. They begin with the connective tissues that come up from your tailbone, and they end in a variety of places on your ribs and vertebrae. Even though you're trying *not* to move any of the joints of your spine when you do deadlifts, the muscles responsible for moving your vertebrae will get much bigger and stronger as you advance through the workouts in this book.

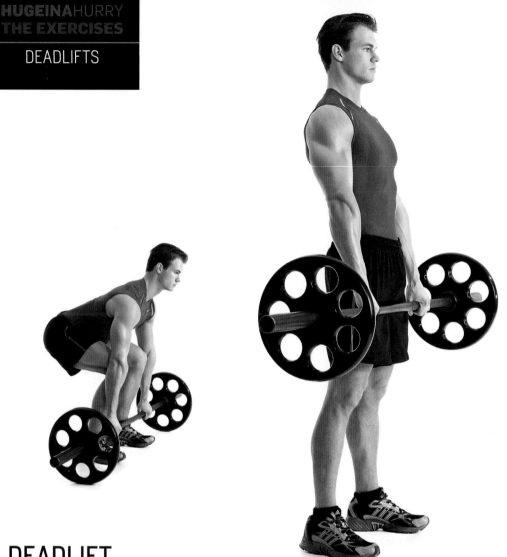

DEADLIFT

WHERE IT IS: Get Ready; Get Big, Phase 1; Get Even Bigger, Total-Body HFT; Get Strong, Phase 1; Get Even Stronger, Phases 1 and 2; Get Lean, Phases 1A, 2A, and 3A

PREP: Load a barbell and set it on the floor. Stand with the bar in front of your shins and your feet shoulder-width apart, toes pointed straight ahead. Squat down and grab the bar with an overhand grip, your hands just outside of your legs. Drop your hips as far as you can with your feet staying flat on the floor. Tighten your core and straighten your back so that your body forms a straight line from your neck to your pelvis. Advanced lifters, especially those with powerlifting experience, will tend to deadlift with their legs relatively straight and their hips farther from the floor, but everyone else will do better with their hips lower and knees bent.

UP: Suck air into your stomach and hold it as you pull the bar straight up from the floor. Pull until your hips and knees are completely straight, with your shoulders pulled back. Exhale when you finish these actions, not before.

DOWN: Push your hips back, keeping your back flat, as you get the bar to the floor as quickly as possible without dropping it. When you're using superheavy weights and doing just two or three reps, regrip the bar and reset your body from head to toe before you do the next rep.

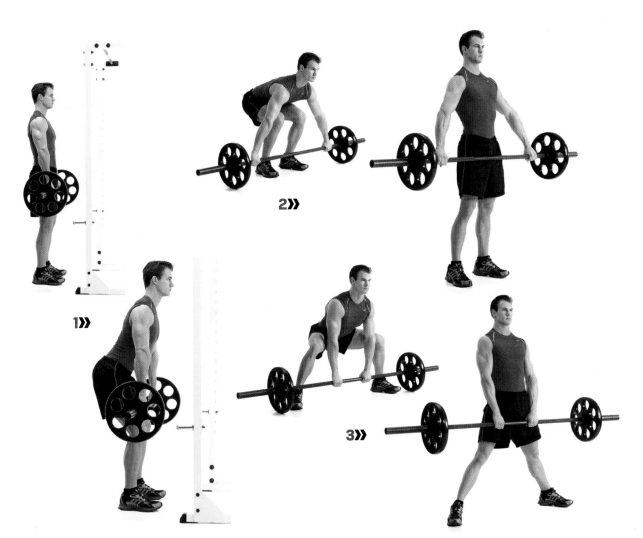

2》

1》

3》

VARIATIONS:

1》 SUPRAMAXIMAL DEADLIFT

WHERE IT IS: Get Even Stronger, Phase 1

HOW TO DO IT: Use a load that's approximately 20 percent more than your one-rep max. Start with the barbell resting on the pins of a power cage at mid-thigh level. Unrack the load, push your hips back slightly to lower the barbell 3 to 4 inches, and hold.

2》 SNATCH-GRIP DEADLIFT

WHERE IT IS: Get Even Bigger, HFT for Arms

HOW TO DO IT: Grab the barbell overhand with your hands as far apart as your arm length allows. Everything else is the same. This variation forces you to squat down lower to begin and end each repetition, and it offers a unique challenge to your trapezius and the rest of the muscles supporting your shoulder girdle.

3》 SUMO DEADLIFT

WHERE IT IS: Get Even Stronger, Phase 3

HOW TO DO IT: Widen your stance as much as possible, with your feet angled out slightly. Grab the barbell overhand with your hands between your legs. The movement is the same. When you deadlift sumo-style, your torso is more vertical, which puts more emphasis on your thigh muscles, particularly those in your inner thighs.

DEADLIFT
(CONTINUED)

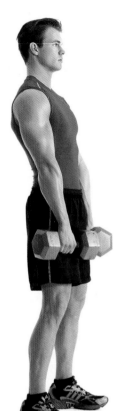

4»

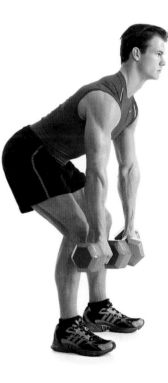

4» DUMBBELL ROMANIAN DEADLIFT

WHERE IT IS: Get Big, Phases 1A, 2A, and 3A; Get Even Bigger, HFT for Arms, HFT for Other Muscle Groups, and Total-Body HFT; Get Strong, Phases 1A, 2A, 3, and 3A; Get Even Stronger, Phases 1A, 2A, and 3A; Get Lean, Phase 2

HOW TO DO IT: Stand holding dumbbells in front of your thighs, palms turned toward your body. Your feet should be shoulder-width apart, toes pointed forward. Start the movement by taking a deep breath, then holding it as you push your hips back, allowing your torso to bend forward. Let your knees bend slightly. Lower the weights until they're just past your knees, then push your hips forward to return to the starting position, and exhale at the top. Keep your core tight and back flat throughout the movement.

A note on terminology: This is not a "stiff-legged" deadlift, in which you bend forward without pushing your hips back, thus keeping your legs straight. Any time you see "Romanian" in front of a deadlift variation, you're supposed to start the movement with your hips moving back, allowing your knees to bend. Some trainers use the two terms interchangeably, but there is a difference.

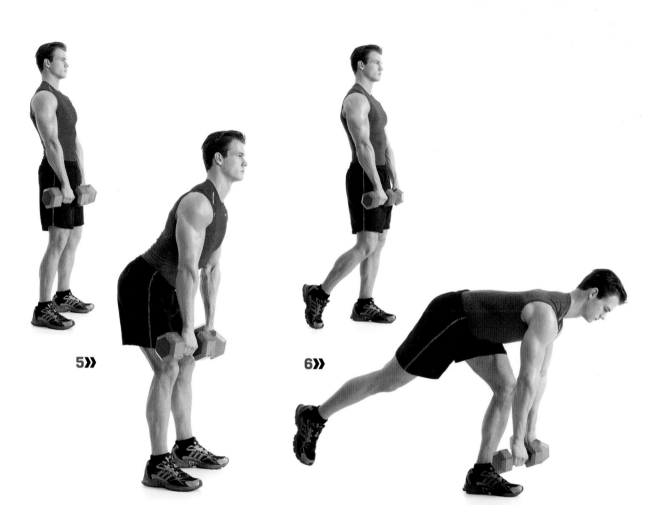

5» **6»**

5» FAST PARTIAL DUMBBELL ROMANIAN DEADLIFT

WHERE IT IS: Get Even Stronger, Phase 2

HOW TO DO IT: Start at the top position, push your hips back, and lower the dumbbells until they're a few inches above your knees.

6» DUMBBELL SINGLE-LEG DEADLIFT

WHERE IT IS: Get Big, Phase 2; Get Even Bigger, HFT for Other Muscle Groups; Get Strong, Phases 2 and 3; Get Even Stronger, Phase 2; Get Lean, Phases 1 and 3

HOW TO DO IT: As with all single-leg exercises, you want to start with your weaker or nondominant leg. But to keep the description simple, I'll just assume everyone starts with his left leg. So: Stand with your feet shoulder-width apart, holding dumbbells at your sides, palms turned toward your body. Lift your right foot up behind you, a few inches off the floor, with your right thigh perpendicular to the floor. Push your hips back and allow your torso to bend forward, while keeping your abs tight and back flat. Your left knee should bend slightly. Bend forward as far as you can while keeping your lower back flat. Return to the starting position. Complete all your reps with that leg and then repeat with your other leg.

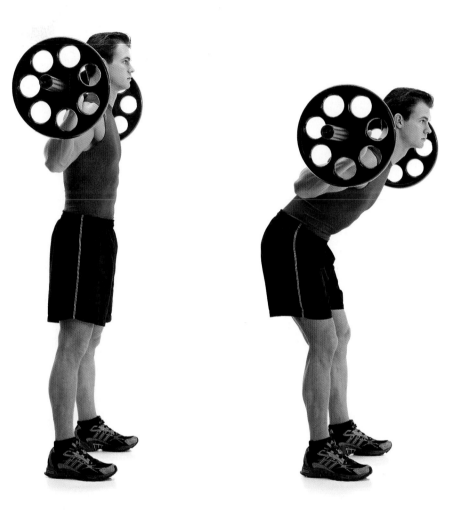

GOOD MORNING

WHERE IT IS: Get Strong, Phase 2; Get Lean, Phase 3

PREP: You'll need to set up in a squat rack (also called a power rack or power cage). Set the barbell on pins at shoulder height. Duck your head under the bar and pull your shoulder blades back to form a shelf-like ridge with your upper-back muscles. Set the bar on that ridge, and grab it overhand with as wide a grip as you can manage. Lift it off the pins and take two steps back. Set your feet shoulder-width apart, take a deep breath, and hold it as you tighten your abs and back.

DOWN: As in a Romanian deadlift, described earlier, push your hips back, allowing your knees to bend slightly, as your torso bends forward. Go down as far as you can while keeping your back flat.

UP: Push your hips forward as you lean back into the bar and return to the starting position, exhaling when you get there.

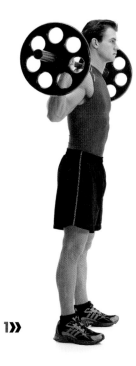

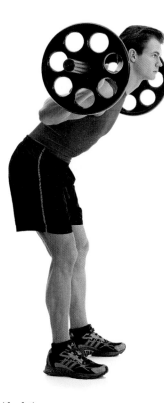

1»

VARIATIONS:

1» FAST PARTIAL GOOD MORNING

WHERE IT IS: Get Even Stronger, Phase 1

HOW TO DO IT: Use the first half of the range of motion—from the top position to where your torso is about 45 degrees relative to the floor.

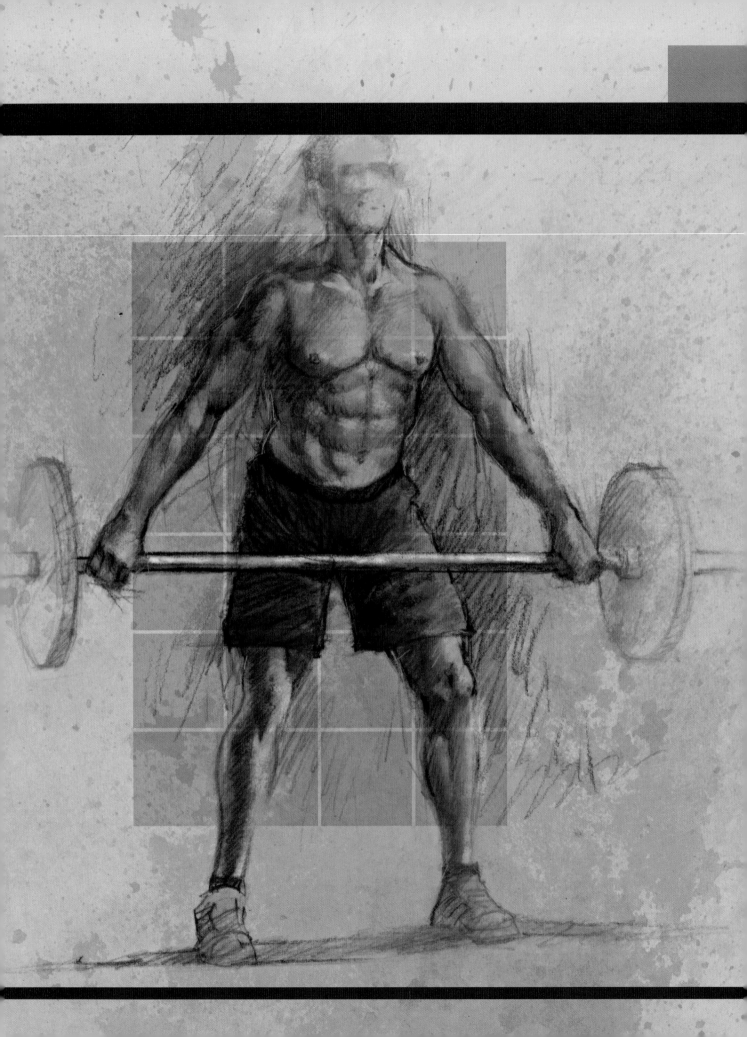

CHAPTER 19

POWER EXERCISES

These exercises are usually classified as "Olympic lifts," even though just one of them, the snatch, is the actual lift contested in the actual Olympics. The others—overhead squat, jump shrug, clean, power clean—are variations on or components of the snatch and clean and jerk.

Both Olympic lifts start with a deadlift, an exercise that's so important to the *Huge in a Hurry* workouts that it merits its own chapter. But instead of stopping where you stop a traditional deadlift—feet flat, barbell resting against your thighs—you power past that point into what's called "triple extension." Your hips and knees are "extended" (which is to say, you're standing up straight) but you're also up on your toes (thus extending your ankle joints) and shrugging your shoulders to propel the bar upward at maximum velocity. In my programs, you'll practice that part of the Olympic lifts with an exercise called the jump shrug.

The next step is to bend your arms as you pull the bar up to the level of your chest, a move that you'll learn in an exercise called the high pull. Superficially, if you were to do it slowly, it would look like an upright row. But when you do it with maximum force, it looks like a continuation of the jump shrug.

At the point when you've generated maximum momentum and the bar is rising up past your chest, you duck under the bar and go into a deep squat. If you're doing a clean and jerk, you "catch" the bar on the front of your shoulders as you descend into your squat. That's how we get the front squat, which you learned in Chapter 17—it's a component of the Olympic clean and jerk, minus all the action it takes to bring the bar to your shoulders, and minus all the action that follows as you jerk the bar overhead. For the record, I also skipped the jerk for this book (I use the push press instead, which offers the same benefits but is easier to learn), although if there's ever a sequel (*Massive in a Millisecond*?), I might use the jerk there.

That entire process, with the barbell starting on the floor and ending up on the front of your shoulders while you descend into a squat, is an exercise called the clean. You'll also learn a variation called the power clean, which is the same except you catch the bar with your body going into a quarter squat, rather than going all the way down.

If you're performing a snatch, you don't catch the bar on your shoulders. Instead, the momentum you generate with the triple extension and high pull drives the bar all the way overhead, and you catch it with straight arms while descending into a full squat. You'll recognize this as the bottom position of the overhead squat, which you also learned in Chapter 17.

Three of the five exercises in this chapter are included in Get Lean, my fat-loss program. Why do Olympic lifts help you burn off excess body fat? Think back to Chapter 14, when I described five key elements of successful fat-loss training. Number two on the list is "increase the metabolic cost of each exercise." Trust me on this: Of all the exercises you can do in the weight room, nothing requires more focus and effort than Olympic lifts, and nothing jacks up your heart rate in quite the same way.

These lifts do have a learning curve. That's why I cautioned against starting off with Get Lean unless you have a lot of lifting experience, and why it comes last in *Huge in a Hurry*. If you do my programs in the order in which they appear, you'll learn to do deadlifts, front squats, and high pulls in the early phases of Get Big, and you'll get to try power cleans in Phase 3 of that program. You'll add jump shrugs in Phase 1 of Get Strong, followed by overhead squats in Phase 3.

Finally, in the second and third phases of Get Lean, you'll learn to do cleans and snatches. By that point, you'll not only be lean, strong, and muscular, you'll also be a complete lifter, a master of the weight room and a member of the iron elite.

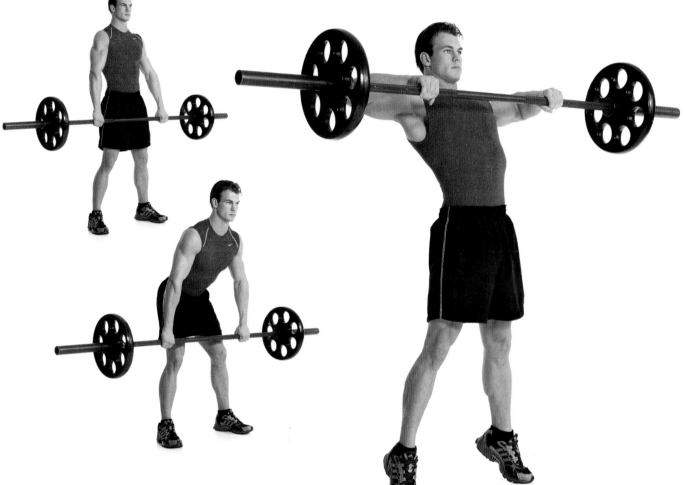

HIGH PULL

WHERE IT IS: Get Big, Phase 1; Get Even Bigger, HFT for Arms and Total-Body HFT; Get Strong, Phases 2 and 3; Get Lean, Phases 2A and 3A

PREP: You'll start this exercise with the bar off the floor. It's easiest if you set it up in the squat rack on pins, but you can also set it up on the floor and then lift it to the starting position. Either way, you'll grab the barbell with an overhand, shoulder-width grip, set your feet shoulder-width apart with your toes pointing straight ahead, and hold the bar at arm's length in front of your thighs, as if you've just finished a deadlift.

DOWN: Take a deep breath, tighten your abs, push your hips back, and lower the bar until it's just above your knees.

UP: Thrust your hips forward and pull the bar up toward your chest, lifting your elbows high and rising all the way up on your toes as you lean your entire body back. Exhale and immediately drop down into the next repetition.

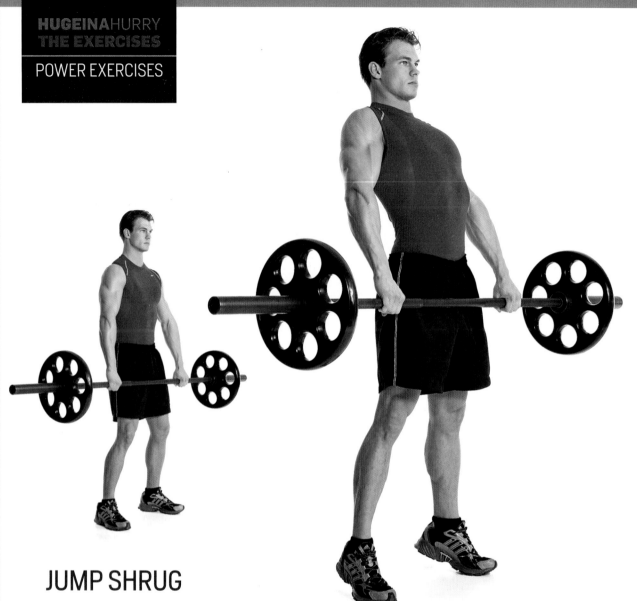

JUMP SHRUG

WHERE IT IS: Get Strong, Phase 1

PREP: Grab the barbell with an overhand, shoulder-width grip. Set your feet shoulder-width apart, toes pointed forward. Tighten your abs, push your hips back, and hold the bar with straight arms at mid-thigh level.

UP: Take a deep breath, then thrust your hips forward as you shrug your shoulders and rise all the way up on your toes, leaning your entire body back and keeping your arms straight.

DOWN: Exhale as you drop back down to the starting position.

Note: Aside from the obvious difference between the jump shrug and high pull—you bend your arms in the latter but keep them straight in the former—there's also a slight difference in how and where you start the exercise. You lower the bar to the top of your knees to start a high pull, then quickly and powerfully reverse the motion to pull it up toward your chest. But in a jump shrug, you start from a dead hang, with the bar at mid-thigh level. This slight difference makes the jump shrug more of a size- and strength-building exercise for your upper traps, while the high pull emphasizes total-body strength, power, and muscularity.

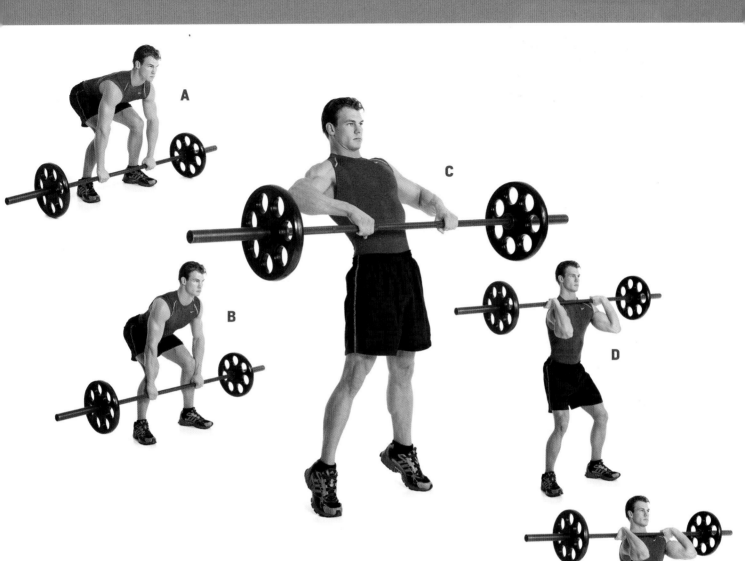

POWER CLEAN

WHERE IT IS: Get Big, Phase 3

PREP: Set up as you would for a deadlift: shoulder-width stance, toes pointing straight ahead, overhand grip, arms just outside your legs, back straight, abs tight, neck and head aligned with your back (A).

FIRST PULL: Take a deep breath, then stand as you pull the bar off the floor, thrusting your hips forward (B).

SECOND PULL: As your hips and knees are straightening, shrug your shoulders and rise up onto your toes as you pull the bar up past your abdomen, with your entire body leaning back (C).

CATCH: Push your hips back and drop into a quarter squat as you catch the bar on the front of your shoulders, rotating your arms under it so your elbows point forward, your upper arms are parallel to the floor, and the bar rolls back from your palms to your fingers (D).

FINISH: Stand up with the bar on your shoulders, and exhale (E). Drop the bar to the floor by rolling it back to your palms, rotating your arms so they're back over the bar, and pushing your hips back as the bar descends. It should come to a full stop on the floor as you reset your stance and grip for the next repetition.

POWER CLEAN
(CONTINUED)

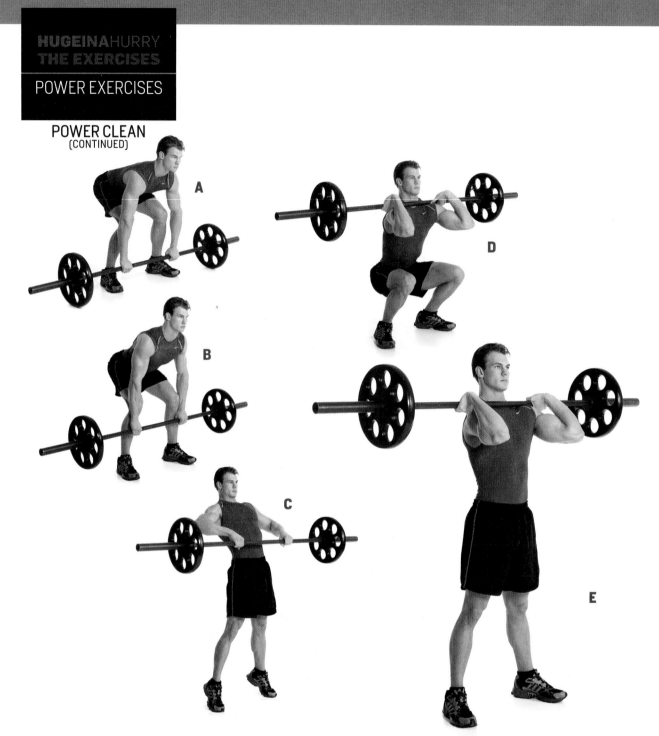

A

B

C

D

E

VARIATION:
CLEAN

WHERE IT IS: Get Lean, Phase 2

HOW TO DO IT: Much as it pains me to describe the clean as a variation of the power clean—the truth is the opposite—for our purposes it helps to start with the power clean, which has a shorter range of motion and is thus easier to learn. The difference with the clean is that you're going to descend into a full squat as you catch the bar on your shoulders. It's like a front squat, only with a lot more momentum from a barbell that's moving fast. So you have to pay special attention to your core; it has to be tight to keep your lower back in its natural arch.

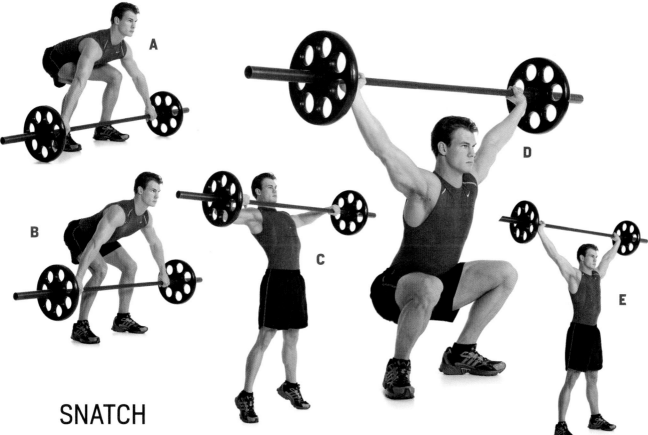

SNATCH

WHERE IT IS: Get Lean, Phase 3

PREP: Set up as you would for the snatch-grip deadlift, described in the previous chapter: With your feet shoulder-width apart and toes pointing forward, squat down and grab the bar with an overhand grip that's as wide as your arm length allows. Tighten your abs and straighten your back (A).

FIRST PULL: Suck air into your stomach, hold your breath, then stand as you pull the bar off the floor, thrusting your hips forward (B).

SECOND PULL: As your hips and knees are straightening, shrug your shoulders and rise up onto your toes as you pull the bar up toward your chest, keeping your elbows high as you lean your entire body back (C).

CATCH: As the barbell moves upward, squat down underneath it, rotating and straightening your arms so you catch the bar overhead (or slightly behind your head) with straight arms. You'll end up in the bottom position of the overhead squat, shown in Chapter 17 (D).

FINISH: Stand up with the bar overhead, and exhale (E). Lower the bar to your chest, then slide it to the floor.

Key point: You want to squat down far enough that you indeed catch the bar while your arms are already straight; if you catch it halfway, you'll end up doing a shoulder press to finish the movement. There's nothing wrong with that, but it's a different exercise. If you don't feel comfortable doing the snatch, you can substitute the overhead squat instead.

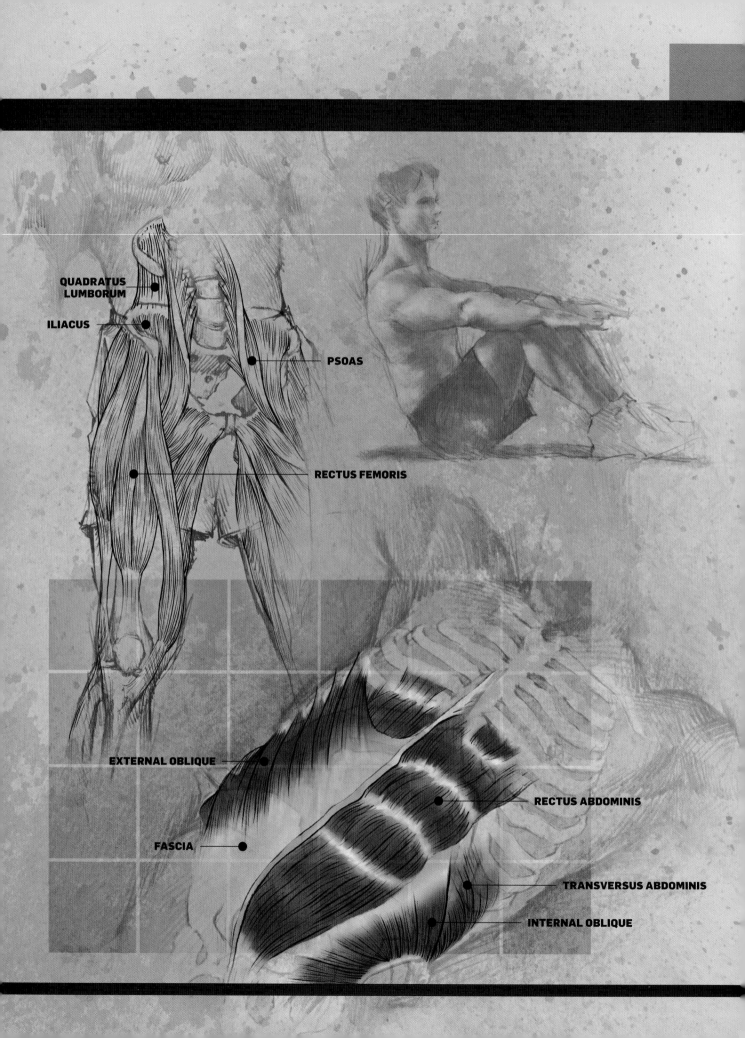

QUADRATUS
LUMBORUM

ILIACUS

PSOAS

RECTUS FEMORIS

EXTERNAL OBLIQUE

RECTUS ABDOMINIS

FASCIA

TRANSVERSUS ABDOMINIS

INTERNAL OBLIQUE

CHAPTER 20

ABDOMINAL EXERCISES

I confess: I don't obsess over abs. If you're doing total-body workouts that include a full spectrum of multi-joint, big-muscle exercises, your abs are entirely capable of taking care of themselves. They get ferociously strong when you do exercises like deadlifts and squats (particularly front squats). They engage on shoulder presses and standing rows, and their work increases when you do single-arm versions of those exercises.

However, there are certainly times when you want to give your abs some special attention, building their size to bring out their ripples and contours. That's why I include so many ab exercises in the Get Lean program, and why it's worth knowing what these muscles are and how they work.

All these muscles act on your spine to bend it or twist it, or—and this is really the most important function of all—to *prevent* it from bending and twisting. So let's look at the key players.

MIDDLE AND LOWER TORSO

I never know whether to laugh or cry when I see books, magazine articles, and even infomercials promising a visible six-pack. Whether or not you can see the individual segments of your **RECTUS ABDOMINIS** is almost entirely dependent on your genes and body-fat percentage. It has little to do with your exercise selection. The traditional crunch, the exercise of choice in these programs, is one of my least favorite exercises. The belly-squeezing motion has almost nothing to do with the functional role of the muscle you're targeting.

The rectus is a very strong muscle, uniquely cross-hatched with thick bands of connective tissue called **FASCIA**. Whether you can see it or not when you take off your shirt, your rectus acts as a kind of crossroads for every action your body performs. It engages with your **EXTERNAL OBLIQUES** when you do anything involving torso rotation—which includes practically every movement in every sport.

When you're not twisting—when you're actively trying to prevent your spine from shifting out of its strongest position in exercises such as deadlifts and squats—your rectus and obliques work together to hold everything in place, along with the two layers of muscle beneath them: your **INTERNAL OBLIQUES** and **TRANSVERSUS ABDOMINIS**.

The classic crunch, technically speaking, is a movement called "spinal flexion," meaning you deliberately pull your lower back out of its natural arch—its strongest, safest position—and force it to straighten out into a much weaker, more vulnerable position. Why anyone thinks it's a good idea to train your body to weaken itself is beyond me.

I prefer to train the abdominal muscles in the opposite direction, forcing them to *lengthen* in exercises like walkouts and rollouts, rather than to shorten in crunches and situps. That way, you're training your muscles to respond to real-life challenges, protecting your back by forcing it to stay in its strongest position, instead of training it to shift into its weakest posture. As a bonus, you engage all the muscles responsible for keeping your skeleton together, including those in your lower, middle, and upper back. In Get Even Bigger, I recommend the barbell rollout to develop your lats, even though it's most often used as an ab-training exercise.

HIPS AND PELVIS

On the other hand, I *do* like to train the hip flexors, the muscles that pull your thighs up toward your torso. These include your **PSOAS MAJOR**, which connects your thigh bone to your lower back, and the **ILIACUS**, which links your thigh to your pelvis. A deeper muscle, the **QUADRATUS LUMBORUM**, links your pelvis to your spine, giving it a key role in keeping your lower back safe.

Other hip-flexing muscles include your **RECTUS FEMORIS** (a dual-purpose muscle that's also part of the quadriceps group), **SARTORIUS** (a triple-purpose muscle that helps you lift your leg forward, bend and turn your knee inward, and lift or turn your thigh outward), and **TENSOR FASCIAE LATAE**, an outer-hip muscle that helps you lift your leg forward or out to the side.

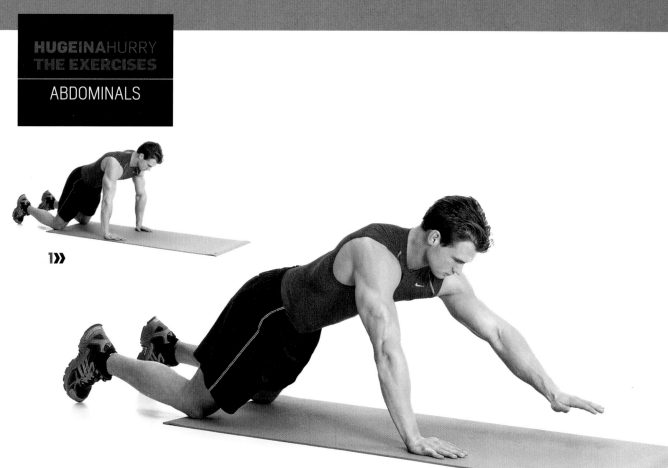

WALKOUTS AND ROLLOUTS

PREP: You'll want to do these on a carpeted floor, preferably one with some padding. And even with a padded, carpeted floor, you might want to put an extra towel or mat under your knees to avoid irritation. The knobbier and more battered your knees, the more padding you'll want.

You'll start most of these exercises from the same basic position: knees on the floor, hands either on the floor or resting on an ab wheel or barbell, back flat, abs tight, neck and head aligned with your back.

OUT: Walk or roll your hands out as far forward as possible, keeping your core tight. Stop the movement as soon as you realize you can't go any farther and still maintain the natural arch in your lower back.

Your hips will shift forward as you move out, and the farther your hands go, the closer your hips will get to the floor. Don't push yourself too far the first few times you try these exercises; over time, your range of motion will increase, and as it does, the strength and stability of your core muscles will improve dramatically.

IN: Walk or roll your hands back to the starting position.

VARIATIONS:

1» HAND WALKOUT

WHERE IT IS: Get Lean, Phase 1

HOW TO DO IT: Start on your hands and knees, with your hands flat on the floor and directly beneath your shoulders. Walk out as far as you can without any change in your lower back.

WALKOUTS AND ROLLOUTS
(CONTINUED)

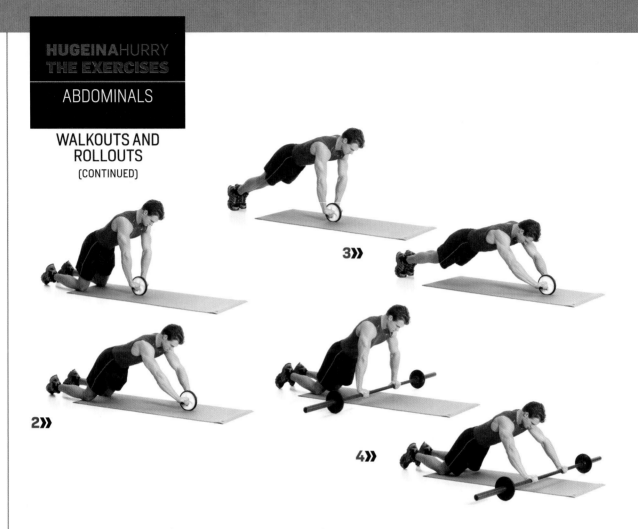

3»

2»

4»

2» AB-WHEEL ROLLOUT FROM KNEES

WHERE IT IS: Get Lean, Phase 2

HOW TO DO IT: Same as on page 271, only with your hands on an ab wheel directly below your chest. Be extremely careful the first few times. The wheel sometimes rolls faster than you expect it to. (This is why it's better to do this on a padded and carpeted floor rather than on wood or concrete.)

As you pull the wheel back to the starting position, you'll feel muscles in your shoulders and arms working, along with your core.

3» AB-WHEEL ROLLOUT FROM TOES

WHERE IT IS: Get Lean, Phase 3

HOW TO DO IT: Start on your toes with your body bent forward at the hips and your hands on the ab wheel directly below your

chest. *Carefully* roll out as far as you can while keeping your core tight. This is a terrific exercise, but it may be as challenging as anything in this book. If you can't master it, it's perfectly fine to continue doing the ab-wheel rollout from your knees, or substitute the barbell rollout, shown next.

4» BARBELL ROLLOUT

WHERE IT IS: Get Even Bigger, HFT for Other Muscle Groups

HOW TO DO IT: Load your barbell with a 5-, 10-, or 25-pound plate on each side. Grab the bar with your hands slightly beyond shoulder width. Start from your knees, with your arms straight and the bar beneath your eyes. The rollout part is the same, except you'll find it's a bigger challenge to pull the bar back to the starting position. (That's why I suggest it as an exercise for your lats in Get Even Bigger.)

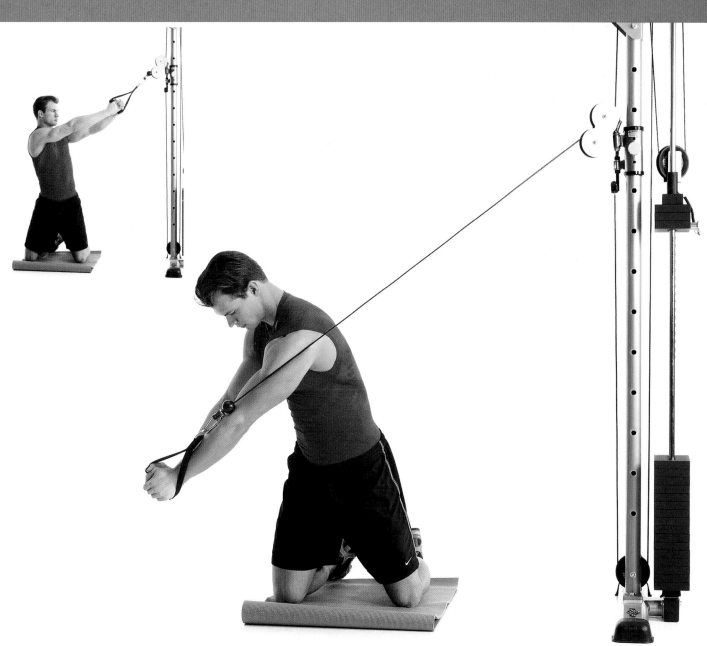

CABLE WOODCHOP ON KNEES

WHERE IT IS: Get Lean, Phase 1

PREP: Set the cable pulley to a position that's just above your head when you're kneeling alongside it. Attach a D-shaped handle. Kneel with the cable pulley to your dominant side. Reach up and grab the handle with both hands, rotating your shoulders and head toward it. Start with your arms straight and tension on the cable.

DOWN: Pull the handle down and across your body to your weaker side while keeping your arms straight.
Your torso should twist to your weaker side, while your head follows your hands from start to finish. Pull until your hands are just outside your nondominant knee.

UP: Return to the starting position, again keeping your arms straight. Finish all your reps, then switch sides and do the same number of reps twisting to your dominant side.

CABLE WOODCHOP
(CONTINUED)

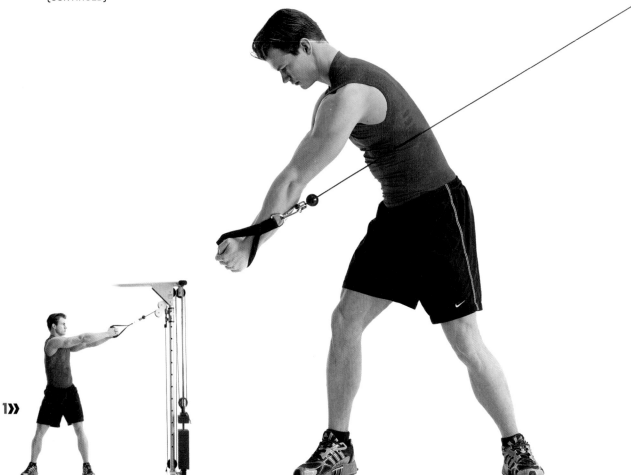

1»

VARIATION:

1» CABLE STANDING WOODCHOP

WHERE IT IS: Get Lean, Phases 2 and 3

HOW TO DO IT: Move the cable pulley to its highest position and attach a D-shaped handle. Stand with the cable pulley to your dominant side. Reach up and grab the handle with both hands, rotating your shoulders and head toward it. Split your stance so that your feet are about shoulder-width apart but your nondominant leg is forward and your stronger leg is back. Pull the handle down and across your body to your weaker side while keeping your arms straight. The rest is the same, except you may need to turn on your dominant foot, with the heel coming off floor. The key is for your shoulders to twist while your abdomen and hips turn as a unit. Pull the handle all the way to the outside of your nondominant knee. Finish all your reps, then switch sides and do the same number of reps twisting to your dominant side.

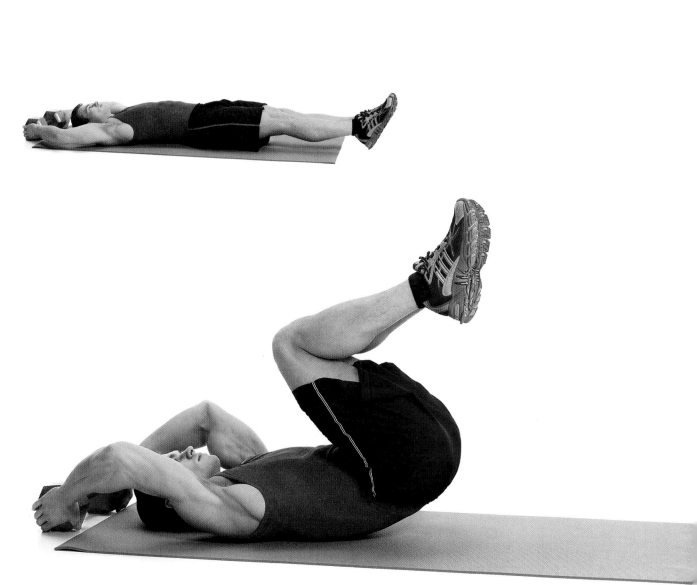

REVERSE CRUNCH

WHERE IT IS: Get Lean, Phase 1

PREP: Lie on your back on the floor with your legs straight. With both hands, hold on to a secure structure behind your head. Attach ankle weights or hold a dumbbell between your feet for added resistance.

UP: Pull your knees into your chest and roll your hips up.

DOWN: Reverse the movement, ending with your legs straight and heels touching the floor.

REVERSE CRUNCH
(CONTINUED)

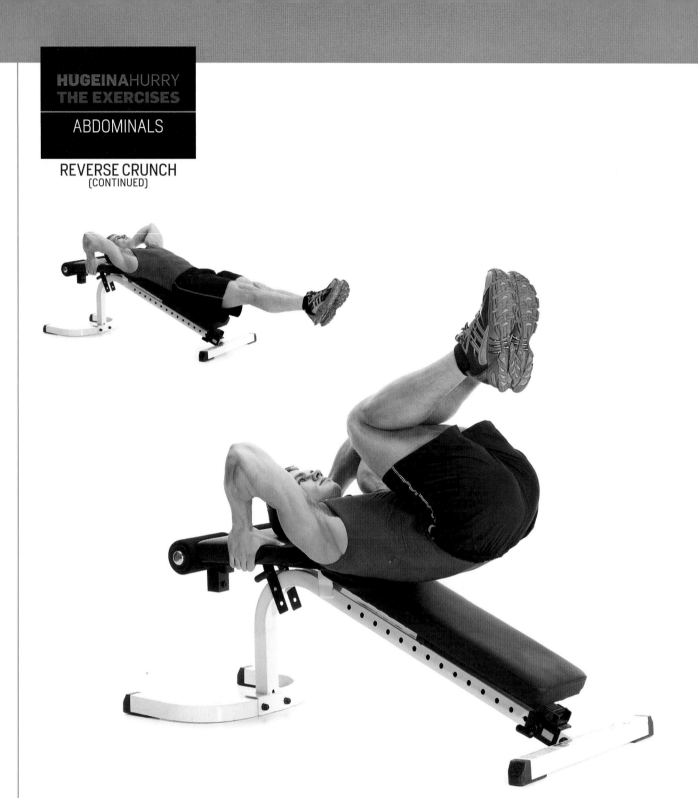

VARIATION:
REVERSE CRUNCH ON SLANT BOARD

WHERE IT IS: Get Lean, Phase 2

HOW TO DO IT: Lie on your back on a slant board or decline situp bench, with your head higher than your legs. Your legs should be straight. With both hands, hold on to a secure structure behind your head. If necessary, attach ankle weights or hold a dumbbell between your feet for added resistance. Pull your knees into your chest and roll your hips up. Reverse the movement, ending with your legs straight and heels touching the floor.

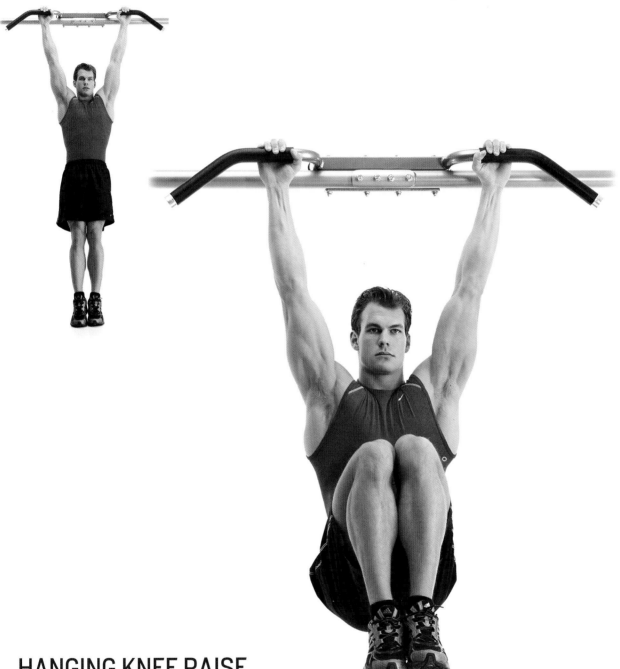

HANGING KNEE RAISE

WHERE IT IS: Get Lean, Phase 3

PREP: Hang from a pullup bar with your palms facing forward and your legs straight. If you need extra resistance, attach ankle weights or hold a dumbbell between your feet.

UP: Pull your knees into your chest and roll your hips up.

DOWN: Reverse the motion, being careful to control the descent so you minimize swinging on the bar.

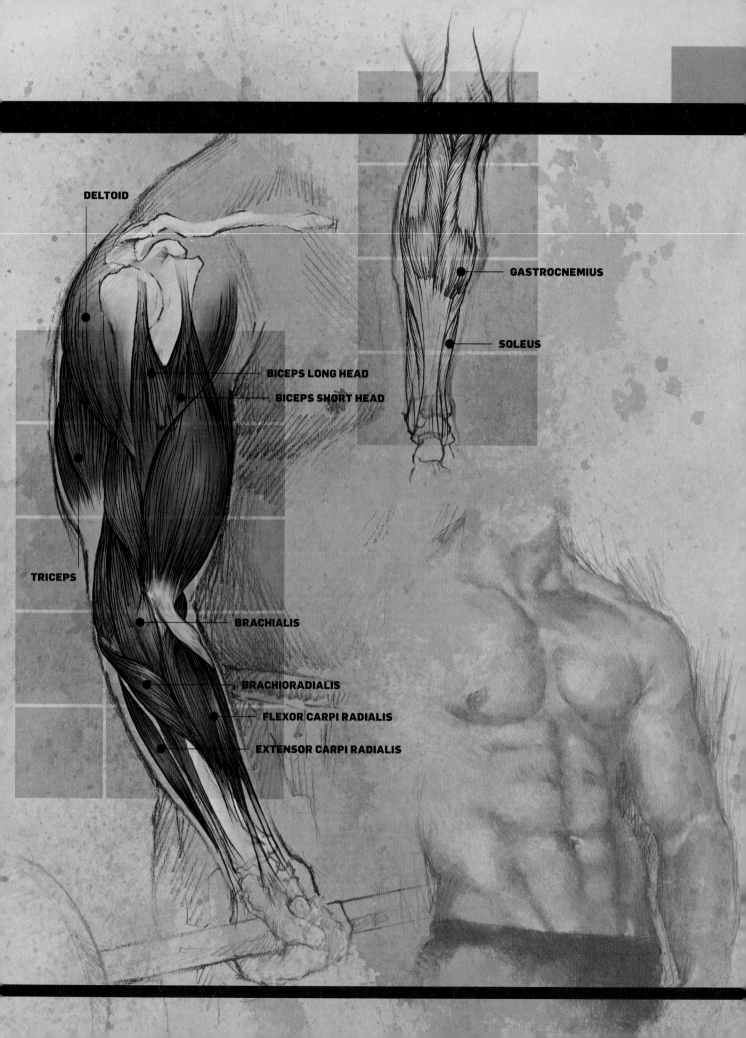

DELTOID

GASTROCNEMIUS

SOLEUS

BICEPS LONG HEAD

BICEPS SHORT HEAD

TRICEPS

BRACHIALIS

BRACHIORADIALIS

FLEXOR CARPI RADIALIS

EXTENSOR CARPI RADIALIS

CHAPTER 21

SPECIALTY AND SINGLE-JOINT EXERCISES

Most of the exercises in this chapter are found in Get Even Bigger, which features my high-frequency training method for developing specific muscle groups that lag behind others. The rest are single-joint movements that appear as the fourth exercise in the Get Big programs. Since most of the exercises in this chapter are simple and straightforward, you probably won't refer to it nearly as often as you'll reference the chapters on squats, deadlifts, pulls, and pushes.

But there's always a chance someone will pick up the book and open to this chapter without reading anything else, which means I feel obligated to repeat my main themes.

The total-body workouts in *Huge in a Hurry* are based on three exercises: upper-body pull (such as a chinup or row), upper-body push (a dip or chest or shoulder press), and either a squat or deadlift variation. So when you use some of these single-joint exercises in the Get Big workouts, it should be with the understanding that they're the fourth movement in a three-movement system. They're extra. That doesn't mean you shouldn't do them as they appear in my workouts. It just means they're the least important components.

If you decide to try the high-frequency programs in Get Even Bigger, that's a different story. The whole point there is to impose extra stress and fatigue on select groups of muscles. Since you're already doing compound exercises three times a week in your total-body workouts, these single-joint exercises allow you to work the targeted muscles without interfering with your overall recovery.

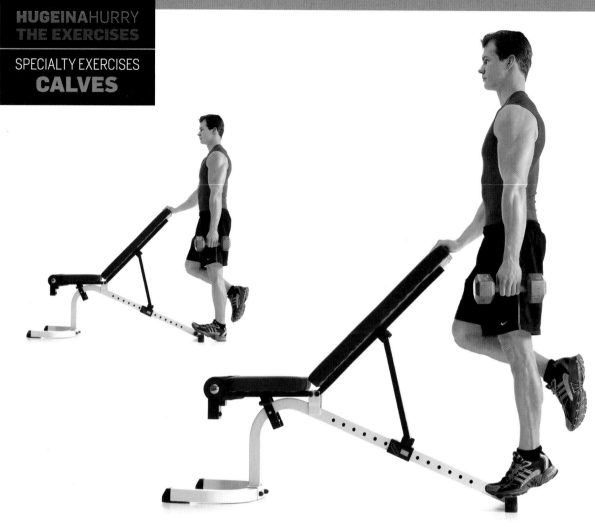

STANDING SINGLE-LEG CALF RAISE

WHERE IT IS: Get Big, Phases 1, 2, and 3; Get Even Bigger, HFT for Other Muscle Groups

PREP: Grab a dumbbell and hold it in your left hand as you stand on the ball of your left foot (assuming you're right-side dominant) on a low step. The base of an adjustable weight bench works perfectly. Just lift the bench's pad until it's vertical, and rest your free hand on the top of the bench for balance. Your right foot is lifted slightly—just enough so it's above the floor and not touching the step.

DOWN: Lower your left heel as far as possible while keeping your left leg straight.

UP: Push your big toe down into the step and lift your left heel as high as possible. Finish all your reps with your left leg, then switch legs and repeat.

VARIATIONS:

1» SEATED SINGLE-LEG CALF RAISE

WHERE IT IS: Get Even Bigger, HFT for Other Muscle Groups

HOW TO DO IT: Grab a dumbbell or weight plate, and sit on the edge of a bench or chair with the ball of one foot on a board or low step. Set the weight on your corresponding thigh, just above the knee. Move your other foot away (it doesn't matter where). Lower and lift your heel, as described for the standing calf raise. Finish all your reps with that leg, then switch legs and repeat.

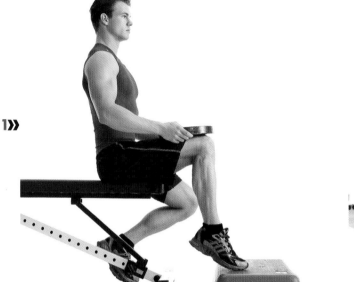

1»

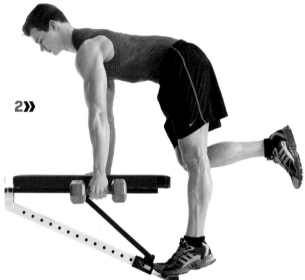

2»

2» SINGLE-LEG DONKEY CALF RAISE

WHERE IT IS: Get Even Bigger, HFT for Other Muscle Groups

HOW TO DO IT: Have you ever seen those pictures of Arnold-era bodybuilders doing donkey calf raises? One guy is bent forward like he's getting a prostate exam, and the other sits astride his hips. If you didn't know what they were doing, your imagination could come up with some colorful possibilities.

The purpose of the donkey calf raise is to put your calves into a prestretch position, making them work harder to lengthen and contract. If you're willing to invest that much time in calf development, it's actually a pretty good exercise, although I prefer the single-leg version. If nothing else, you won't need a bodybuilder sitting on your hips for it to be effective.

You need a sturdy step, and something that supports your weight as you lean forward with your torso parallel to the floor. (You can do this in the gym by leaning forward into an upright on a squat rack, or at home by putting your working foot on the bottom step and your hands on a higher step. In the latter example, you won't be able to get your torso parallel to the floor, but it's better than nothing.) Set the ball of your left foot (assuming you're right-side dominant) on the step, raise your right foot just far enough to get it out of the way, hold a dumbbell in your left hand, and use your right hand to hold on to something for balance. After that, you know the drill.

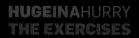
SINGLE-LEG HOP

WHERE IT IS: Get Even Bigger, HFT for Other Muscle Groups

PREP: Stand on your left leg (assuming you're right-side dominant) with your right foot a few inches off the floor, just high enough to get it out of the way. Hold a dumbbell in your right hand for added resistance.

UP: Now jump into the air, pushing down with your left toes while keeping your left leg as straight as possible. The less you bend the knee of your working leg, the harder you'll work your calf muscles.

DOWN: Land. Do all your reps with your left leg, then switch the dumbbell to your left hand and hop on your left leg.

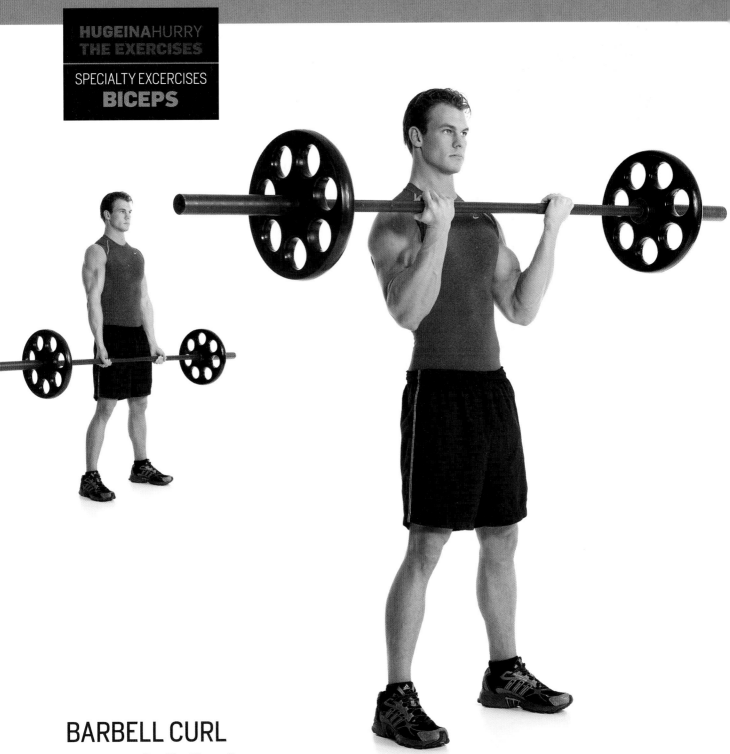

BARBELL CURL

WHERE IT IS: Get Big, Phase 2

PREP: Hold a barbell at arm's length in front of you with an underhand, shoulder-width grip. Tighten your abs and glutes and make sure your neck and head are aligned with your back (*not* contorted to allow you to observe your bulging biceps in action).

UP: Curl the barbell up while keeping your elbows at your sides. Stop right before you lose tension in your biceps.

DOWN: Lower the bar to the starting position.

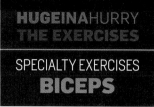
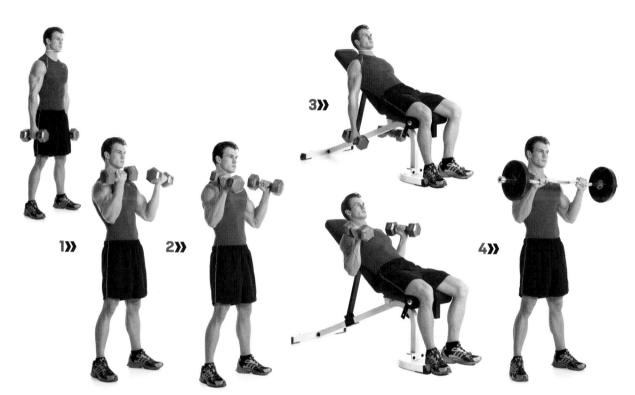

1»

2»

3»

4»

VARIATIONS:

1» DUMBBELL CURL

WHERE IT IS: Get Even Bigger, HFT for Arms

HOW TO DO IT: Stand holding dumbbells at arm's length at your sides, palms facing in. Keep your elbows at your sides as you curl the dumbbells, turning your palms up as you do.

2» HAMMER CURL

WHERE IT IS: Get Big, Phase 1; Get Even Bigger, HFT for Arms

HOW TO DO IT: Same start as the previous exercise, but instead of turning your hands to a palms-up position as you lift, keep your palms facing each other throughout the lift.

3» INCLINE HAMMER CURL

WHERE IT IS: Get Even Bigger, HFT for Arms

HOW TO DO IT: Lie on your back on a 45-degree incline bench. The movement is the same, except your arms will be slightly behind your torso. That changes the range of motion. Don't pull your arms forward (toward your torso) as you lift—keep them behind you. Otherwise, it turns into more of a challenge for your shoulders than for your biceps.

4» EZ-BAR REVERSE CURL

WHERE IT IS: Get Big, Phase 3; Get Even Bigger, HFT for Arms

HOW TO DO IT: Grab an EZ-curl bar with an overhand grip. Your hands will be diagonal, with your thumbs higher than your pinkies. Stand holding the bar at arm's length in front of your thighs. The rest is the same as any other curl.

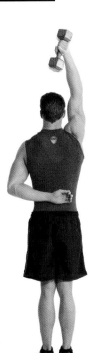

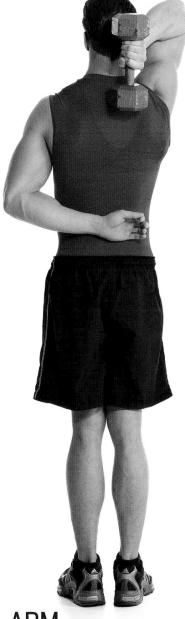

DUMBBELL STANDING ONE-ARM TRICEPS EXTENSION

WHERE IT IS: Get Big, Phase 1

PREP: Grab a dumbbell with your weaker or nondominant hand (probably your left if you're right-handed). Stand holding it straight overhead, palm facing in. Hold your nonworking arm behind your back.

DOWN: Bend your elbow to lower the dumbbell back and behind your head until it touches your upper back. Keep your upper arm as close to your ear as possible.

UP: Extend your arm overhead while keeping your upper arm close to your ear. Complete all your reps with that arm, then repeat with the other arm.

DUMBBELL STANDING ONE-ARM TRICEPS EXTENSION
(CONTINUED)

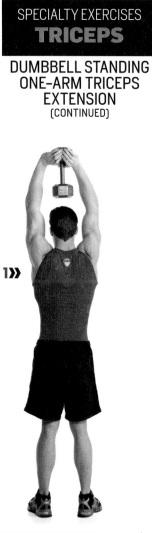

1»

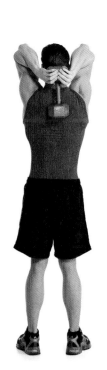

2»

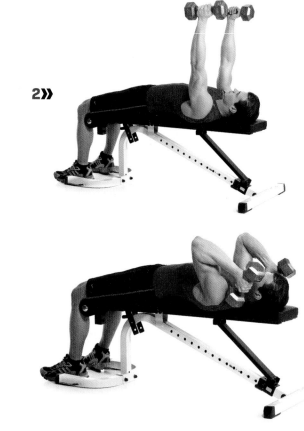

VARIATIONS:

1» DUMBBELL STANDING TRICEPS EXTENSION

WHERE IT IS: Get Even Bigger, HFT for Arms

HOW TO DO IT: Stand holding a single dumbbell overhead with both hands, starting with your arms straight. Bend your elbows to lower the dumbbell back and behind your head until it touches your upper back, then lift it back overhead. Keep your upper arms as close to your ears as possible throughout the lift.

2» DUMBBELL LYING TRICEPS EXTENSION

WHERE IT IS: Get Even Bigger, HFT for Arms

HOW TO DO IT: Grab two dumbbells and lie faceup on a flat bench, holding the weights over your chest with straight arms, your palms facing each other. Lower the weights down past your ears, then back to the starting position. Try to keep your elbows from flaring out.

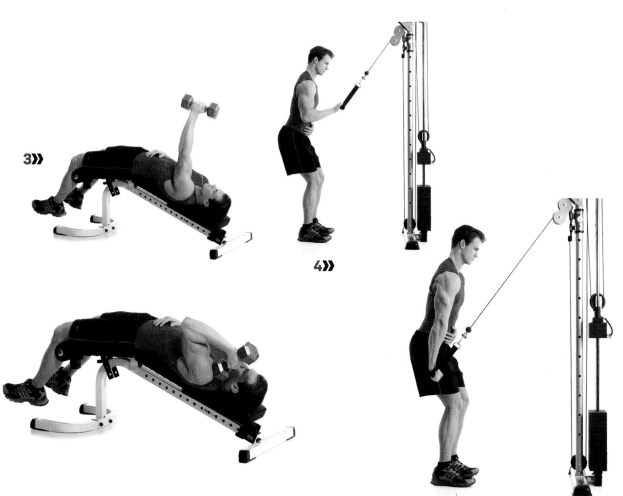

3》

3》 DUMBBELL DECLINE ONE-ARM TRICEPS EXTENSION

WHERE IT IS: Get Big, Phase 2

HOW TO DO IT: Grab a dumbbell with your nondominant hand and lie faceup on a decline bench. Hold the dumbbell over your chest with your arm straight and palm facing in. Put your nonworking hand on your stomach. Lower the weight down past your ear, then back to the starting position. Try to keep your elbow from flaring out. Complete all your reps with that arm, then repeat with the other arm.

4》 CABLE ONE-ARM TRICEPS PUSHDOWN

WHERE IT IS: Get Big, Phase 3

HOW TO DO IT: Set a cable pulley to its highest position and attach a D-shaped handle. Stand facing the pulley, and grab the handle palm-down with your non-dominant hand. Unlike the other triceps extensions described here, you'll start with the elbow of your working arm bent 90 degrees. (As with the biceps curls described earlier, you want to keep your working elbow tight against your side.) Place your nonworking hand on your stomach. Press the handle down, then return to the starting position. Complete all your reps with that arm, then repeat with the other arm.

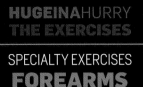
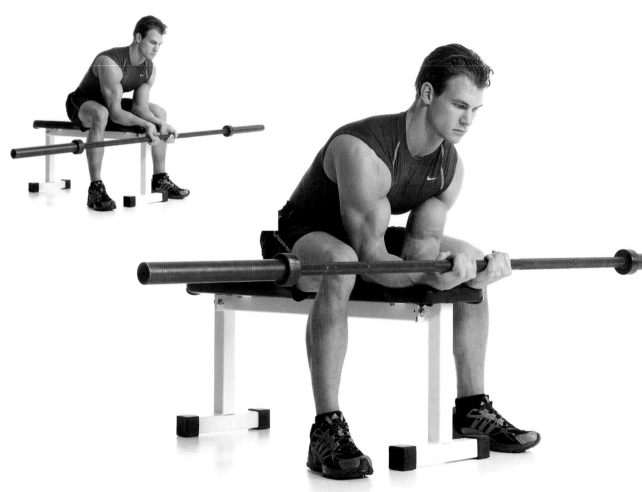

BARBELL WRIST CURL

WHERE IT IS: Get Even Bigger, HFT for Other Muscle Groups

PREP: There are lots of ways to set up for this exercise. All of them accomplish the same thing, since the exercise is so simple that it's almost impossible to do it wrong. (I'm sure some 15-year-old somewhere has managed to hurt himself doing wrist curls; I'm just saying it's not easy to be that foolish.)

Here's my favorite setup.

UP: Grab a barbell with a narrow, underhand grip and sit on a bench with your forearms between your legs and resting flat on the bench. Your hands and wrists hang off the end of the bench.

DOWN: Moving only at the wrists, lower your hands as much as possible without lifting your forearms off the bench.

UP: Curl your hands up toward you as far as possible, again moving only at the wrists and without lifting your forearms off the bench.

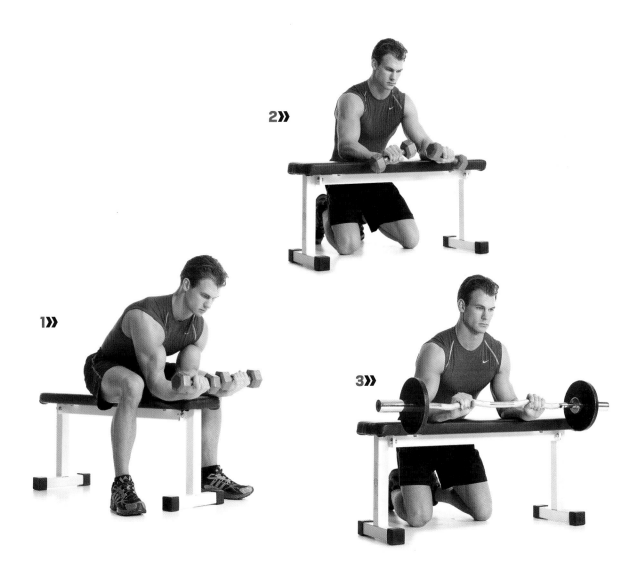

VARIATIONS:

1» DUMBBELL WRIST CURL

WHERE IT IS: Get Even Bigger, HFT for Other Muscle Groups

HOW TO DO IT: Same as for the barbell version, except you hold a dumbbell in each hand.

2» DUMBBELL REVERSE WRIST CURL

WHERE IT IS: Get Even Bigger, HFT for Other Muscle Groups

HOW TO DO IT: Same as for the dumbbell wrist curl, only this time you have your palms down.

3» EZ-BAR REVERSE WRIST CURL

WHERE IT IS: Get Even Bigger, HFT for Other Muscle Groups

HOW TO DO IT: Same as for the dumbbell reverse wrist curl, except you use an EZ-curl bar with an overhand grip and your thumbs higher than your pinkies.

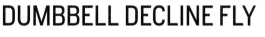

DUMBBELL DECLINE FLY

WHERE IT IS: Get Even Bigger, HFT for Other Muscle Groups

PREP: Grab two dumbbells and lie faceup on a decline bench, with your feet hooked under the supports. Hold the dumbbells straight up over your chest with your palms facing your feet.

DOWN: Lower your arms out to the sides as far as your shoulder mobility allows, keeping your arms as straight as possible.

UP: Pull the weights back to the starting position, following the same trajectory.

Note: Other exercises suggested for your chest in Get Even Bigger, including two pushup variations, are shown in Chapter 16.

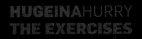
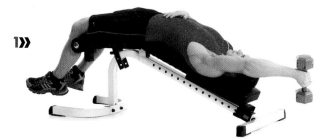

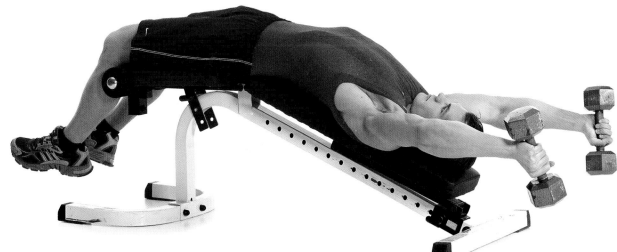

DUMBBELL DECLINE PULLOVER

WHERE IT IS: Get Even Bigger, HFT for Other Muscle Groups

PREP: Grab two dumbbells and lie faceup on a decline bench. Hold the dumbbells straight up over your chest with your palms facing each other.

DOWN: Lower the dumbbells back behind your head, keeping your arms straight and palms facing each other, with the same distance between your arms throughout the movement.

UP: Pull the dumbbells back to the starting position, following the same trajectory.

VARIATION:

1» DUMBBELL DECLINE ONE-ARM PULLOVER

WHERE IT IS: Get Even Bigger, HFT for Other Muscle Groups

HOW TO DO IT: Same as the bilateral version, holding a single dumbbell over your chest in your weaker or nondominant hand. Your nonworking hand should rest on your stomach. After you complete all the reps on one side, switch to the other side.

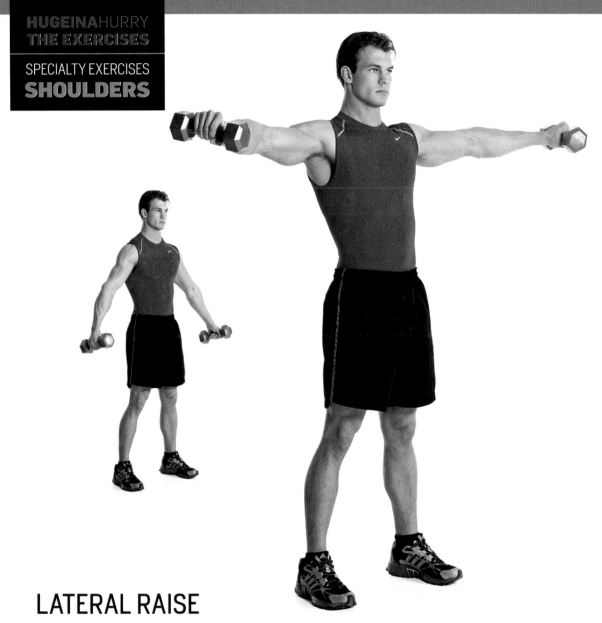

LATERAL RAISE

WHERE IT IS: Get Even Bigger, HFT for Other Muscle Groups; Get Even Stronger, Phase 1

PREP: Stand with your feet shoulder-width apart, holding dumbbells at arm's length at your sides, your palms facing each other.

UP: Lift the dumbbells up and out to the sides while keeping your arms relatively straight (a slight elbow bend is okay) until your arms are parallel to the floor.

DOWN: Lower the dumbbells about halfway—you want your arms at an angle that's about 45 degrees, relative to the floor. Do all your reps within that range of motion, which keeps maximum tension on your shoulder muscles.

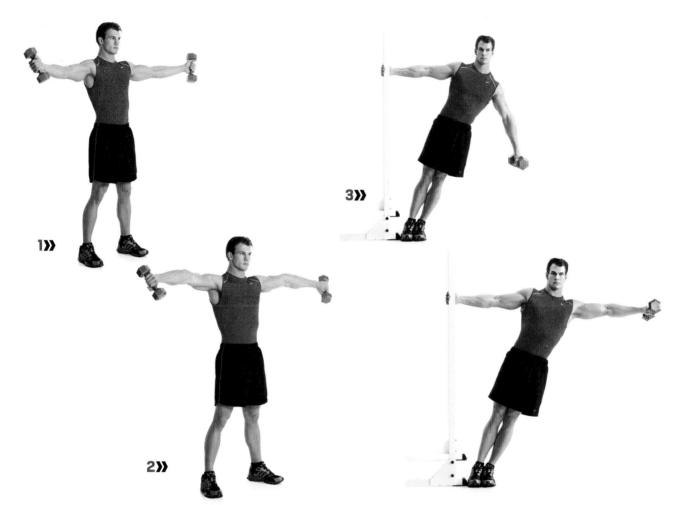

VARIATIONS:

1» LATERAL RAISE WITH THUMBS UP

WHERE IT IS: Get Even Bigger, HFT for Other Muscle Groups

HOW TO DO IT: Same as for the lat raise except your palms are facing forward, with your thumbs higher than your pinkies.

2» LATERAL RAISE WITH PINKIES UP

WHERE IT IS: Get Even Bigger, HFT for Other Muscle Groups

HOW TO DO IT: Same as for the lat raise except your palms are facing back.

3» LEAN-AWAY LATERAL RAISE

WHERE IT IS: Get Even Bigger, HFT for Other Muscle Groups

HOW TO DO IT: Grab a dumbbell with your left hand (assuming you're right-hand dominant), and with your right, grab onto something solid—the post of a squat rack works perfectly. Stand close to the post, then lean away from it to your left; you want your right arm parallel to the floor, with your body diagonal to it. Hold the dumbbell at arm's length straight down from your shoulder, perpendicular to the floor, with your palm facing your body.

Lift the dumbbell up and out to the side until your left arm is parallel to the floor, then lower it halfway, as described for the lateral raise. Finish your reps with your left arm, then switch sides and repeat with your right.

HUGEIN**A**HURRY
THE EXERCISES

SPECIALTY EXERCISES
SHOULDERS

LATERAL RAISE
(CONTINUED)

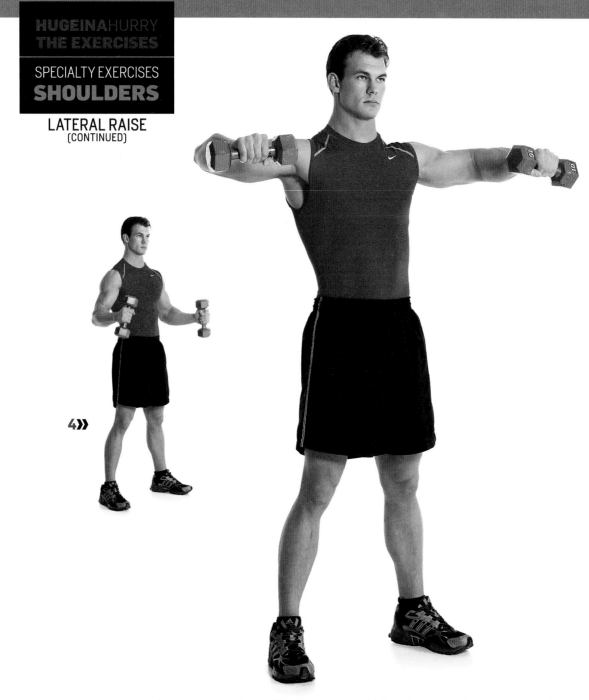

4»

4» L-RAISE

WHERE IT IS: Get Even Bigger, HFT for Other Muscle Groups

HOW TO DO IT: Same as the lateral raise, except you start with your elbows bent 90 degrees and your palms facing each other. Lift your elbows up and out to the sides until your upper arms are parallel to the floor, keeping the same 90-degree bend. Lower the dumbbells about a third of the way, until your upper arms are at 60 degrees relative to the floor, and do the rest of your reps in the set from that starting point.

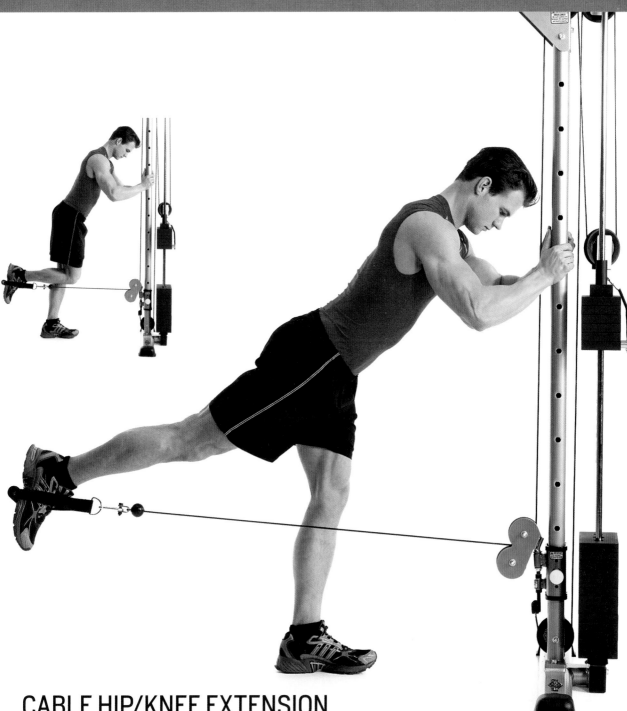

CABLE HIP/KNEE EXTENSION

WHERE IT IS: Get Even Bigger, HFT for Other Muscle Groups

PREP: Set a cable pulley on its lowest position and attach a foot strap. Stand facing the pulley and place the strap around the bottom of your nondominant foot. Take one step back, then lift your working leg, with your thigh parallel to the floor and your knee bent 90 degrees.

DOWN: Pull your leg down and behind you, with your knee straightening by the time your leg is past the plane of your body. Your foot shouldn't touch the floor.

UP: Pull that leg back to the starting position. Finish all your reps with that leg, then switch the foot strap and repeat the set with your other leg.

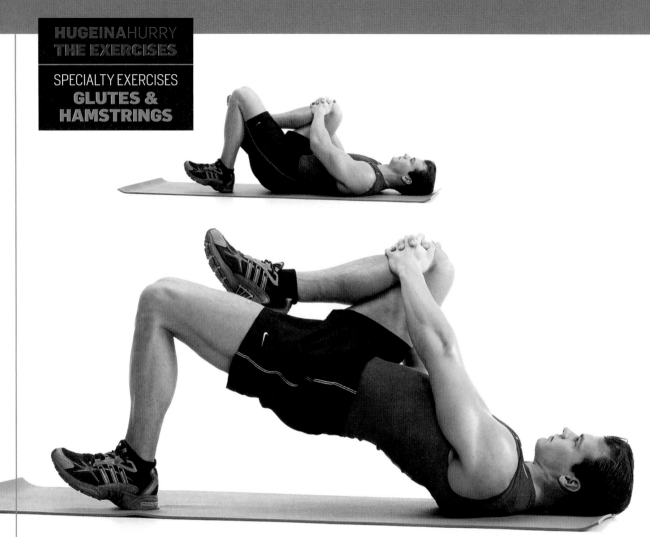

SINGLE-LEG BRIDGE

WHERE IT IS: Get Even Bigger, HFT for Other Muscle Groups

PREP: Lie faceup on the floor with your knees bent and feet flat. You want your heels as close to your glutes as possible. Pull your right knee (assuming you're right-side dominant) into your chest and hold it with both hands just below the knee. Now lift the toes of your left foot so your left heel is the only part of your foot that's on the floor.

UP: Squeeze your glutes and lift your hips as high off the floor as possible, arching your back at the end.

DOWN: Lower your hips, stopping just before they touch the floor. Do all your reps with your left leg, then switch legs and repeat.

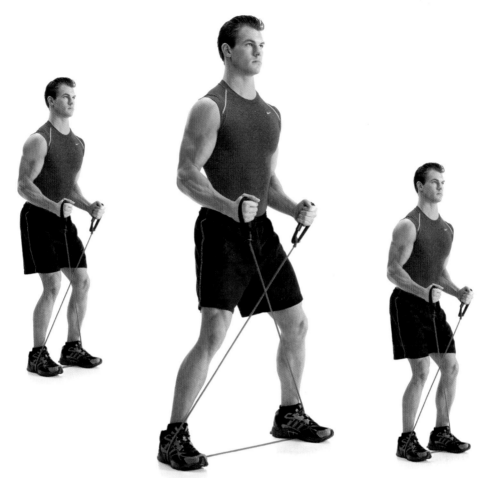

HIP ABDUCTION WITH BAND

WHERE IT IS: Get Even Bigger, HFT for Other Muscle Groups

PREP: You'll need a stretch band for this one. (Just about any fitness-equipment store will have bands.) Hold an end of the band in each hand, with the middle of the band on the floor. Step on the band with both feet. You want your feet shoulder-width apart, your toes pointed ahead, and the band under the arches of both feet. Make sure there's an equal amount of band on both sides. (If it's off-center, adjust so it's not shorter or tighter on one side.) Throughout the exercise, you want to hold it so there's no slack in the band at any point.

Now switch hands with the ends of the band, so it crosses in front of your knees. Push your hips back just a bit, allowing a slight bend in your knees—imagine that you're in a good defensive position in basketball, only with your elbows in at your sides, arms bent.

START: Step to the left with your left foot without changing your posture. Your toes stay pointing straight ahead. Now step the same distance to the left with your right foot. If you stepped 12 inches with your left, step 12 inches with your right.

FINISH: Reverse the movement: Step to the right with your right foot, then step the same distance to the right with your left foot. This should put you back in the spot from which you started. That's one repetition.

Key point: There should be tension in the band throughout the movement.

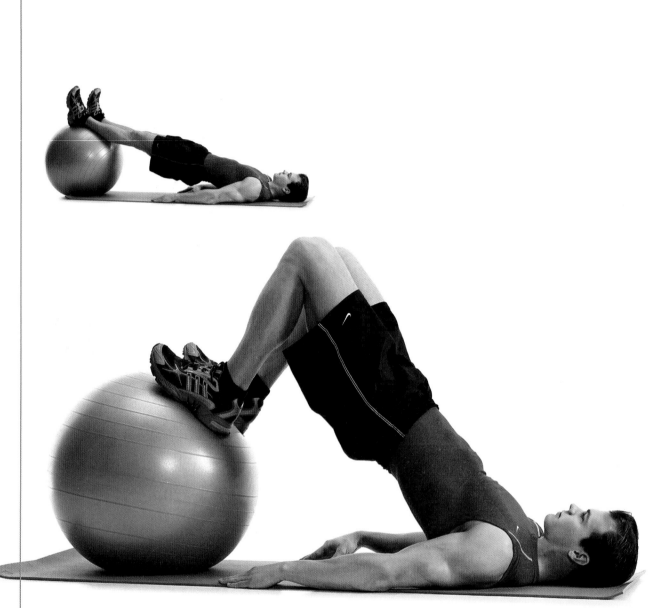

SWISS-BALL LEG CURL

WHERE IT IS: Get Even Bigger, HFT for Other Muscle Groups

PREP: Grab a Swiss ball; the size doesn't matter, although it's easier to learn the movement on a smaller ball (45 or 55 centimeters versus 65 or 75 centimeters). Whatever size you use, make sure it's fully inflated. Lie faceup on the floor with your heels resting on the ball, your legs straight, and your feet pointed straight up. Lift your hips, tighten up your core, and set your body in a straight line from ankles to shoulders.

IN: Pull your heels toward your glutes as far as possible, raising your hips as you do. At the end, your body should form a straight line from knees to shoulders.

OUT: Roll back to the starting position; don't let your hips sag below the plane of your ankles and shoulders.

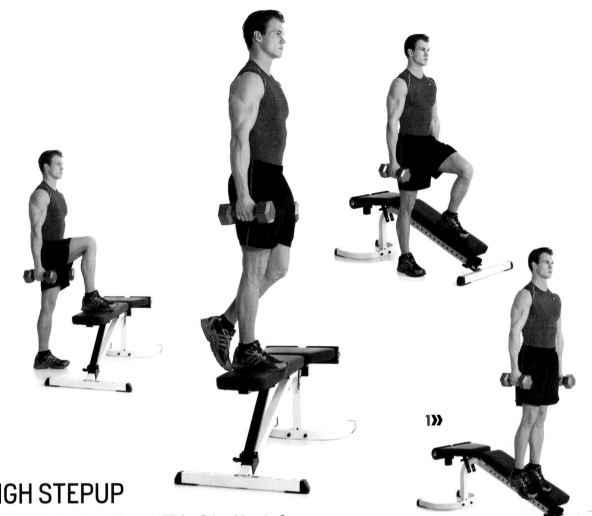

HIGH STEPUP

WHERE IT IS: Get Even Bigger, HFT for Other Muscle Groups

PREP: Grab a pair of dumbbells and stand in front of a step, bench, or box that's at knee level. Place your nondominant foot flat on the step, holding the dumbbells at arm's length at your sides. Both your feet should point straight ahead.

UP: Push down through your foot on the step, lifting yourself up until that leg is straight and your other foot is also on the step.

DOWN: Reverse the motion, keeping your nondominant foot on the step while stepping down with your other one. Do all your reps with your nondominant leg, then repeat the set with your other foot on the step.

Key point: You want all the power for this exercise to come from the leg that's on the step, so avoid helping out by pushing off with your trailing leg. It's there strictly for ballast.

VARIATION:

1» STEPUP ON DECLINE BENCH

WHERE IT IS: Get Even Bigger, HFT for Other Muscle Groups

HOW TO DO IT: Grab a pair of dumbbells and stand with a decline bench to your left. Hold the dumbbells at arm's length at your sides. Place your nondominant foot on the decline with your toes lower than your heel. Now do stepups as described above.

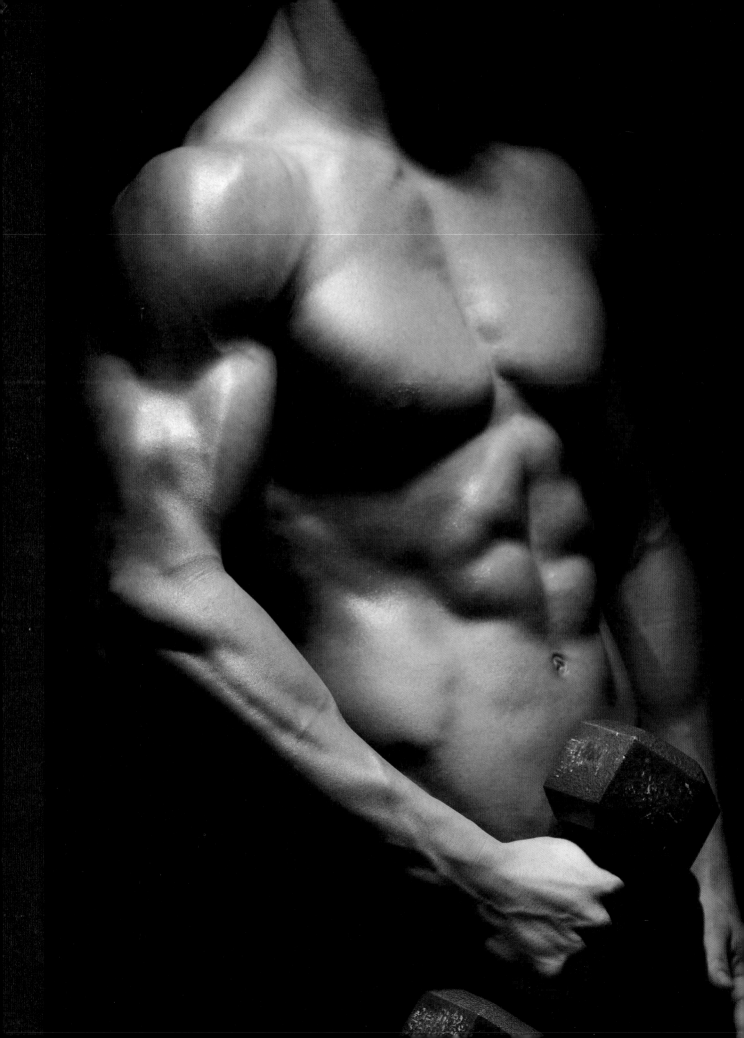

PART 5: THE FUEL

CHAPTER 22

FEEDING YOUR MUSCLES...
AND YOUR BRAIN

To most of us, the word *energy* has multiple meanings, some vague, some specific. If you have a great workout, you probably attribute it to the energy you had at the time. If you feel good one day at work or school but tired or listless the next, you point to "energy" as the culprit—you had enough, or you didn't. Sometimes we describe family, friends, teachers, and co-workers in terms of their energy. Your economics prof in college was "a real low-energy guy." He was better than Ambien if you needed to catch up on sleep. But your current boss is driving you nuts with his oversupply of that same resource; he's like the Energizer Bunny with stock options.

In my world, *energy* has a single, extremely specific meaning: fuel. Food, in other words. It has no subjective meanings, no nuance, no value attached to it aside from the simple math you need to calculate how much energy is contained in any given unit of food.

And yet, I think it's important for us to think about food both ways: as measurable units of fuel, and as chemicals with specific powers to affect our "energy" at any particular moment.

This chapter will start with the basics: how we measure energy, and how it applies to you. Then I'll get into the fun stuff about how food triggers or shuts down the hormones that matter to muscleheads like us, including some insight into the ways nutrients and hormones affect both mood and muscle. The specifics—what you should and shouldn't eat to reach your goals—are the subject of the next chapter.

CALORIES:
THE MEASURE OF A MEAL

In science, we measure food two different ways. The first is with kilocalories, which in casual conversation becomes the simpler and shorter "calories." A calorie is a unit of energy. So when someone tells you that a pound of fat has 3,500 calories, what they're really saying is that it contains 3,500 units of energy. Which means . . . well, what does it mean?

All human activity requires energy, which as I already said is measured in calories. Your brain and heart and all the other working parts use energy at every moment of your life. They use more energy when you're awake than asleep, more when you're moving than when you're sedentary, and much more when you're working out.

Your body also uses energy at a faster clip after you're finished working out, as it gets busy refueling and rebuilding your muscles. Your energy use likewise ramps up after you eat, during digestion. That means it takes energy to process the energy you've thrown into your stomach.

Thus, you should think of *food, energy,* and *fuel* as three words that mean the exact same thing to your body.

And that brings us back to calories, the units of food/energy/fuel that keep your body running. Your body prefers to use the food you eat as its main source of fuel. That's how it maintains homeostasis, which is to say your current weight, metabolic rate, and ratio of fat

to muscle. In science, we say you're in "energy balance" if you're not gaining or losing weight. It's a fancy way of saying that all the fuel you need comes from the food you eat.

If you think about it, it's kind of amazing that anybody manages to stay in a state of energy balance. Your energy needs change from day to day, especially if you work out hard several times a week. What you eat, when you eat, and how you eat also affect the amount of energy your body uses. (I'll explain that in more detail in the next chapter.) That's why few of us are in energy balance on an hourly or daily or even weekly basis. But a lot of us maintain our weight over longer periods of time—months and even years. It's what your body wants you to do, and later in this chapter I'll introduce you to the hormones that work to make it happen. The system is great for guys who have hit their ideal body weight, but not so wonderful for those of us who want to gain muscular weight or lose excess pounds of fat.

Now we're back to that pound of fat, with its 3,500 calories' worth of energy. If all you know about energy balance is what you read in newspapers and magazines, you get the impression that all you need to do is eat less and exercise more, and when your body runs out of food to use for fuel, it taps right into that energy-rich pound of fat.

If it were really that simple, you wouldn't need a book like this one. So let's jump into the complexities.

MANAGING YOUR MACROS

Our food supply has three macronutrients: protein, carbohydrate, and fat. Usually, we measure these in terms of their weight in grams. Two macronutrients—protein and carbohydrate—contain 4 calories per gram. Fat, though, has 9 calories. There was a time when nutritionists thought these numbers were really important for weight control, even though we now know they really aren't. What matters is not how much energy each has per gram, but how your body uses that energy. I'll return to that theme throughout this chapter.

PROTEIN

Protein comes from the Greek word *prota*, meaning "of primary importance." That's because your body can't survive without it. It needs protein to build muscle tissue, to help cells communicate with each other, and to serve as a catalyst for various chemical reactions that aren't worth going into here.

You probably think of your muscles as magnificent repositories of protein, but in fact they're mostly water and other fluids. Only about 20 to 25 percent of your muscle mass is actually grade-A protein, while 70 percent, give or take, is liquid. Most of the rest is stored energy from carbohydrates and fat. You also have some minerals in the mix.

All protein isn't created equal. Different types are made of different combinations and quantities of amino acids, the building blocks

of protein. The best are those we call "complete" proteins, meaning they include all 20 of the amino acids you need to build muscle. Your body can actually fabricate 11 of those amino acids from other nutrients. The other nine are what we call "essential" aminos, and they have to come from food. Three of those nine are branched-chain amino acids (BCAAs), and they're the most important of all for building the muscle you want. You find complete proteins in food that comes from animals: meat, poultry, fish, eggs, and dairy products. Very few nonanimal products have complete proteins, which is why you need to combine several of them in the same meal—beans and rice, say—to get the entire set. (Soy is the best-known vegetable source of complete proteins, and I'll explain in the next chapter why you want to avoid it whenever possible.)

When you eat protein, your body breaks it down into its components and then rebuilds those components into functional muscle tissue. The process is called protein synthesis, and it goes on continuously, day and night, throughout your body. Training accelerates the process, of course, but it goes on even if you don't work out.

Experts have widely divergent opinions on how much protein you need, mostly because there are so many ways to define "need." To some, it's the minimum required for survival, which isn't much. Eat a chicken breast and you're covered for the day. To others, it's the amount required for homeostasis, to stay exactly where you are. Put another way, it's the amount you need to avoid losing muscle tissue, which, as I said, your body breaks down and builds up throughout the day no matter how much or how little exercise you get. By that definition, a typical nonexerciser could eat more than enough protein from a typical American diet without giving it any thought.

Yet another type of expert looks at how much protein guys like us actually use. This is where it gets interesting. The process involves measuring the amount of protein going in, and subtracting what comes out. (I'll spare you the details.) The difference, in theory, is the amount of protein your body can actually use. Most experts agree this number is a little less than 1 gram of protein for every pound of body weight.

I round up, like every ambitious muscle-head, and say that the best starting point is 1 gram per pound per day. You might be able to use a little more than that, but I doubt if any of us could actually tell the difference. You don't want to overshoot in any substantial way for two practical reasons: First, your body will use the excess as a source of energy, which you don't want; your body is made to run on a combination of fat and carbohydrate, and protein is strictly a last-resort energy source. Second, if you're eating that much protein, you're not eating foods that provide benefits you won't get from steak and eggs. Beef and eggs have a nice array of vitamins and minerals, along with their high-quality amino acids and perfectly useful fats, but can't remotely replicate all the healthful nutrients you find in fruits and vegetables.

CARBOHYDRATES

Your body likes to keep things as simple as possible. That's why it loves to run on carbohydrates: During digestion, all carbs are broken down into glucose (some more easily than others), the energy source your body can use for fuel with the fewest metabolic hurdles.

You always have some glucose in your bloodstream; you'd die if you didn't. But you rarely have enough to keep you going for 3 hours between meals, and you certainly don't have enough for a hard workout. That's when your body turns to the next simplest source of energy: carbohydrates stored in your muscles and liver, in the form of glycogen. Again, it never completely runs out of those energy stores, but it does manage them carefully. When the supply starts to run low, it turns to the fat you have stored in your fat cells. (You also keep some fat in your muscle cells, but not a lot.) And if you're ever at the point when that energy starts to run out, your body turns to the last resort: the protein you've accumulated in your muscles.

There are two ways to get your body to use more fat for energy:

▶▶ Become really good at endurance exercise, training your body to use fat so it hangs on to more of its precious glycogen.

▶▶ Give your body fewer carbs to work with, forcing it to use fat more readily.

The latter strategy, as you certainly guessed, is the one I advocate for you. It brings with it a major bonus: When you give your body fewer carbs, you reduce its production of insulin. And that means you're less likely to store fat in the first place.

Here's why: **Insulin** is your body's equivalent of an air-traffic controller. Its job is to keep your blood vessels clear and open to traffic. When you send nutrients into your bloodstream after a meal, insulin goes to work to get them out of there. It has three places to store that food:

›› Your muscle cells, where of course you want protein and carbs to go;

›› Your liver, which it uses to store glycogen if your muscles don't need it; and

›› Your fat cells, which take whatever is left over after your muscles and liver have all they can handle.

Any time you eat carbohydrates, insulin is released. (It's also released by protein and fat, but carbs are what really set it off.) You need some insulin to pull glucose and amino acids out of your bloodstream and into your muscles—which of course happens when you train with weights. Bigger muscles store more glycogen and protein than smaller muscles. This is one of the reasons strength training helps you stay lean: More nutrients go into your muscles, leaving fewer to get stored in your fat cells. Training also makes your muscles more receptive to insulin, the metabolic equivalent of a big "welcome" sign.

The amount of insulin you produce with any given meal is proportional to the amount of carbohydrates in the meal, and how fast they reach your bloodstream. You have two key windows of opportunity to get protein and carbs into your muscles: your first meal of the day, and the meal that immediately follows your workout. That's when muscle tissue needs and wants those nutrients, so your best strategy for building bigger muscles is to use food and insulin to your advantage at those two key moments.

At other times of the day, insulin can do more harm than good by pushing nutrients into fat cells, which of course is the last thing you want. Since insulin is a storage hormone, nothing comes out of storage while it's at work. If you tend to store fat around your midsection, you can safely assume that your body is producing too much insulin. You need a strategy for getting what you need when you need it, and for avoiding the wrong carbs at the wrong time.

Specifically, you want to eat fast-acting carbs—raisins and bananas are good examples—in the 1-hour window following a workout. You need whatever carbs and protein you eat in that hour to get into your bloodstream as quickly as possible, for two big reasons:

›› Fast-acting nutrients cause your body to release more insulin, and release it faster, than slower-digesting foods.

›› Since your muscles are most receptive to insulin in that hour, they'll make good use of those carbs and protein.

At other times, you want slower-digesting carbohydrates, particularly those with a lot of fiber, like vegetables and black beans. Because they take a while to make their way into your bloodstream, your body generates less insulin in response. The less insulin you have, the less urgency there is to pull the nutrients out of your bloodstream. So, some will be used as fuel, some will get stored in your muscles, and relatively little will end up warehoused in your fat cells.

The best way to slow down digestion, and thus limit the mischief insulin can perpetrate on your body, is to include fat and protein in every meal, along with carbohydrates. Fat and protein are slower to digest, and leave you feeling fuller longer. One exception: the meal you eat immediately after your workout. Since you want to speed up digestion at that moment, you avoid fat.

Ideal carbohydrate sources are vegetables and fruits, along with beans whenever practical. Starches and grains—a category that includes breads, cereals, pasta, rice, and potatoes—should be minimized. They offer too many calories in proportion to their nutritional value.

Vegetables are the best carbs of all. They provide:

>> Fiber, which keeps food moving through your system more efficiently, and also helps you feel full longer between meals;

>> Antioxidants, which fight disease-causing chemicals called free radicals;

>> Anti-carcinogens, which help prevent cancer; and

>> Enzymes, to help your body use the protein in your meals.

Fruit offers many of the same benefits, but it also has more calories (almost all of which come from carbohydrates) and tends to be faster-acting. I'll discuss all this in more detail in the next chapter, but for now I'll just say that fruit is important, but the amount you should eat depends on your goals.

FAT

I won't say that any of the three macronutrients is more important than the others, but fat is by far the most underrated. Some fats are essential, meaning your body can't make them from other fats. You have to get them from food and supplements.

These essential fats increase your HDL, the "good" cholesterol. They help you use fat for fuel, fight inflammation, and improve the health and efficiency of your nervous system, and they might even make your muscles more sensitive to insulin. Believe me, I could add a lot more to this list, but I think you get the point.

I talk about the best and worst fats in detail in the next chapter, but for now I want to focus on saturated fat. It's not an essential fat, but it's still an important one that, in my view, has been unfairly demonized. The main reason is the widely held belief that saturated fat raises your cholesterol levels, particularly your levels of LDL, the "bad" cholesterol.

But consider this: In a 12-week study at the University of Connecticut, overweight men and women on a low-carb diet actually reduced their LDL more than a matched group on a low-fat diet. This was despite the fact that the low-carb group ate a lot more saturated fat.

Another important finding of the study:

The low-carb group ended up with lower levels of triglycerides in their blood than the low-fat dieters. Triglycerides are the form of fat our bodies use for fuel. We store some in our muscles, but most of the triglycerides we use for activity come either from the food we eat—in other words, we use them before they're stored in our fat cells—or from the fat cells themselves. The really important thing to know about triglycerides is that they're linked to heart disease and diabetes. The more you have floating around in your blood, the higher your risk. A 40-year study by the University of Hawaii showed that people who had low triglycerides in middle age had the best chance to live more than 85 years without suffering from a major disease.

Obviously, this book is about building bigger muscles, not longevity. But I bring this up for two reasons: First, overall health is important to all of us. Second, having the right kinds of fat in your diet—one of the essential fats I mentioned earlier, along with saturated fat, plus another muscle-friendly type that I'll discuss in the next chapter—is crucial to getting those bigger muscles.

The biggest reason we fear fat, beyond the misguided and simplistic notion that it makes us fat, is because we've been told it will give us heart disease. Specifically, experts have told us that dietary fats raise the levels of cholesterol in our blood. I've already mentioned the two main types of cholesterol: LDL, which you already know is the bad one, and HDL, the good one. For

decades, most doctors, nutritionists, and researchers agreed that foods containing relatively high amounts of cholesterol would increase the cholesterol in your blood. So they warned us about egg yolks, meat, poultry, seafood, and dairy products.

But there's a big problem with this belief: If you don't eat foods with cholesterol, your body will make its own supply. Your liver can manufacture several times more cholesterol than you could ever eat. In fact, every cell in your body can make it. Cholesterol provides the essential components of cell membranes, acts as an antioxidant, and helps you digest dietary fats.

All of which is nice, of course, but for us it pales in importance to the cholesterol-testosterone connection. Cholesterol is the only substance your body can use to make its most important muscle-building hormone. With that in mind, let's shift the conversation from food to hormones, and the role these chemical messengers play in the muscle-building process.

MUSCLE-BUILDING MESSENGERS
Along with helping you turn that steak you ate into muscle, testosterone also increases libido, boosts your mood, improves your immune function, and protects your bones against osteoporosis. The simplest way to keep your testosterone levels up is to eat enough cholesterol, which is a major goal of the nutrition plan in the next chapter.

While testosterone has its biggest impact on your muscle tissue, **growth hormone (GH)** stimulates every cell in your body. If you inject synthetic growth hormone on a regular basis (something I'd discourage), almost everything will get bigger, including your skull and internal organs. Growth hormone also helps you regulate body fat and recover from workouts. You'll get your biggest dose of GH about an hour after you fall asleep at night, but the dose you generate with training will do more to enhance your physique.

Insulin-like growth factor (IGF-1) is a derivative of GH, and it helps regulate cell growth, particularly in muscle and nerve cells. It has its own derivative, called mechano growth factor, or MGF. This is the part of IGF-1 that seems to respond to training by helping to repair muscle damage. One intriguing possibility is that it may activate satellite cells within our muscles, which manufacture proteins that make bigger muscle fibers.

Cortisol is the anti-testosterone. While testosterone increases protein synthesis, cortisol shuts it down. It's also the anti-insulin: It pulls amino acids out of muscles, turns them into glucose, and allows them to be used for fuel. You're particularly vulnerable to cortisol-induced muscle breakdown when you're stressed, starved, or short of sleep.

The easy and obvious ways to limit cortisol include eating enough food, eating it frequently, and getting plenty of sleep. Just about anything else you do to relax your body and mind will help you keep your hard-earned muscle tissue.

FROM MOUTH TO BRAIN

The hypothalamus is a small region at the base of your brain that regulates your feelings of hunger and satiety. Scientists have shown that they can make a laboratory animal obese or lean by manipulating different parts of its hypothalamus. Since you aren't a lab rat, you have to use your diet to manipulate your own brain, with the goal of making your key appetite-regulating hormones work for you, rather than against you.

Here's a brief overview of the key players.

EMPTY STOMACH

Ghrelin: This hormone is produced in the stomach 20 to 30 minutes before eating. The trigger for release is unclear, but it may signal the brain that it's ready for a meal.

FULL STOMACH

Stomach and intestinal distention: When you're full, your stomach distends and transmits nerve signals to your brain to decrease appetite.

Liver: Receptors in the liver send signals to your brain indicating that ingested food is being broken down.

Insulin and glucose: Circulating levels of insulin from the pancreas, along with glucose from the food itself, tell the brain that you now have a readily available supply of energy.

CCK and PPY: These peptides are produced by the intestines and are secreted into the bloodstream after a meal to tell the brain to decrease appetite.

SLEEP YOUR WAY TO BIGGER MUSCLES

If you want a better physique—and, of course, you wouldn't be reading this book if you didn't—you know you need to exercise. You almost certainly realize that you need to eat the right foods at the right times, and in the right quantities. You probably know that sleep matters as well; you can't recover sufficiently from one workout to the next unless you get enough of it. But I'd be surprised if you've considered the importance of naps.

Sleep has five stages, two of which happen during a 20-minute nap. The first stage relaxes your brain and facial muscles. The second stage relaxes all the rest of your muscles throughout your body. Not only does a postworkout nap help you jump-start the recovery process, it can also reduce your levels of cortisol, the stress hormone that eats away at your muscle tissue.

Longer naps offer even more benefit, particularly if you're short on sleep for any reason. Sleep loss reduces your levels of leptin, a hormone that puts a brake on your appetite, and increases ghrelin, which makes you hungrier. Catch up on your sleep with a nap, and you rebalance those hormones.

The downside to longer naps is that you go beyond the first two sleep stages, leaving you groggy and disoriented when you wake up. (Especially if you have one of those dreams about showing up at work in your underwear.) But there's rarely a need to go beyond 20 minutes. You'll feel better, look better, and probably be mentally sharper for the rest of the day. Plus, you'll be in good company: Albert Einstein, John F. Kennedy, and Lance Armstrong are among the most famous enthusiastic napsters.

Not only does your gut talk to your brain when it's hungry or full, your fat cells also jump in on the conversation. And make no mistake about this: The brain takes their calls.

This is still a new area of research. Until the mid-1990s, nutritional science thought of fat cells as inert blobs of grease. Since then, researchers have identified some dozen hormones generated by fat cells. Collectively, they're known as adipokines.

The first hint came decades ago, when researchers observed a puzzling syndrome in obese mice: They were hungrier than normal-weight mice but also had slower metabolisms. It doesn't take a PhD to figure out that if you eat more calories and burn less, you'll get fat. What puzzled the scientists was why these particular mice would get stuck with such a lousy genetic predisposition.

Jeffrey Friedman, MD, PhD, and his colleagues at Rockefeller University finally identified the culprit in 1994. They also discovered that the gene was predominantly active in fat cells; it regulated a hormone that worked in normal-weight mice, but not in the obese ones.

The researchers named the protein "leptin," from the Greek root *leptos*, for "thin." Once leptin was injected into the obese mice, they ate less, moved around more, and consequently lost weight. The same gene mutation was soon identified in some unlucky humans. When they were injected with leptin, they lost fat, just as the mice had.

The existence of leptin was interesting enough; nutrition scientists immediately sensed a breakthrough in their understanding of obesity, and a possible way to reverse it. But even more important was evidence that fat cells were more complex than anyone had previously assumed.

Then, as now, the most important question is this: What do we do with this information?

First off, you want to keep your body's natural leptin production as high as possible. Leptin levels drop when you're dieting, triggering a cascade of events that cancel out whatever benefits you're getting from cutting calories. Hunger increases, and your metabolism slows down. That's why a lot of people believe that dieting just makes you fatter in the long run.

This probably doesn't apply to you right now, but it could if you finish off the *Huge in a Hurry* workouts with a fat-loss phase to bring out the details in the muscles you worked so hard to build. You'll need to cut calories, but you also have to ensure you don't undermine

your goals by shutting down your leptin production.

The best strategy is to have a day each week when you eat more calories, including a "cheat" meal. You want the cheat meal to have plenty of calories from all three macronutrients—carbs, protein, and fat. Pizza and cheeseburgers are good examples (although having both in the same meal is overkill).

Second, you want your body to be sensitive to the effects of the leptin you produce, just as you want your muscles to be sensitive to insulin. Many obese people produce plenty of leptin, but their cells aren't sensitive to it. Lucky for us, exercise increases your sensitivity to leptin. So as long as you're following the training and nutrition programs in this book, you'll get all the benefits leptin has to offer.

BRIDGING THE GAP BETWEEN BODY AND MIND

I know I've hit you with a lot of information in this chapter, some of which may not be immediately useful to you. But I can sum it up simply enough: Everything you eat affects your brain. If you feel good, it's because you gave your brain and body the nutrients they need. If you feel rotten, you threw your hormones out of whack by ingesting the wrong nutrients at the wrong time.

With that in mind, let's move on to the specifics of my nutrition plan.

CHAPTER 23

WHAT TO EAT
AND WHEN TO EAT IT

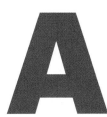colleague of mine, Chris Shugart, was asked about the importance of nutrition. "Diet is much, much more important than training," he said. "Not really a secret, just something that's underestimated and overlooked. It took several experiences for me to accept this fact. One of them was when I gained 10 pounds of mass using a Chad Waterbury program. Then I turned around a few months later, changed from a mass diet to a cutting diet, and lost 10 pounds of fat . . . using the same Waterbury program. This made me realize that while good training has to be there, it's the *diet* that drives the results."

He's right. You could follow one of the fat-loss training programs in this book and gain fat if you don't eat right. And the muscle-building workouts will never help you gain as much size as you want, as fast as you want, unless you give your body the nutrients it needs when it needs them most. Nobody argues that a good training program isn't important. It's crucial. Your results, though, are maximized or limited by your diet.

Is it possible to lose some body fat and build a little muscle with a crap diet? Sure, if you're young and getting so much exercise that you burn off more calories than you eat. College basketball players are good examples. But for most of us it's just not possible to do that much exercise. Nor should you have to. You'll *always* get better results, regardless of your age or energy expenditure, if you make your diet work for you rather than against you.

Experts differ on the best nutritional parameters for muscleheads. As you know, I'm not a nutritionist. But the guidelines I lay out in this chapter have worked for most of the athletes and clients I've trained or consulted with, and they've certainly worked for me over the years.

WHAT TO EAT

In the previous chapter I discussed why you need carbohydrates, protein, and fat, as well as the effects each has on the hormones you want to maximize and minimize. Now it's time to put that advice into practical guidelines.

PROTEIN

Ideal sources: grass-fed beef, free-range poultry, salmon, mackerel, shellfish, wild game, and whole eggs.

Good sources: Cheese, yogurt, and milk are good options for those who aren't lactose-intolerant. (Cheese, including cottage cheese, is almost always a better option than yogurt and milk, though, since it contains fewer carbs.) Protein powders made with the two main milk proteins, whey and casein, are staples of postworkout nutrition for most muscleheads.

FAT

Ideal sources: avocados, extra-virgin olive oil, macadamia nut oil, ground flaxseeds, and mixed nuts. (All of the other fat you need will come from the ideal protein sources.)

Good sources: extra-virgin coconut oil, flaxseed oil, and butter.

CARBOHYDRATES

Ideal sources for gaining muscle: all fruits and vegetables, including sweet potatoes and yams; oatmeal; and quinoa.

Ideal sources for losing fat: berries and fibrous vegetables.

Each meal should consist of carbohydrates, protein, and fat, with one exception: You want to minimize fat in your postworkout recovery meal. (The same advice applies to preworkout meals, for those of you who need them; I'll discuss that later in the chapter.) That's the one time of the day when your goal is to maximize the action of insulin. Carbs and protein help you, but fat doesn't.

How much of each micronutrient you should consume depends on your weight, as well as your goals. You can make the details as simple or complex as you want. I prefer to keep things simple. In my experience, most guys never have to worry about counting calories, as long as they follow the basic nutritional principles I'm about to describe.

I'll start with the most basic of all: Eat protein, fruits, and vegetables every 3 hours while awake.

I wish I could stop here. I wish everyone

could stick to that one simple principle. I wish I could make that wish come true because 90 percent of you would transform your bodies, and improve your health, faster than you ever imagined. But I'm a realist and I know that it would be difficult for most of you to make it work without more details. So let's fill in the blanks.

Let's say that you wake up at 7 a.m. and go to bed at 11 p.m., and that you eat your first meal as soon as you get up. (If you don't already do that, you absolutely must start.) That gives you 16 hours for six meals—or, more accurately, three meals and three snacks.

Even though I can't see you as you read this, I know from experience that a lot of you are rolling your eyes at the thought of eating six times a day. The words "yeah, right!" are probably on your mind, if not actually spoken aloud. I've seen that look, and heard those words, from my clients. Inevitably, though, clients who groan at the idea of eating six times a day get tripped up by that very issue. They'll do fine with breakfast, lunch, and dinner. What they eat in between those meals, or what they *don't* eat, inevitably comes back to bite them on the ass.

The irony here is that the three daily snacks are the easiest meals to get right. They're the easiest to prepare and keep track of. We aren't talking about slaving over a hot stove to prepare a gourmet meal. Downing a single piece of fruit and a serving of vegetables is easy. The only trick is to get enough protein. So let's start there.

THE PROTEIN DILEMMA

I recommend 1 gram of protein per pound of body weight per day, with each gram coming from a complete protein source whenever possible. This is the *minimum* requirement. It's better to eat a little extra protein than to cut it close and miss out on some potential benefits.

Here's a look at how to meet that minimum, assuming three meals and three snacks per day:

BODY WEIGHT (POUNDS)	TOTAL PROTEIN PER DAY (GRAMS)	PROTEIN PER MEAL (GRAMS)	PROTEIN PER SNACK (GRAMS)
100–150	100–150	20–30	15–20
150–200	150–200	30–50	20
200+	200+	50–60	25

Let's look at practical examples. I'll start with the assumption that you weigh 175 pounds. If you're bigger or smaller, it's easy to adjust the numbers I use to fit your own targets.

Your goal is 20 grams of protein per snack. Chances are, you'll need to eat at least two of those snacks outside your home, assuming you're either employed full-time or in school. But even if you're a lazy bum living off a bogus insurance settlement, you probably value convenience. The easier a snack is to put together, the more time you can spend doing . . . whatever it is you do.

Some easy ways to get 20 grams of protein:

>> 3 ounces of natural cheese (that is, not American or other processed cheeses)

>> 3 ounces of turkey breast

>> ¾ cup of low-fat cottage cheese

A slightly more exotic option is salmon jerky, which can be found at wildsalmonjerky.com.

Like I said, snacks are simple and easy, as long as you anticipate your need and plan accordingly. Convenient, high-quality protein sources are rare, but their opposite—nutritionally useless snacks and sweets—are everywhere. That's what trips so many people up. A little planning prevents a lot of Little Debbies and nacho-cheddar potato chips.

A lot of lifters turn to protein powders and bars. They're easy and convenient to use. If the choice is between a protein bar and a Snickers bar, of course I'd choose the former over the latter. But protein bars often use nasty, undigestible chemicals called sugar alcohols to cut down on their carbohydrate count, and protein powders often include lots of real or artificial sugars to improve their taste. That's why I think you can avoid making that choice and come out ahead.

Meal-replacement powders are a slightly better option than bars. The best ones have a combination of two milk proteins, whey and casein, which provide the full spectrum of amino acids and digest slower than pure whey protein. I confess I'm not a big fan of

protein powders as meal replacements outside the context of postworkout recovery drinks. (I'll discuss pre- and postworkout drinks in a bit.) But if they're your best or only option, use them.

Even incomplete proteins are better than nothing. If your only protein source is a handful of mixed nuts, that still beats the microwave popcorn or Three Musketeers.

WHAT COUNTS, WHAT DOESN'T

I'm absolutely convinced that the protein in your diet—the right kind, the right amount, the right timing—is more important than any other nutritional consideration. So I want you to count protein grams until you get the hang of it.

But I don't want you to count anything else. Don't worry about fat grams; the fat in the protein sources I recommend takes care of itself. Don't count grams of carbohydrate; the only way carbs will hurt you is if you stray too far from the recommendations in this chapter. And, most of all, don't count total calories. In my experience, calorie counting has three big pitfalls:

>> Nobody can do it for long; unless you're obsessive-compulsive, it quickly becomes too much of a chore.

>> Even if you tried, you couldn't do it with the kind of accuracy the word "counting" implies.

>> It's a waste of time for most people, since your nutritional needs aren't constant. They fluctuate for any number of reasons, and no

one can predict how many calories he'll need on any given day. Your appetite does a surprisingly good job of regulating this for you, as long as you allow it to.

You could make some of the same arguments about protein grams. Certainly, you can't count them accurately in some situations, especially in restaurants. Then there are family and communal meals, at which you're all sharing the main course. Even if you prepared a meal that contains a mix of macronutrients—a soup or stew, for example—you can't really know how many grams of protein you put on your own plate. And your body's need for protein fluctuates from day to day as well.

But no system is perfect, and of all the ones I've read about or tried, counting protein grams works best for me, my clients, and the people I turn to for advice. The number is smaller—few of you will need more than 200 protein grams a day—and you'll find fewer variables.

Really, the only trick is to remember how much protein there is in a few categories of food that you'll typically eat. Soon you'll be able to plan and prepare meals and snacks without stopping to add up how much protein is in any given portion of any given food. Master that skill, and the rest of the diet—especially fat and total calories—falls into place.

Most high-quality protein sources have similar amounts of protein—about 7 grams per ounce. That applies to beef, poultry, seafood, and cheese. A large egg also has 7 grams.

So if you weigh 175 pounds and shoot for 40 grams of protein per meal, all you really need are some visual cues and fourth-grade math skills to calculate your options.

Three ounces of meat, fish, or poultry is about the size of a deck of cards. That's 21 grams of protein, roughly. Now picture a steak the size of two decks of cards—side-by-side, in the case of a sirloin; on top of each other, if it's a fillets. That's six ounces, giving you 42 grams of protein.

An ounce of cheese is about the size of two dice. Six ounces—42 protein grams—is 12 dice.

Eggs are easiest of all: Six of them give you 42 grams of protein. An omelet with five eggs and 1 ounce of cheese gets you to the same place.

GETTING YOUR CARBS RIGHT

My advice on carbs is simple: Have one serving of fruit and one serving of vegetables with each meal and snack. A serving of fruit is an apple, banana, orange, peach, or pear, or a cup of berries or melon.

You don't have to be nearly that precise with vegetables, which have very few carbs. You'd have to eat 6 cups of broccoli to equal the carbs in one banana. Just don't eat too few carbs. A serving of most vegetables is about half a cup, or the size of a light bulb. Six spears of asparagus or seven or eight baby carrots will get you there. A serving of salad greens is a cup.

Beans aren't technically vegetables—they belong to a category of plant foods called legumes—but they have a lot of the same qualities. They're rich in fiber, slow to digest, and packed with nutrients. They also tend to be relatively high in protein. It's not complete protein, but it's still good for your health and your muscles. My favorites are black beans and lentils. A serving is a third of a cup; eat as many as you want, as often as you want.

Once you get beyond fruits, vegetables, and beans, there's one more category of carb-rich plant food: grains and starches. You should avoid grains and starches as much as possible—which, unfortunately, isn't easy. We're talking about the most prominent sources of carbohydrates in our diets.

Because grains haven't been in the human diet as long as other food sources, a lot of us don't handle them particularly well. The problems include allergies, digestive issues, and excess body fat. The latter, of course, is the most serious to a guy who's working hard to improve his physique.

I know you can't avoid grains altogether, especially when a sandwich is your only choice for lunch. A bowl of oatmeal in the morning is perfectly okay, and you certainly won't ruin your waistline with an occasional baked potato.

Just stick with fruits, vegetables, and black beans most of the time, and you'll be amazed at how much better you look and feel.

THE FAT OF THE LAND

You're probably wondering why I haven't mentioned fat very much so far. It's not because I consider it a trivial subject—I don't. But it's different from the other two in that our biggest concern is with type, rather than quantity. With protein, "type" is easy. Your goal is to get complete proteins, and you know you can find them in animal products such as beef and dairy. The trick is getting enough of them, meal after meal and day after day. With carbohydrates, the issue of quantity is reversed; you want to minimize calories from carbs without losing the substantial health benefits of fruits and vegetables.

Quantity isn't an issue with fat. You want to get about a third of your calories from fat, and that happens almost automatically when you eat the protein sources I recommend. But getting the right combination of saturated, monounsaturated, and polyunsaturated fats is as difficult as it is crucial to the health of your heart, brain, muscles, and joints.

The most important are omega-3 fatty acids, one of the two main types of polyunsaturated fats. They've been linked to bigger muscles, less body fat, and prevention of just about any disease you can think of. They're also increasingly rare in the foods we eat, compared with the foods our ancestors enjoyed. To get them these days, you must either eat a lot of fish or use supplements that contain fish oil. Your goal is to get two key fats: docosahexaenoic acid (DHA) and eicosapentaeonic acid (EPA). Both are necessary for optimal health, but DHA is the superstar. If fatty acids were basketball players, DHA would be Michael Jordan to EPA's Scottie Pippen.

DHA is the most abundant essential fatty acid in your brain. It's been shown to offset cancers and various neurological disorders, including Alzheimer's. Plus, it's been shown to reduce blood triglycerides, which is important for cardiovascular health.

This is not to say that EPA isn't important. It helps reduce inflammation—another key to preventing cardiovascular disease—and it's been shown to decrease the rate of some mental problems, including schizophrenia.

Together, DHA and EPA work to keep your good hormones up and bad hormones down. I'll spare you the details (I'd have to walk you through a biochemistry lesson to explain all the mechanisms) and ask you to take my word on this: These fats play hard at both ends of the court.

I wish I could say that all omega-3 supplements are more or less equal, but they're not. There's a risk of mercury contamination, and some don't have much DHA and EPA. My favorite is Carlson's liquid fish oil. It's made from deep-water Norwegian fish, which have high concentrations of DHA and EPA with low risk of contamination. Plus, it's purified and put through rigorous testing for impurities by an independent agency. The only drawback to Carlson's is that it must be refrigerated after you open the bottle. You can avoid that by

getting Carlson's fish oil capsules, but you need to swallow a lot of them to get the same amount of the key fats.

The simplest way to figure out how much omega-3 you need is to focus on DHA; EPA will take care of itself. Here's how much daily DHA you need, based on body weight.

BODY WEIGHT (POUNDS)	DHA PER DAY (MILLIGRAMS)
100–150	2,000
150–200	3,000
200+	4,000

Each teaspoon of Carlson's liquid fish oil contains 500 milligrams of DHA. Since there are 3 teaspoons in each tablespoon, a 175-pound person would need to take 2 table-spoons per day. Regardless of your body weight, I recommend splitting your fish oil into two doses per day, spaced as evenly apart as possible. Most of my clients take their fish oil with breakfast and dinner.

If you're taking fish oil capsules, you have a three-step process:

>> See how much DHA there is per serving. Let's say it's 300 milligrams.

>> Divide your daily target by that number. In our 175-pound guy, that's 10 servings.

>> Multiply by the number of capsules each serving includes. If the label says a serving is two capsules, you need 20 capsules per day.

>> Take half—10 capsules—with breakfast, and 10 more at dinner.

The other main type of polyunsaturated fat is omega-6, which most of us get too much of unless we're careful to avoid it. Soybean and vegetable oils have a lot of it, and you find those oils everywhere you look.

But there is one type of omega-6 fat that you should seek out: gamma-linolenic acid (GLA). Unlike the most common omega-6 fat, called linoleic acid, GLA is thought to have anti-inflammatory properties, and it might help stave off certain cancers. Most high-quality GLA supplements contain 240 milligrams per softgel. Here's how many you should take:

BODY WEIGHT (POUNDS)	GLA PER DAY (240-MILLIGRAM SOFTGELS)
100–50	4
150–200	6
200+	8

As with fish oil supplements, I recommend splitting your daily target into two servings. Again, having them with breakfast and dinner is easiest.

Monounsaturated fats are also important, since they've been linked to higher testosterone levels in men. Fortunately, they're easy to include. A handful of mixed nuts will give you plenty, since you're already getting a lot from meat and other protein sources. You can also add some sliced avocado to a salad.

As for saturated fat, you don't have to worry about getting too little or too much with the protein-rich foods I listed earlier.

ROTATE YOUR RATIONS

In ancient times, before our ancestors knew how to grow food, much less preserve it against spoilage, humans got a wide variety of food. They had access to wild fruits, nuts, and seeds, along with whatever they could catch in the water or kill on land. Plus, they got nutrients from whatever the fish or game typically ate. Since they were more worried about survival than about the size of their waistlines, they ate all parts of the animals they killed, including the fat-rich brains and bone marrow.

You'd think, with all the choices of foods we have now, that our diets would be even more varied than those of our cave-dwelling forebears. Paradoxically, we have the opposite problem: We can eat so much from such a small range of our favorite foods that we end up overfed and undernourished. In particular, I see this repetitive cycle with protein and carbs.

The easiest way to get variety in your carbs is to pay attention to color. In any given week, you want a variety of green vegetables (peppers, spinach, broccoli, lettuce), as well as fruits and veggies that are red, orange, blue, and purple.

Protein sources differ nutritionally as well. Turkey, grass-fed beef, eggs, and dairy products offer vitamins and minerals that you won't find in the others. To various degrees, those foods are rich in B vitamins (which help the nervous system perform better in sports and exercise, improve your body's ability to use fat for energy, and promote muscle growth by making it easier for your body to process the protein in your diet), calcium and phosphorus (which promote faster muscle reactions), and vitamin D (which helps your body absorb and use calcium and phosphorus).

One last thought about food choices: Avoid anything that makes you feel worse after you eat it. It doesn't matter if it's the most nutritious food on the planet; if it doesn't sit well in your stomach, it's a poor choice for you. Believe me, I speak from experience. Oranges and red peppers are packed with vitamins and minerals, but I can't eat them because they make me feel fatigued and nauseated. Sometimes these problems come from allergies (to strawberries or shellfish, for example), and sometimes you feel bad because your body just doesn't have the enzymes it needs to digest certain foods. You might also just hate the taste or texture of something.

That's why I have an aversion to diet plans that get too specific about which foods to eat when. If the plan includes something you hate, or to which you have an intolerance, the whole thing comes apart. And yet, I wouldn't be doing you any favors if I gave you a bunch of dietary guidelines without at least providing a sample menu.

Here, for demonstration purposes only, is a sample 1-day eating plan for a 175-pound lifter:

7 A.M. MEAL

5 whole eggs, cooked however you like

1 ounce cheese

$\frac{1}{2}$ cup green vegetables (chopped up as part of an omelet, for example)

1 cup blueberries

1 tablespoon Carlson's liquid fish oil

3 GLA softgels

10 A.M. SNACK

3 ounces cheese

1 apple

Celery sticks (handful)

1 P.M. MEAL

6 ounces grilled salmon

Spinach salad with sliced avocado or walnuts, drizzled with olive oil

1 orange

4 P.M. SNACK

$\frac{3}{4}$ cup cottage cheese

1 cup pineapple, mixed into the cottage cheese

Mixed nuts (handful)

7 P.M. MEAL

6 ounces grass-fed beef

6 spears asparagus

1 cup raspberries

1 tablespoon Carlson's liquid fish oil

3 GLA softgels

10 P.M. SNACK

3 ounces free-range chicken breast

Carrots (handful)

1 cup blackberries

PRE- AND POSTWORKOUT NUTRITION

In my experience, a typical lifter falls into one of three nutritional traps:

>> Mediocre overall diet, doesn't do anything special pre- or postworkout.

>> Eats crap throughout the day, but thinks he makes up for it with protein shakes after his workouts.

>> Tries to follow an extreme low-fat or low-carb diet because he thinks it's healthy, and ends up eating too much of everything out of boredom and frustration.

If you simply follow an eating plan like the one I just outlined, without any special adjustments before or after your workouts, you'll be better off than most muscleheads. You'll get everything you need to help you recover from—and thus benefit from—your hard work. You'll have protein for muscle repair and growth, carbs and fat to replenish energy stores, and enough overall calories to allow you to get bigger and stronger.

Still, you can do better. Your muscles are uniquely receptive to nutrients immediately after a workout. That's why, to no one's surprise, I recommend whey protein powder and fast-acting carbohydrates as soon as you finish training.

My choice for a postworkout meal is different from most: raisins with whey protein powder. Creatine is recommended, but optional.

Let's discuss them one at a time:

Whey protein, mixed with water, digests faster than whole-milk proteins, which include a mix of whey and casein. It has high concentrations of branched-chain amino acids (BCAAs), the proteins that are the most valuable for building muscle.

Raisins are an alkaline food, which means they offset acids. Since workouts acidify your muscles and other tissues, you need something alkaline to help restore balance. The more acidic your body is, the harder it is to build muscle. Plus, raisins digest quickly, helping to replenish the glycogen used up in your workout. One caution: Use only organic raisins. Nonorganic raisins are made from grapes that have some of the highest levels of pesticides you'll find.

Creatine speeds up recovery and is linked to improved strength and muscle mass. I prefer micronized creatine.

On the days you work out, just swap the following postworkut meal for one of the snacks you'd ordinarily have that day:

POSTWORKOUT FEEDING

BODY WEIGHT (POUNDS)	RAISINS	WHEY PROTEIN	CREATINE*
100–150	¼ cup	20 grams	3 grams
150–200	⅓ cup	30 grams	4 grams
200+	½ cup	40 grams	5 grams

* Recommended, but optional

If for some reason, you can't eat raisins or if you can't find organic raisins, go for organic grape juice instead. You can mix it with your protein and creatine. The one catch is that grape juice has so many carbs that you'll need to dilute it like this:

BODY WEIGHT (POUNDS)	GRAPE JUICE	WATER
100–150	4 ounces	4 ounces
150–200	6 ounces	4 ounces
200+	8 ounces	4 ounces

"BUT WHAT IF I'M A HARDGAINER?"

"Hardgainers" are guys who struggle more than most lifters to put on solid muscular weight. Most of them are young and skinny, but not all. Some are older and still thin, despite years of dedicated lifting. Others are young but not exactly skinny; they just put on fat more easily than muscle.

True hardgainers—as opposed to guys who just haven't lifted long enough or hard enough to see results, or who worry so much about their abs that they never eat enough to build muscle where it matters—know that the dilemma can't be solved with calories alone. Usually the problem is appetite. They just aren't hungry enough. If they force themselves to eat more one day, they end up eating less the next day or the day after as their appetites adjust to the sudden influx of calories. For the nonskinny hardgainers, more food usually results in more body fat.

But there's a way to add calories that works for almost every hardgainer with whom

I've consulted: Add a preworkout meal. The easiest option is whey protein and fast-acting carbs 20 to 30 minutes before you hit the weight room. You can supercharge that meal by adding extra BCAAs to the mix.

The protein and carbs trigger an insulin release, something you normally don't want before a workout. For a lot of lifters, pre-workout insulin leads to additional fat, rather than muscle. But a hardgainer usually benefits from that extra boost. The insulin pushes nutrients into his muscles while he's training, and the extra BCAAs keep protein synthesis as high as possible.

Here's how it would look:

PREWORKOUT FEEDING FOR HARDGAINERS ONLY

BODY WEIGHT (POUNDS)	CARBS	WHEY PROTEIN	BCAAS
100–150	½ banana*	10 grams	5 grams
150–200	1 banana	20 grams	8 grams
200+	1 banana	30 grams	10 grams

* It doesn't have to be a banana; organic raisins, grape juice, or an orange will work just as well.

POSTWORKOUT FEEDING FOR HARDGAINERS

BODY WEIGHT (POUNDS)	RAISINS	WHEY PROTEIN	CREATINE	BCAAS
100–150	¼ cup	20 grams	3 grams	5 grams
150–200	⅓ cup	30 grams	4 grams	8 grams
200+	½ cup	40 grams	5 grams	10 grams

earlier, the
. t a lack of "fine-
-tune what hasn't yet
. That's why I want you to
this: You won't try to tweak your
.n until you've given it at least 2 weeks
work. That is, you follow my recommendations for protein, carbs, and fat as closely as
you can, along with my suggestions for
postworkout nutrition (and preworkout nutrition, for hardgainers).

I'd prefer that you wait 4 weeks, but
experience tells me a lot of guys will decide
it's not working long before that. Fortunately,
there's a lot you can learn in 2 weeks. No
single indicator gives you all the information
you need, but if you use a combination of
them—scale weight, circumference measure-
ments, performance, mood—you can make
some reasonable assumptions about how
it's going.

The most obvious sign of trouble is when
your body does the opposite of what you
intended—you lose weight when you're
trying to bulk up, or you gain fat when
you're trying to lose it. The solution is usually
pretty simple: Eat fewer carbs when you're
trying to lose fat, and more when you can't
gain muscle.

Manipulating that one variable alters two
important body-changing mechanisms:

>> The total calories you consume

>> The effect of insulin on where those calories
end up

Here's a sample fat-loss plan for our 175-pound
lifter:

7 A.M. MEAL

5 whole eggs, cooked however you like

1 ounce cheese

$\frac{1}{2}$ cup green vegetables (chopped up
as part of an omelet, for example)

1 cup blueberries

1 tablespoon Carlson's liquid fish oil

3 GLA softgels

10 A.M. SNACK

3 ounces cheese

Celery sticks (handful)

1 P.M. MEAL

6 ounces grilled salmon

Spinach salad with sliced avocado
or walnuts, drizzled with olive oil

1 orange

4 P.M. SNACK

$\frac{3}{4}$ cup cottage cheese

Mixed nuts (handful)

7 P.M. MEAL

6 ounces grass-fed beef

6 spears asparagus

1 cup raspberries

1 tablespoon Carlson's liquid fish oil

3 GLA softgels

10 P.M. SNACK

3 ounces free-range chicken breast

Carrots (handful)

You'll notice I didn't change the protein or
fat. I simply removed a serving of fruit from

three of the six meals. (Worth mentioning: I didn't omit any carbs from breakfast, since that's one time when your body can put them to full use. The other time, of course, is immediately after a workout.) That removes a couple hundred calories from the daily total, and it also blunts the effects of insulin three times a day.

If you need to lose a lot of fat—10 pounds or more—cut fruit from all meals except breakfast and the one you have postworkout. Berries are the ideal choice for breakfast, since they're high in nutrients but low in calories.

The biggest problem with a calorie-cutting diet is that it can throw off your hormonal balance within a week or two. Specifically, you can get burned by leptin, an appetite-regulating hormone. As you slip into a caloric deficit—burning more calories than you take in—your body produces less leptin, with the goal of increasing your appetite until you get back into balance. But it's easy enough to keep this mechanism in check. Just add fruit back into every meal once every 7 days.

You should also have a "cheat meal" on the day you're adding the extra fruit. Have pizza for dinner, or a bowl of ice cream for dessert. Don't worry about undoing all your hard work. The extra calories will give you a temporary metabolism boost while taking the edge off the cravings that build up whenever you're maintaining such strict dietary discipline. Meanwhile, your reinvigorated leptin will slow down your appetite.

WHAT TO DRINK

Your body looks and functions best when fully hydrated. Your muscles, being about 70 percent fluid, look stronger and fuller when they have the water they need. And if they're even slightly dehydrated, they can't perform at their peak.

But there are good and bad ways to stay hydrated. Fruit juices, non-diet soda, frou-frou coffee drinks, and flavored iced tea can pump sugar into your body by the shovelful. No workout program ever invented can neutralize the damage wrought by such massive infusions of nutrient-free calories.

Water is by far the most important beverage. I recommend drinking $\frac{1}{2}$ ounce per pound of body weight per day. (If you weigh 200 pounds, you need 100 ounces per day.) It's counterintuitive, but drinking so much water actually prevents your body from retaining fluid. You might even boost your metabolism. Even if you don't, you'll at least get some bonus exercise by going to the restroom more often.

I've had clients who were chronically dehydrated when they came to me. I had them drink 2 gallons of water the first day, followed by a gallon each day from that point on. All of them told me they looked and felt better once they were fully hydrated.

How do you know if you're hydrated? Your urine should be clear. If it's not, you need to drink more water.

Another beverage you should have each day is green tea. Its nutrients and antioxidants—

particularly a catechin called epigallocatechin-3-gallate—help you burn fat and support your immune system. If you need more caffeine than green tea provides, go for organic black coffee. Coffee has antioxidants and provides some health benefits, but green tea is a far better choice.

More and more people are hooked on diet cola and other beverages with artificial sweeteners. I don't like them for two big reasons. First, I'm not at all convinced they're safe; diet-soda addicts are conducting a mass-scale chemistry experiment on themselves, and I'm willing to wait until they hit old age to see how it works out. Second, I've never seen a serious diet-soda drinker who didn't have an insatiable sweet tooth. You'd think that the beverages would satiate the need, but I suspect they do the opposite and reinforce or even exacerbate the craving for sweets. To me, it makes more sense to satisfy your cravings with the natural sugar in fruit.

Alcohol is another obvious problem beverage. Beer and mixed drinks are the worst offenders. Red wine, which is low in carbs and rich in antioxidants, is by far your best choice. I don't recommend drinking much of it if you want to stay lean, but a few glasses a week probably won't hurt.

"Green drinks" are becoming more popular. The original green drink was a shot of wheat grass. These days, products such as ProGreens, PaleoGreens, and Greens+ are good sources of important nutrients such as spirulina, barley grass, wheat grass, and chlorella, just to name a few that you may have heard of. (The rest are even more obscure.) If you stick to the recommended servings of fruits and vegetables in this chapter, green drinks aren't mandatory. If not, one or two green drinks a day can help you limit the nutritional deficit.

DON'T EAT (OR DRINK) THIS

It would be wonderful if we could all eat freshly prepared food at every meal, made from all-natural ingredients produced by farmers with exemplary personal hygiene. But that's a fantasy. In reality, we all have to make compromises and buy packaged food from time to time.

When you do, check the labels to make sure none of the foods contain the following ingredients.

HIGH-FRUCTOSE CORN SYRUP (HFCS)

I'm an even-tempered person, but HFCS makes me boiling mad. Here's why.

You know that carbohydrates trigger insulin release. If you're eating right, insulin will pull glucose out of your blood and into your muscle cells, where you can use it for energy. If you're eating wrong, insulin can shuttle glucose into your fat cells. But insulin also stimulates leptin, a hormone that tells your brain when you're full. When you eat or drink something loaded with HFCS, the glucose in your blood shoots up, as you'd expect when you eat so much pure sugar. HFCS is actually a combination of two sugars: glucose and fructose. (Sucrose, better known as table sugar, is made up of the same two ingredients, but with more glucose and less fructose.) The higher concentration of fructose in HFCS blunts the effect of insulin. With less insulin, there's less leptin, and less satiety. You can drink six cans of soda—900 calories of pure sugar—and still feel hungry. Eat 900 calories of anything else, and you'll feel stuffed.

But that isn't the biggest problem. Without insulin, your blood sugar remains elevated. Your liver then converts all that glucose into fat. You wreck your waistline and still feel hungry afterward. Avoid HFCS at all costs.

MAN-MADE TRANS FATS

Some trans-fatty acids—fats that are transformed from other fats—are natural. I single out the "man-made" versions because conjugated linoleic acid (CLA) is a good fat that also happens to be a naturally occurring trans fatty acid, found in meat and cheese. The ones you have to watch out for are usually labeled "partially hydrogenated vegetable oil" or similarly appetizing words. Since they're man-made, your body doesn't metabolize them the same way it metabolizes natural fat sources. That's probably why trans fats have been linked to numerous health problems, including heart disease.

The good news is that food manufacturers have taken most of the trans fats out of their prepared foods, and fast-food restaurants are doing the same. Still, if you see trans fats on a nutrition label, buy something else.

SUGAR ALCOHOLS

A few years back, a new phrase entered the nutritional lexicon: "net carbs." This was a way of distinguishing which carbohydrates in a food labeled "low carb" were actually absorbed into your bloodstream, and which just passed on through. This allowed companies to manufacture a protein bar with 30 grams of carbohydrates, but sell it as having just 6 grams of "net carbs."

The gross carbs—the ones that don't get into your bloodstream—are a man-made combination of sugar and alcohol. You'll see them listed on nutrition labels with names like xylitol, mannitol, and sorbitol.

As you can imagine, your body doesn't respond well to sugar alcohols, just as it struggles to digest any type of food made in a lab. Typical reactions include bloating, diarrhea, and gas. I mean really, really, *really* bad gas. So avoid sugar alcohols, and get your carbs the way nature intended: with fruits, vegetables, nuts, seeds, and beans.

SOY AND XENOESTROGENS

Soy is the most overrated food of my lifetime. For a while it was linked to a long list of health benefits, including cholesterol reduction. Most of these claims were unfounded. Although soybeans themselves include complete proteins—one of the few non-animal foods that do—most soy products, such as tofu, are low in nutrients and offer poorly utilized, incomplete proteins. But people today still consider it a health-promoting food, which is odd since it offers no proven benefits to the entire male gender. It may actually lead to estrogen production—the opposite of what a musclehead needs or wants.

I recommend avoiding anything with soy on the label. But even if you manage that, you can't avoid soy altogether. Soy products are hidden in so many foods today that we all get more of them than we could ever keep track of. Not only is fast food often laced with concentrated vegetable proteins made from soy, but seemingly soyless foods like milk, flour, and various vegetable oils might also include soy. So even though a nutrition label might not indicate any soy at all, there's always a chance that soy has been snuck in as part of another ingredient.

Which brings me to a really nasty class of man-made chemicals called xenoestrogens. They are found in plastics, canned foods, pesticides, and detergents—the complete list is much longer—and have been linked to cancer and several types of hormonal dysfunction. Here are some ways to avoid them:

Use glass and ceramic containers to store your food: I hate to break it to you, but bottled water that comes in plastic containers is not good for your health. If you're going to refrigerate water, keep it in glass bottles. And never heat up your food in plastic containers, since heat releases the chemicals in the plastic, sending them into your food.

Don't buy canned food: Most cans are lined with a plastic coating to keep the food from tasting metallic. Heat and long-term storage can allow the coating to break down, with xenoestrogens passing into your food.

Only buy organic produce: Nonorganic fruits and vegetables are often exposed to pesticides. Beyond the risk of xenoestrogen exposure, pesticides have long been considered carcinogenic—that is, they raise the risk of cancer.

Only buy hormone-free meats: Commercially raised cattle are often given xenoestrogens to fatten them up. This can affect your health in several ways: decreased sperm count, increased estrogen levels, and, potentially, a disrupted metabolism. Before livestock hormones were regulated, people eating the most highly saturated meat and dairy products experienced bizarre reactions. Girls as young as 1 year old started puberty, while boys developed breasts. Those levels of hormones are a thing of the past—the worst offenders were phased out by the 1970s—but they haven't been eliminated entirely. My big point here isn't that your health is immediately imperiled by these hormones, but that you can accumulate more than you think by eating large amounts of foods that contain small amounts of feminizing hormones. Obviously, that's the last thing you want when you're trying to build bigger, stronger muscles.

CHAPTER 24

GETTING READY FOR YOUR CLOSE-UP

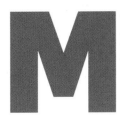y friend Holly used to compete in natural bodybuilding shows. Coached by her husband, she trained hard and had a great physique to show for it. The week before each show, she followed a protocol that manipulated water, sodium, and carb intake . . . and it never quite worked. She entered her contests holding too much water in her skin and not enough in her muscles. That made her look like she had more fat and less muscle than was actually the case.

After the shows, she'd treat herself to pepperoni pizza. The next morning, much to her dismay, she'd look in the mirror and see a better physique than the one she'd starved and dehydrated herself to achieve the night before. Her muscles were bigger and fuller; her skin was tighter and showed more vascularity.

This went on for 2 years—different shows, same outcome.

Finally, in her third year of figure competition, she decided to make one crucial change: Instead of eating pizza after the contest, she treated herself the night before.

And she won.

I'd be willing to bet something similar has happened to you. It usually goes like this: You've been training hard and consistently for weeks or months, with no particular goal in mind except getting stronger and looking better. Your diet has been reasonably clean, and your body-fat percentage is in the low double digits. Then one night you get together with your buddies to watch the biggest game of the year, and you don't even bother restraining yourself. You eat three-quarters of a pizza and wash it down with six of Milwaukee's finest.

The next morning, you wake up with a headache, bleary eyes, a cotton mouth . . . and better abs than you've ever seen on your own torso. You know where you were the night before, and it sure as hell wasn't the gym. And you know what you ate and drank. So why did the Ab Gods choose this particular morning to give you something you've always wanted but never before achieved?

Here's the surprising truth: A fatty, sodium-infused meal, combined with the dehydrating effects of alcohol, can pull water from underneath your skin and shuttle it into your muscles. You look lean and pumped up, even if you feel bloated and beaten down.

Unfortunately, that same pizza and beer probably made your buddies wake up looking like beached whales.

And that brings me to this book's final program. You're 99 percent of the way to the hugeness promised in the book's title, with the bigger, stronger muscles you've built since you started doing my workouts. Now I'll leave you with a diet strategy for displaying what you've accomplished.

A FLUID SITUATION

The problem, as you can see from the anecdote I opened with, is water. You need lots and lots of water to build your body; as I said in the previous chapter, the more you drink, the less

your body will hold in your skin, and the better your muscles will look.

But when you need to peak for a single event—spring break, your wedding day, a bodybuilding contest, a modeling shoot—you have to come up with a strategy to hold even less water in your skin. And if you're a fighter who has to forfeit if you can't make weight, you need to know how to lose some water without sacrificing muscle, compromising performance, or risking your health.

Unfortunately, what I'm about to describe is hard to do (I always tell my bodybuilding and figure clients that training and dieting are the *easy* part), and there's no single way that works for everybody.

Before I get into the particulars, I want to throw out two cautions:

›› If your career depends on achieving peak leanness and muscularity for a single day—or even a single hour if you're a fighter who has to get through a weigh-in—don't attempt this for the first time immediately before that moment of truth. You have to give it a trial run several weeks in advance to make sure it's going to work. That gives you plenty of time to make adjustments if it's not right for you.

›› If you have any medical concerns or considerations that might come into play during a strenuous attempt to go from lean to superlean, talk them over with a doctor, trainer, coach, nutritionist, or any other health or fitness professional who knows you well enough to offer an informed opinion. Make sure it's right for you before starting.

CUTTING WATER FOR FUN AND PROFIT

I always get a chuckle when someone asks me how they can look dramatically better in a week or less. If the person is 20 pounds overweight, the answer is easy: nothing. So the first rule of cutting water is that you need to be pretty lean to make it worth the trouble. For a guy, that means single-digit body fat. For a woman, it won't work unless she's at 15 percent body fat or below.

If that describes you, the following protocol will probably work.

DAYS 4 AND 3 BEFORE EVENT:

Drink 1.5 gallons of water if you weigh 100 to 150 pounds; 2 gallons if you weigh 150 to 200 pounds; 2.5 gallons if you weigh close to 250 pounds. Add a little extra salt to your food. Take a multivitamin/mineral supplement. I recommend Super Nutrition's Perfect Blend, but others might work just as well.

DAY 2 BEFORE EVENT:

Drink half the amount of water you drank on days 4 and 3 (1 gallon if you weigh 150 to 200 pounds). Avoid sodium, although a little is acceptable.

DAY 1 BEFORE EVENT:

Sip on 6 ounces of water throughout the day if you weigh 100 to 150 pounds; 10 ounces if you weigh 150 to 200 pounds; and 14 ounces if you weigh close to 250 pounds. Avoid sodium, which means prepared foods and restaurant meals are out. Eat small meals and avoid heavy foods.

EVENT DAY:

Drink small amounts of water throughout the day. Consume small, frequent snacks, such as trail mix with dried fruit.

Fair warning: If you're cutting water for an event that culminates with lots of alcohol— such as a wedding or your first day of spring break—remember that your alcohol tolerance will be a fraction of what it normally is. Drink responsibly.

CUTTING WATER FOR A BODY-BUILDING OR FIGURE CONTEST

I've seen bodybuilders use protocols that are nothing short of terrifying. Extreme water deprivation paired with powerful diuretic drugs that wipe out key electrolytes can be a lethal combination. Even if you stay out of the emergency room, you're taking too big a risk to your long-term health.

But with better planning and adherence, you should never have to resort to such extreme measures.

DAYS 5, 4, AND 3 BEFORE EVENT:

Drink 1.5 gallons of water if you weigh 100 to 150 pounds; 2 gallons if you weigh 150 to 200 pounds; 2.5 gallons if you weigh close to 250 pounds. Eliminate all carbs except for vegetables. Add a little extra salt to your food on days 5 and 4, but stop salting your food on day 3. Take a multivitamin/mineral supplement.

DAY 2 BEFORE EVENT:

Drink half the amount of water you consumed for days 5, 4, and 3. Your carb-avoidance strategy remains the same. Avoid sodium, which means no packaged foods or restaurant meals. Take a dandelion-root supplement (it's a mild, natural, and safe diuretic), using the dose recommended on the label.

DAY 1 BEFORE EVENT:

This day isn't fun. Sip on 6 ounces of water throughout the day if you weigh 100 to 150 pounds; 10 ounces if you weigh 150 to 200 pounds; 14 ounces if you weigh close to 250 pounds. Avoid sodium. Eat six small meals, including complex carbs and low-fat protein. An ideal meal would be sweet potato with egg whites or skinless chicken breast. This is the one time when you need to measure your carbs carefully: For the entire day, you want to have 100 grams if you weigh 100 to 150 pounds; 125 grams if you weigh 150 to 200 pounds; 150 grams if

you weigh close to 250 pounds. (A baked sweet potato, 5 inches by 2 inches, has about 30 grams of carbs.) Take dandelion root as recommended on the label.

EVENT DAY:

Sip water throughout the day, and eat small, frequent snacks, such as trail mix with dried fruit.

I mentioned this earlier but it bears repeating: You *absolutely must* give this protocol a trial run at least 1 month before your event. Most of my clients have had great success with it, and if it also works for you, you'll know a month before the contest, giving you confidence going into that final week. But if you go through your mock "event day" without the look you wanted, try my friend Holly's method. Eat some pepperoni pizza that night, and see how you look the next day.

If it's the look you'd hoped to achieve, you know what to do before the event. Follow the plan I just described, but eat pizza in your sixth and final meal the night before the contest. Then continue with the contest-day strategy of sipping water and eating small, frequent snacks.

DROPPING AND REGAINING WEIGHT FOR A FIGHT

A fighter is different from a bodybuilder in one crucial way: After he makes weight, he has to go into a ring with someone who can't wait to beat his face to a bloody pulp. But he also has the option of regaining as much as 10 pounds in the 24 hours between the weigh-in and the actual fight. Bodybuilders have to compete while hungry and dehydrated, which has the ironic effect of making them irritable enough to *want* to throw some punches.

A fighter who can successfully make it into his chosen weight class, then quickly regain weight, has two big advantages over an opponent who isn't so determined or clever. Being heavier than the other guy is a plus, which is why we have weight classes in the first place. And if you also have more water and nutrients in your body, you'll be less susceptible to fatigue.

Before I describe the protocol, I want to throw down two rules:

1. The weight-regaining strategy won't work unless you lose the weight the right way. If you use diuretics, or sweat the weight off with a rubber suit in an overheated room, your electrolytes will be out of whack, and your performance will suffer.

2. Ten pounds is the limit. If you drop more than 10 pounds in the days before the fight, or put on more than 10 after weigh-in, you're setting yourself up for a beating.

DAYS 5, 4, AND 3 BEFORE WEIGH-IN:

Drink 1.5 gallons of water if you weigh 100 to 150 pounds; 2 gallons if you weigh 150 to 200 pounds; 2.5 gallons if you weigh close to 250

pounds. Add a little extra salt to your food. Take a multivitamin/mineral supplement.

DAY 2 BEFORE WEIGH-IN:

Drink half the amount of water you consumed for days 5, 4, and 3. Avoid sodium, although you can get away with a little.

DAY 1 BEFORE WEIGH-IN:

Sip on 6 ounces of water throughout the day if you weigh 100 to 150 pounds; 10 ounces if you weigh 150 to 200 pounds; 14 ounces if you weigh close to 250 pounds. Absolutely no sodium can enter your mouth. Eat three small meals, each consisting of just 2 ounces of chicken breast and ¼ cup of berries. It sucks, but at least you'll make weight.

Remember, you *must* try this protocol at least 1 month before your fight to make sure you can lose 10 pounds, or whatever you have to lose to make it through your weigh-in. If you didn't lose enough, here's what you should add in.

On the day leading up to the weigh-in, sit in a sauna for 10 to 15 minutes in the morning, and another 10 to 15 minutes in the afternoon. This is usually enough to drop another pound or two.

If you still need to lose a little more, you can perform 20 to 30 minutes of light activity—just enough to make you sweat. But keep in mind that this is a last resort. Any exercise you do with your body so depleted of water and nutrients will compromise your performance.

BETWEEN THE WEIGH-IN AND THE FIGHT:

Start drinking water right away; you need to drink 2 to 3 gallons over the next 24 hours; you want to be urinating frequently, with the urine coming out clear, before you start fighting.

You also need to eat six or seven small meals spaced at regular intervals, with the first one as soon as possible following the weigh-in. The first three meals should consist of fruit, lean protein, and a little sodium (a bit of salt on your protein at each meal is plenty). Or you can have trail mix with nuts and dried fruit. For your final three meals, eat complex carbs (such as sweet potatoes) along with lean protein. Don't eat anything you aren't accustomed to.

Finally, you must take a multivitamin/mineral supplement.

When the announcer holds up your hand at the end of the fight, remember to thank your nutrition advisor.

INDEX

Underscored page references indicate boxed text and tables. **Boldface** references indicate illustrations.

INDEX

INDEX